NEW THEMES IN
PALLIATIVE CARE

FACING DEATH

Series editor: David Clark, Professor of Medical Sociology,
University of Sheffield

The subject of death in late modern culture has become a rich field of theoretical, clinical and policy interest. Widely regarded as a taboo until recent times, death now engages a growing interests among social scientists, practitioners and those responsible for the organization and delivery of human services. Indeed, how we die has become a powerful commentary on how we live and the specialized care of dying people holds an important place within modern health and social care.

This series captures such developments in a collection of volumes which has much to say about death, dying, and end-of-life care and bereavement in contemporary society. Among the contributors are leading experts in death studies, from sociology, anthropology, social psychology, ethics, nursing, medicine and pastoral care. A particular feature of the series is its attention to the developing field of palliative care, viewed from the perspectives of practitioners, planners and policy analysts; here several authors adopt a multi-disciplinary approach, drawing on recent research, policy and organizational commentary, and reviews of evidence-based practice. Written in a clear, accessible style, the entire series will be essential reading for students of death, dying and bereavement and for anyone with an involvement in palliative care research, service delivery or policy making.

Current and forthcoming titles:

David Clark, Jo Hockley, Sam Ahmedzai (eds): *New Themes in Palliative Care*
David Clark and Jane Seymour: *Reflections on Palliative Care*
Mark Cobb: *Spiritual Issues in Palliative Care*
Kirsten Costain Schou and Jenny Hewison: *Experiencing Cancer: Quality of Life in Treatment*
David Field, David Clark, Jessica Corner and Carol Davis (eds): *Researching Palliative Care*
David Kissane and Sidney Bloch: *Family Grief Therapy*
Gordon Riches and Pamela Dawson: *An Intimate Loneliness: Supporting Bereaved Parents and Siblings*
Tony Walter: *On Bereavement*

NEW THEMES IN PALLIATIVE CARE

Edited by
DAVID CLARK
JO HOCKLEY
SAM AHMEDZAI

OPEN UNIVERSITY PRESS
Buckingham · Philadelphia

Open University Press
Celtic Court
22 Ballmoor
Buckingham
MK18 1XW

email: enquiries@openup.co.uk
world wide web: http://www.openup.co.uk

and
325 Chestnut Street
Philadelphia, PA 19106, USA

First published 1997
Reprinted 1999

Copyright © The editors and contributors 1997

A catalogue record of this book is available from the British Library

ISBN 0 335 19605 5 (pbk)   0 335 19606 3 (hbk)

Library of Congress Cataloging-in-Publication Data
New themes in palliative care / edited by David Clark, Jo Hockley, Sam Ahmedzai.
    p. cm.
Includes bibliographical references and index.
ISBN 0–335–19606–3 (hbk)   ISBN 0–335–19605–5 (pbk)
1. Terminal care.   2. Palliative treatment.   I. Clark, David,
1953– . II. Hockley, J.M.   III. Ahmedzai, Sam, 1950– .
R726.8.N486   1997
616'.029—dc21
97–12123
CIP

Typeset by Graphicraft Typesetters Limited, Hong Kong
Printed in Great Britain by Biddles Ltd, Guildford and King's Lynn

Contents

Acknowledgements

Busy contributors, busy editors and heavily committed secretarial staff have combined to make the production of this collection a good deal of hard work for many people. We thank them all. Our authors, responding to numerous cajolings, pesterings and pleas, have all given great support to the project. Several of them have benefited in turn from other colleagues who have provided additional information and assistance in the preparation of the chapters, together (in some cases) with English language editing. Closer to home we have been grateful for the efficient help of Joan Malherbe and the quiet patience of Jacinta Evans, both at the Open University Press. Jane Seymour produced the index with her usual efficiency. In the hot seat itself has been Margaret Jane who, together with Lesley Keers at the Section of Palliative Medicine, Sheffield University School of Medicine, has been in constant communication with authors, has typed numerous drafts of chapters and dealt with innumerable faxes, emails and telephone calls. The resulting volume has truly been a collective effort and a work of international collaboration which has enriched us all.

David Clark, Jo Hockley, Sam Ahmedzai

Notes on the editors

David Clark was educated at the universities of Newcastle and Aberdeen. Following early postgraduate research in the sociology of religion, his subsequent interests centred upon sociological aspects of family life. While working at the Medical Research Council (MRC) Medical Sociology Unit in Aberdeen in the early 1980s, he began to develop an interest in the sociological aspects of health and illness, which have now become his major research focus. He was appointed Professor of Sociology at Sheffield Hallam University in 1993 and in July 1995 took up the Chair of Medical Sociology at the University of Sheffield. He is currently engaged in a number of studies concerned with health needs assessment and service evaluation relating to the provision of palliative care. He has a particular interest in the historical developments of the modern hospice movement. He is the author and editor of several books on sociological and policy aspects of palliative care, including the successful collection *The Future for Palliative Care* (Open University Press 1993).

Jo Hockley trained as a nurse at St Bartholomew's Hospital, London, in 1970 and then as a midwife. Since 1978 she has specialized in palliative care – first as a charge nurse at St Christopher's Hospice, London, and more recently setting up palliative care teams within the acute hospital setting. She has published extensively on this aspect of palliative care development. She obtained her MSc at the University of Edinburgh and is currently a senior clinical nurse specialist on the Palliative Care Team at the Western General Hospital, Edinburgh.

Sam Ahmedzai took up the Chair of Palliative Medicine at the University of Sheffield in December 1994, based at the Royal Hallamshire Hospital. He was Associate Director of the Trent Palliative Care Centre since its inception and became Director in December 1994. His previous position, for nine years, was Medical Director of the Leicestershire Hospice (LOROS) and Honorary Consultant in Palliative Medicine. Other positions held are editor-in-chief for *Progress in Palliative Care*, associate editor for *Quaderni di Cure Palliative* and member of the Protocol Review Committee of the European Organization for Research and Treatment of Cancer (EORTC). He has published over fifty articles in journals, ten chapters in textbooks and contributed to several teaching videos.

List of contributors

Professor Barbro Beck-Friis, Borensberg, Sweden

Dr Kenneth Boyd, Institute of Medical Ethics, Edinburgh Royal Infirmary, Department of Medicine, Edinburgh, UK

Gilly Burn, World Health Organization, Sir Michael Sobell House, Oxford, UK

Professor Jessica Corner, Centre for Cancer and Palliative Care Studies, Institute of Cancer Research, Royal Marsden Hospital, London, UK

Nessa Coyle, Supportive Care Program, Department of Neurology, Memorial Sloan-Kettering Cancer Center, New York, USA

Dr Carol Davis, Countess Mountbatten House, Moorgreen Hospital, Southampton, UK

Dr Giorgio Di Mola, Research and Documentation Center, Fondazione Floriani, Milan, Italy

Dr Robert Dunlop, St Christopher's Hospice, London, UK

Calliope Farsides, Centre of Medical Law and Ethics, King's College, London, UK

M. Dulce Fontanals, Unitat de Cures Palliatives, Hospitalet de Llobregat, Barcelona, Spain

Eve Garrard, Centre for Contemporary Ethical Studies, University of Keele, UK

Dr Rob George, Camden and Islington Community Health NHS Trust, Palliative Care Team, London, UK

Dr Xavier Gómez-Batiste, Unitat de Cures Palliatives, Hospitalet de Llobregat, Barcelona, Spain

Pauline Heather, Research and Evaluation Division, Employment Service, Sheffield, UK

Dr Roger W. Hunt, Southern Community Hospice Programme, Daw House Hospice, Repatriation General Hospital, Daw Park, South Australia

Dr Jane M. Ingham, Palliative Care Program, Georgetown University Department of Medicine, Lombardi Cancer Center, Washington, DC, USA

Professor Jacek Łuczak, Palliative Care Department, Karol Marcinkowski University of Medical Sciences, Poznań, Poland

Professor Ian Maddocks, Southern Community Hospice Programme, Daw House Hospice, Repatriation General Hospital, Daw Park, South Australia

Dr Karen Mallett, Palliative Medicine Section, Department of Surgical and Anaesthetic Sciences, University of Sheffield, UK

Dr Helen Malson, Department of Psychology, University of East London, UK

Francesc Martinez, Unitat de Cures Palliatives, Hospitalet de Llobregat, Barcelona, Spain

Dr Bren Neale, School of Sociology and Social Policy, University of Leeds, UK

Dr David Oxenham, Fairmile Marie Curie Centre, Edinburgh, UK

Dr Margaret Robbins, School of Social Sciences, University of Bath, UK

Jordi Roca, Unitat de Cures Palliatives, Hospitalet de Llobregat, Barcelona, Spain

Pere Roige-Canals, Unitat de Cures Palliatives, Hospitalet de Llobregat, Barcelona, Spain

Frances Sheldon, Department of Social Work Studies, University of Southampton, UK

Dr Neil Small, Trent Palliative Care Centre, Sheffield, UK

Dr Jan Stjernsward, Global Cancer Concern, London, UK

Dr Jo Sykes, Department of Palliative Medicine, Bristol Oncology Centre, UK

Elisabeth Valles, Unitat de Cures Palliatives, Hospitalet de Llobregat, Barcelona, Spain

David Whynes, Department of Economics, University of Nottingham, UK

Series editor's preface

The rapid expansion of interest in cancer and palliative care has become a significant feature of health care development in recent times. Within only a few decades the care and treatment of people with cancer has been subject to wide-reaching and rapid change, much of it driven by advances in biomedical science. Increasingly, however, enthusiasm for aggressive, curative treatments has been tempered by a growing awareness of and interest in the psychosocial aspects of cancer, linked to an understanding of the place of the disease within late modern culture, or what Frank (1995) calls 'remission society'. At the same time, the progress made by hospices and the emerging specialty of palliative care has thrown into relief the plight of people with other chronic, life-limiting illnesses who might also benefit from a similar approach. In a period of such rapid development in palliative care it is important therefore to have informed commentary which can stimulate policy making, practice innovation and related research.

Palliative care is an exciting field in which to be involved and one surrounded by many challenges. In part this is a specialty which gets to the very limits of medicine, dealing with some of the sickest people in society and facing the personal, social and societal implications of human mortality. Within it lies the possibility of understanding individual suffering inside a wider cultural, spiritual and structural context. Palliative care must therefore grapple with questions about the meaning of illness and the narratives which might accompany it, as well as the ways in which these are differentiated within specific groups in society. Listening to the voices of sick people and their carers is an important feature of this and has a high priority within clinical practice, in service planning and in research.

Palliative care also faces challenges relating to service organization as it seeks to develop patterns of delivery which can be sensitive to individual needs and preferences and yet at the same time make these available on an equitable basis. High quality physical and psychosocial care is central to this approach, but how can it be delivered across large and highly segmented populations via both specialist and mainstream services? These questions of equity have been thrown into relief by the success of hospice services, often working within the independent sector, but where coverage can be limited.

It is a hallmark of palliative care that it seeks to promote a multi-disciplinary approach which integrates the efforts of a wide range of health and social care providers. It therefore has a good deal to teach us about the ways in which professions operate within the medical division of labour, how they might work together and about how collaboration can take place across the artificial boundaries of 'health' and 'social' need. At the same time we must also be aware of the tensions and difficulties which can occur between professionals in different occupational cultures and explore ways in which these might be overcome.

All areas of health care are being encouraged to look to the evidence-base which supports practice. Of course this poses many problems for palliative care. These can perhaps be most easily overcome in relation to pain and symptom management. But in palliative care, quality of life is an important focus of care and often it is the *process* of care which is more significant than the *outcome*. New research methodologies and technologies are therefore being developed to give a more sophisticated understanding of quality of life and its connection to the outcomes of care. Considerable progress has also been made in areas of clinical and organizational audit and in service evaluation. Nevertheless, palliative care research must deal with complex problems of research design, sample selection and attrition, together with the ethical considerations which underpin these.

Finally, there are questions of resource allocation and the ability of palliative care to make its case against the competing claims of other health care specialties. Of course, palliative care is an area which has strong emotional associations, but these alone will not be sufficient to sustain development without substantial endorsement by politicians, policy makers and the professions.

Such issues form the backdrop to all of the volumes in this series and will be addressed in varying ways by different authors. The editors of *New Themes in Palliative Care* have sought to provide an excellent introduction to the series by producing a collection of chapters which is wide-ranging in character and which sets out the current parameters of a fast-changing field. The collection places a strong accent on multidisciplinary perspectives, it is international in orientation and gives due weight to the interconnections between ethics, policy, research and practice. It will serve as a useful introduction to newcomers in palliative care, but also has much to say on current debates and dilemmas in the specialty which will be of interest to those already knowledgeable in the field who wish to further extend their understanding.

David Clark

Reference

Frank, A. (1995) *The Wounded Storyteller*. Chicago: University of Chicago Press.

Introduction

Palliative care is moving through exciting times, as is appropriate to the early history of a specialty. Month by month we are conscious of new writings, expert reports, innovative conferences, all of which are seeking to capture and formalize a range of developments in clinical practice and in service provision. Even for those centrally involved, it becomes difficult to maintain a detailed overview of research findings, current debates and emerging ideas. For these reasons, to have called this collection *New Themes in Palliative Care* runs certain risks. What is reported as new here, some of our contributors have observed, may be orthodox and mainstream by tomorrow, if indeed it has not already sunk without trace. Our purposes in producing this volume should therefore be explained.

Books on palliative care which incorporate perspectives from policy, service development and clinical practice are still comparatively rare. Yet it is only at the conjunction of these three areas that we can form a detailed view of how palliative care is developing and where it may be going. We are fortunate therefore in having contributors to this book who share that viewpoint and who in the chapters that follow repeatedly demonstrate its importance. Our book is aimed at all of those people who are involved in the development of palliative care, regardless of their particular training, professional background or role. Palliative care prides itself on an inclusive approach which is multidisciplinary, takes seriously the views and concerns of patients and informal carers, makes use of voluntary labour, and enjoys communal and societal support. This complex mosaic of interests, preoccupations and perspectives can create enormous challenges, not least to professionals deeply involved with the views and concerns of their host discipline. We try to shed light on these from a multidisciplinary perspective throughout the book. Unidisciplinary concerns remain important, of course, but they are not the focus here.

As editors, we ourselves represent different disciplines, each making a contribution to palliative care. So the preoccupations of nursing, medicine and the social sciences run through every chapter to be found here. In several cases we have asked authors from differing backgrounds to work together in addressing a particular subject. This is no easy task and presents both challenges and opportunities in engaging with the baseline assumptions of a particular discipline. Good examples of this can be found, for example, in Part III of the book, where physicians variously have combined with specialists in social work, nursing, and medical ethics to focus on a range of clinical issues. Elsewhere, we have contributions from health service research, philosophy, sociology and health economics, as well as from those involved in strategic planning and management. Typically, most of our contributors will have multiple responsibilities and involvements in the development and delivery of palliative care services. It is this juxtaposition of patient care, together with service issues, questions of resource allocation, research, evaluation and education that we have sought to capture. We take the view that it is possible to understand what is happening in palliative care only by engaging with the dynamic interplay between all of these factors. We trust that readers will share in this viewpoint and derive benefit from the combination of material presented here.

In preparing the book we have had in mind in particular a student readership. Around the world, there is now a multiplicity of educational provision in palliative care. This may range from occasional input into an undergraduate or basic training course, to specialist programmes at advanced level. Students wishing to learn about very recent developments in palliative care face certain difficulties. Much discussion of new development is taking place in a small number of specialized journals, at specialist conferences or in the 'grey' literature of working party reports, newsletters and information bulletins of various kinds. These are important settings for the exchange of ideas among experts, but are typically less successful in communicating with a wider audience. From the outset, therefore, our book has been concerned to bring new themes and ideas in palliative care to a broader readership, including those still in training and in particular those engaged in higher level studies.

We have also worked hard to give the book a strongly international perspective. The world grows smaller, but there is still often great reluctance to learn from the approaches, knowledge and insights of other cultures and contexts. Our contributors have done excellent work in drawing attention to diverse models of care, modes of organization and varying policy contexts. Palliative care is still very underdeveloped in many parts of the world and several chapters here deal with strategic approaches for addressing this, while also respecting local cultural and ethical systems. We hope that reading these chapters will promote understanding across settings and help to foster and build on the international links that are already such a strong feature of the world of palliative care.

Finally, a few words about how the book is organized. Edited collections can be indigestible at times and even the rich array of the smorgasbord can be offputting without a little guidance on menu selection. Of course, we hope that most people will want to read the whole of this book, but for those who do not, we have provided a detailed introduction and summary for each of the book's three parts. In addition we have listed, for each part, our own impression of the key themes and further questions which seem to arise from it. Part I deals with questions of policy, ethics and research in palliative care. Part II focuses on a variety of innovations in service development around the world. Part III concentrates on new thinking in clinical practice. Each part of the book is interrelated in some way and many chapters share overlapping concerns. No part or chapter necessarily precedes another, so in whatever order it is read we hope that our book will be informative, challenging and, on occasion, provocative.

David Clark, Jo Hockley, Sam Ahmedzai

PART 1

Policy, ethics, evidence

Introduction to Part I

In this first part of the book three interconnected issues are explored, from a variety of perspectives. Drawing on their current work in health services research, in health economics and philosophy, the authors examine questions of policy, ethics and evidence. We begin therefore with a wide focus, at the societal level, in the belief that this forms the essential context in which subsequent sections, concerned with service development and clinical issues, can be understood. This is not to consider matters of policy as in any way logically prior to the organization and delivery of health care, but it does nevertheless acknowledge that, increasingly, health policy is the *only* framework in which services are able to function and health care can be delivered. Policy making is of course always an imprecise, empirical process. Policy outcomes are necessarily complex, often difficult to forecast and subject to innumerable influences, predictable and unpredictable. In this sense they have something in common with the outcomes of palliative care. As the authors show here, the extent to which providers of palliative care can engage with the preoccupations of policy and policy makers will be a crucial factor in shaping the future direction and form of the specialty. Within this policy context, two crucial elements are identified.

The first of these relates to the question of evidence. Health policy in many countries is now hungry for evidence. This takes a variety of forms. There are calls for evidence of need before a service or intervention is offered. There is the demand for evidence of effectiveness, from the macro level of the health system, to the micro level of the individual clinical procedure. Then comes the injunction to demonstrate efficiency through the avoidance of wasteful practices or profligacy with resources. Increasingly there is also an expectation that services can be seen to be available equitably within the population. This adds up to a complex matrix which aspires to a clear fit between need, demand and supply, contained within available resources.

In the following chapters we see how this relates to palliative care. We gain a sense of the range of issues involved in thinking about an 'evidence-based' approach to the delivery of palliative care and we are reminded throughout that we are in only the foothills of this endeavour, with many high peaks yet to be scaled. Research is a crucial factor in this. Palliative care has been perhaps particularly inclined to ignore the importance of research, certainly in relation to other specialties of similar age, such as oncology or pain management. The development of a wide-ranging and multidisciplinary programme of palliative care research is therefore crucial to a more evidence-based approach. In this sense research should not be seen as an esoteric pastime or luxury to be indulged. It may well prove a crucial determinant of the future development of palliative care. Indeed, research may have a vital role in moving palliative care from its current place on the margins, to a position of central influence within health care philosophy, organization and practice in the twenty-first century.

Beyond evidence, but closely linked to it, lies the second key element, the domain of value and judgement. It is not necessary to enter into a detailed study of the sociology of knowledge to recognize that 'facts' can rarely be taken as unproblematic representations of some aspect of the world. 'Knowledge', 'findings', 'results' – these are more typically contingent, partial, temporary statements which are challengeable, even malleable in character. So we must interrogate 'evidence', not only with an eye to the rigour with which it has been produced, but also with regard to the value position of those who produce it. Most importantly of all, where evidence is an unreliable guide, we must replace it with rational thinking and ethically sound judgements. Such is the case with debates about euthanasia, a topic that appears at several points in this book. It is difficult to imagine a situation in which any body of 'evidence' could be assembled to make a conclusive case either for or against euthanasia. Instead we must consider it in relation to what can be argued to be ethically sound practice. This may conflict with personal or spiritual convictions, making judgements even more painful and challenging. We are fortunate to have in the following chapters the views of authors who recognize such complexities and are prepared to engage with them.

The first of these, Margaret Robbins (Chapter 1), begins with a discussion of the three 'Es': economy, efficiency and effectiveness. Robbins calls into question the simplistic assumptions upon which evidence of these has been assembled and assessed, but she also reminds us that until recently palliative care has been unconcerned with such questions, satisfied with the letters of grateful relatives and the warm glow of community acceptance. There is an important point here that we cannot presuppose a shared understanding of what constitutes effectiveness, efficiency or economy. The production of worthwhile evidence about palliative care, she contends, will derive from a methodological pluralism which allows research techniques and perspectives to be adopted which are most suitable to the question at hand. This seems particularly important in palliative care, with its commitment to caring for the 'whole' person through attention to physical, psychological, social, spiritual and material factors. Methodological pluralism should not, however, be an excuse for methodological mediocrity and can be championed only where there is an adherence to rigour within the chosen methods.

One of the problems which continues to bedevil the measurement of effectiveness in palliative care is the very wide range of services in existence – a point which is reinforced throughout this book. This does not, however, explain the bewildering absence of recent studies attempting some fairly obvious comparisons or assessments, for example of the effectiveness of hospices against community hospitals, or the added value produced by the presence of a specialist palliative care nursing/advisory service.

Of course, effectiveness can occur only when the service provided is closely tailored to need. A recent emphasis within health policy, especially in countries which have moved towards the separation of purchasing and providing functions in health care, has been upon health needs assessment as a basis for strategic planning, service development and contracting. This is something which Clark and colleagues explore in more detail in Chapter 4. Here, Robbins highlights some of the prospects and barriers to needs assessment as a rational basis for action. Recent approaches to this subject have favoured a model which combines epidemiological data, with comparisons of service utilization (locally and nationally), together with the views of service users and providers. This seems to offer a robust and sophisticated procedure for effective assessment. Underpinning it are lingering concerns about how need is to be conceptualized, however, and indeed whether or not it constitutes a sound basis upon which to develop strategy, especially when resources are limited. Farsides and Garrard (Chapter 3) raise a similar point when considering whether certain palliative care needs, for example, those which are predominantly physical in character, will predominate over others, such as the psychological. Robbins's careful assessment of the principles underpinning needs assessment is also linked to a pragmatic observation that, in many countries where some form of palliative care is now available, needs assessment cannot begin from first principles and must necessarily be conducted in relation to the services which are currently in place – a point echoed in Chapter 10 by Gómez-Batiste and colleagues.

Robbins's conclusion, that palliative care requires a clearer set of clinical definitions, is a theme also identified by David Whynes in Chapter 2. He too draws attention to the different modalities of palliative care and highlights the distinctions which can be made between care settings. For Whynes, though, an immediate starting point is the overriding dilemma for health care systems and the government policies that underpin them – the potential for expenditure to spiral out of control, making cost containment a major priority. There can be two responses to this dilemma: constrain demand, leading ultimately to rationing, or contain treatment costs by greater efficiency in delivery. However unpalatable these considerations may seem, they are of major importance to palliative care. As Whynes points out, the move in the twentieth century towards a norm of death in institutions has created a major drain on the public purse. In the USA, hospice care has been shown to be a cheaper alternative to conventional care in hospital, but there are indications that changes in the clinical workload of hospices are shifting their cost profile in the direction of hospitals.

The lack of agreed modalities for palliative care in end-stage disease, Whynes emphasizes, makes for difficulties in comparison. Moreover if economic analysis is restricted to formal costs, two sources of bias are introduced. First, such an approach overlooks the contribution made by volunteers to palliative care services, and second, the major contribution of informal carers in the home is ignored. Despite these difficulties, which imply that a 'reduction' in costs may occur simply because some element has been transferred out of the organization (to volunteers or informal carers), Whynes does consider three possibilities for reducing the high cost of dying. These comprise: more use of advance directives which would not only respect patients' wishes but also reduce expenditure; further efficiency gains through, for example, shorter courses of chemotherapy and radiotherapy; and finally, the reduction in levels of 'futile' treatment. Such cost reductions would require greater clarity in the procedures that follow when it is accepted that death is going to occur. They would also require greater agreement on 'proper' palliation modalities. Finally, they would need to give a higher priority, even than that currently witnessed in palliative care, to the views and preferences of patients in treatment and palliation decisions.

It is apparent from such discussions that a strong ethical component enters into questions of policy, planning and resource allocation for palliative care. Calliope Farsides and Eve Garrard (Chapter 3) tackle these issues from the viewpoint of professional philosophers. They recognize that the 'relative detachment' of this position is one that shelters them from the face to face ethical dilemmas experienced by health professionals on a daily basis. Nevertheless they make a strong case for the importance of ethically sound principles as a guide to resource allocation and planning in health care. These authors begin by focusing on one of the less widely explored principles of medical ethics: the concept of *justice*.

A central preoccupation here is the allocation of resources both *to* and *within* health care. Farsides and Garrard see this at the macro level (of national governments), at the intermediate level (of comparison between specialties and services) and, finally, at the micro level (of the individual patient). They are sceptical that tools such as the Quality Adjusted Life

Year (QALY) can be of much help with these problems as they relate to palliative care, where the goal of the intervention is unlikely to be anticipated years of life with a given quality of health. That is, we should add, at least while palliative care continues to be synonymous with end-stage disease; should it be further extended (as many of its practitioners now advocate – see Part III) to include the earlier stage of disease progression and to be integrated within the period of more 'active' treatment, then the QALY may indeed have some greater relevance.

Farsides and Garrard argue that there is justification for the provision of palliative care on ethical and moral grounds – that the 'good death' is in some sense a fundamental human right. This still leaves questions at the intermediate level, however: what should be the priorities for resource allocation here? The authors suggest that, typically, the alleviation of pain has been a priority. This may display a preoccupation with organic disease, but it is likely to score highly on measures of efficacy. Palliative care, of course, seeks to go beyond physical care to include psychological, spiritual and social dimensions. But what if these are deemed unaffordable, within the limits of scarce resources? This has important implications at the micro level of the individual patient. For if the psychological distress is left untreated, the patient may well feel that life is no longer worth living. In such a situation, Garrard and Farsides argue, a patient's request for voluntary euthanasia would have to be treated with sympathy and respect (though they do not suggest that this would necessarily mean acceptance). They conclude with a warning against illiberalism on this issue on the part of palliative care providers.

Chapter 4, by David Clark and colleagues, brings us back to some of the policy issues identified by Robbins. In this case the authors begin with an exploration of the purchasing cycle, examining the theoretical model which begins with health needs assessment and proceeds through strategic planning and service specifications to contracting and quality assurance. It is just such a model that palliative care developments are having to operate within in those countries which have developed a 'quasi-market' for health care. The authors focus on the impact of this in the British context and present evidence on the ways in which recent 'reforms' of the National Health Service (NHS) have been viewed by palliative care providers. They show that the high level of independence enjoyed by the early voluntary hospices in the UK has been circumscribed by moves towards a mixed economy of health care in which hospices must function as providers in a potentially competitive environment. Hospice and palliative care services have therefore had to make major adjustments to the contract culture of health care in the 1990s. The authors conclude that this has been done with some success, but they also present concerns that the introduction of health reforms in the UK may not be working unequivocally for the benefit of palliative care.

New themes and key questions in Part I

- The future of palliative care is more than ever tied into a wider agenda for health and social care policy; this means that palliative care is likely to be judged against success criteria which are generalized across a wide range of services and interventions. In this setting palliative care must be able to stand comparison with other specialties and be assessed in similar ways. It is clear that special pleading, based on the 'unique' character of the activity, is not a viable option. How can the culture of palliative care come to terms with these issues?
- The developing science of health needs assessment has a considerable role to play in the further consolidation of palliative care. Whereas a good deal of service provision, particularly in the west, has been based upon emotive appeals, health needs assessment provides opportunities to delineate the parameters of need in local populations in relation to epidemiological evidence, existing provision and stakeholder preferences.
- The development of health needs assessments in palliative care is a welcome step forward, but what is to be done when studies point to conflicts of view in the perspectives of providers and users of services?
- The role of research is crucial if palliative care is to adopt an evidence-based approach which goes beyond the consensus views of experienced clinicians. Huge obstacles exist to the creation of a rigorous research culture in palliative care, but at the same time multidisciplinary collaboration and openness to a variety of research methodologies and traditions augur well for progress in the future.
- Recent work in defining the precise character of palliative care services and interventions must be maintained if confusion about the aims and practices of the specialty is to be addressed. Why does palliative care continue to suffer from definitional problems and in what ways might these be overcome?
- Cost containment measures will exert increasing pressure on palliative care; it may be that palliative care can respond positively to these in ways which acknowledge that by developing a more sophisticated understanding of the relationship between 'care' and 'cure' it is possible to promulgate a more rational and more humane approach to *all* health care. How can palliative care rise above its own internally focused deliberations to make this wider contribution?
- Resource allocation and ethical issues will increasingly be linked to one another. Here too palliative care can play a wider role by identifying and formalizing models which are ethically defensible. Again, by addressing issues at the extremes of medical ethics (such as euthanasia and physician-assisted suicide), lessons can emerge which are relevant to the whole of health care.

1 Assessing needs and effectiveness: is palliative care a special case?

MARGARET ROBBINS

The 1980s onwards have seen some spectacular ideological debates about the need to control public spending in the health and social services in the face of what appears to be runaway demand for services. In the UK, for example, market mechanisms (albeit in shadowy and quasi form) have been widely introduced as a means of resource management. These mechanisms have brought with them a rhetoric of 'E-ism' – more economy, efficiency and effectiveness, and possibly less equity and equality. Two concepts which have achieved considerable popularity among health planners are effectiveness and needs assessment (Allsop 1995): the former representing the idea that health services should indeed deliver what they promise, and in a way which constitutes value for money and health gain; the latter that the legitimate health care requirements of populations for such effective health services can be quantified in a way that can allow rational health care planning and prioritization. Theoretically, it has seemed comparatively simple to postulate the existence of discernible and measurable 'needs' for health care on the one hand, and their satisfaction (according to various measures of utility) by cost-efficient, acceptable services on the other.

The urgency to establish the *need* for *effective* services as a cornerstone of rational health planning and provision has been born out of the combination of the recent public expenditure crises, hand in hand with spiralling health care costs and the increasing demand for health care in many national populations. In the UK, changes in health service organization and the introduction of the 'internal market' have brought the devolution of policy and planning responsibility to district purchasing agencies, which in turn are working within clearer budget frameworks (Øvretveit 1995). It has thus become more important to plan and provide health care according to explicit priorities, which in some sense provide a moral defence for the inevitable shortfalls between supply and demand. Very few services escape the spotlight of resource management; specialist palliative care services are no exception (see Clark and colleagues, Chapter 4 in this volume).

Specialist palliative care services are now being provided in a different economic and political climate from the one in which they first established themselves in the mid-1970s. Many people have pointed out the extraordinary growth of this sector of care, fuelled by the input of national cancer charities, and tremendous local initiative (Goddard 1989; Eve and Smith 1994). The difficulties that the comparatively unbridled proliferation of hospices over the late 1970s and 1980s have brought, plus the lack of overall regulation and planning, have also been alluded to (Lunt and Hillier 1981; Clark 1993). The establishment in the UK of the National Council for Hospices and Specialist Palliative Care Services (NCHSPCS) in the early 1990s was an important step forward in providing a national voice for the sector at a time of great upheaval and change in the health services generally. However, given the pattern of its growth and the disparateness of its constituencies, the palliative care sector challenges the exercise of 1990s-style needs assessment and health care commissioning.

This chapter examines the concepts of effectiveness and needs assessment as they apply to palliative care services. It begins with a discussion of effectiveness and the evaluation research which has addressed this concept, and then moves on to examine the question of needs for palliative care, and whether they can be assessed at a population level. In conclusion, questions are raised about the integration of voluntary and statutory funding for the support of this sector of care, and how far this is likely to affect future planning.

Effectiveness

A preamble

The availability of 'evidence' concerning the effectiveness of health care interventions has become increasingly crucial as cost-containment policies demand clearer demonstration of 'value for money'. Underlying much of the new rhetoric on evidence-based health care is an assumption that health care can be delivered in a rational manner (Sackett and Rosenberg 1995); that, for example, the relationship between an effective service, the evidence showing its effectiveness, and resulting levels of service provision is achievable in a stepwise fashion. The reality is more complex, however, and the question of effectiveness is itself multilayered and approachable from a number of directions.

Quality and strength of evidence are of course matters of concern in the assessment of effectiveness. Anecdotal evidence from one satisfied patient or client tends rightly to count for less than the evidence produced by a study representing the experiences of a large, randomly selected sample. It is clear from an emerging debate in health services research, however, that there are complementary methods of allocating evidential strength (Fitzpatrick and Boulton 1994). This debate has already surfaced and become commonplace in the social service and social policy literature in relation to evaluation research (Smith and Cantley 1985; Cheetham *et al.* 1992), but given the dominance of the biomedical research tradition in the health services, it seems to have gained ground here only since the early to mid-1990s (Klein 1996). The debate centres around the appropriateness of using experimental and quasi-experimental methods of evaluation in situations where the independent variables involved in a service are difficult both to identify and to measure, and where the dependent variables (the outcomes) are likewise complex and multifaceted. When it is difficult to quantify the inputs and the consequences of an intervention or service, then a highly reductionist and formulaic approach is unlikely to yield results which are of use to policy and practice.

Coulter (1991) outlines four levels of evaluation which need consideration in the health context:

- the evaluation of specific treatments
- the evaluation of patterns of care for particular patient groups
- the evaluation of organizations
- the evaluation of health systems.

(Coulter 1991: 116)

This is a useful distinction to make since these different levels imply an increasing amount of heterogeneity and complexity in the type of health service under consideration. While it is unwise to be prescriptive about the fit between the evaluative strategy, and the level of health context, it is likely that primary evidence derived from experimental and quasi-experimental methods of evaluation should give ground to evidence derived from more naturalistic methods, such as pluralistic (or stakeholder) evaluation (Smith and Cantley 1985) as the health service context becomes less focused and less quantifiable. While evidence from randomized controlled trials might be taken as gold-standard for certain specific treatments, service evaluation requires a multi-method approach (Ong 1993), and the capacity to reconcile conflicting types of qualitative and quantitative evidence.

Such methodological pluralism has not been substantially recognized in the type of evidence used for assessing effectiveness. Health care purchasers are encouraged to regard evidence coming from experimental and quasi-experimental methods of evaluation as being superior to other types. For example, the District Health Authority (DHA) Needs Assessment Series (Stevens and Raftery 1994) adopts, with modifications, the scale developed by the United States Preventive Services Task Force for assessing quality of evidence. This scale rates evidence obtained from at least one properly organized randomized controlled trial highest, and evidence obtained from the opinions of respected authorities based on clinical experience, descriptive studies or reports of expert committees very low, just scraping above evidence deemed to be inadequate owing to problems of methodology, or conflict in evidence (Stevens and Raftery 1994: 24).

A number of points can be made about this. First, evidence of effectiveness is always likely to be stronger from research carried out in a rigorous manner than that which is weak, whichever research design is used. *If* it can be assumed that the most appropriate research design has been carried out for a specific evaluation then the notion of 'hierarchy' is misplaced. Experimental designs are not always appropriate, practical or ethical, therefore evidence derived from alternative designs is not in any sense inferior. Second, any attempt to classify the evidence gained from naturalistic research methods alongside poorly conducted quantitative research shows a lack of understanding of naturalistic research. Third, it is incumbent upon naturalistic researchers to explain the characteristics of rigorous and weak naturalistic research, thus providing a research design rating, against which individual studies can be judged.

It is worth highlighting the existence of this epistemological debate, since much of the jargon of health services research assumes that the meanings attached to terms like 'evidence' and 'effectiveness' are essentially shared, and that most health services are amenable to basically the same kind of investigation. This is too simple an assumption, particularly when it comes to the level of service, organization and policy evaluation. A difficulty that many health purchasers and planners are currently facing is the requirement that provision of services should be based on evidence of effectiveness; asking about the effectiveness of existing services, many of which have developed in an incremental fashion over many years, subject to local pressures, is not something that can be easily answered. The challenges surrounding the evaluation of specialist palliative care services are a case in point.

The effectiveness of specialist palliative care services

Are specialist palliative care services effective? Do they represent good value for money and contribute substantially to health gain in the population? Many health care purchasers would of course like to have a 'yes' or 'no' answer to this question, since palliative care is provided by many non-specialists across a broad range of settings. To many planners it is unclear to what extent specialist services duplicate the care already provided by NHS providers, and to what extent they offer a qualitatively different and valuable service. As well, it is unclear whether the models of care developed over recent years represent the most efficient models of delivering palliative care to the largest number requiring such care. Hospices developed as centres of specialist services (inpatient, home care, day care, and so on) largely out of the directly controlling ambit of health authorities, and it has been since the advent of contracting that a much more formal element has been introduced to the relationship between specialist services and health care purchasers (Clark *et al.* 1995a; Clark *et al.* 1995b). Because on average, independent hospices receive 35 per cent of their income through contracts with district purchasers (Higginson 1995), they have become fair game in the commissioning process and the setting of priorities.

From where might district purchasers find evidence of the effectiveness of specialist palliative care services? Recourse to the research record does not furnish a glittering array of sources. Service level evaluations using experimental and quasi-experimental approaches have not been able to demonstrate incontrovertible superiority of specialist services over generalist (non-specialist) services, although studies focusing on specific palliative care interventions (certain procedures used for some patients requiring palliative care, some of the time, in specific settings) have demonstrated that patients have had better symptom control, or have been more satisfied, or their relatives have been more adjusted/satisfied than non-specialist care (Goddard 1993; Higginson 1995; Johnston and Abraham 1995). At the level of cost analysis, studies have drawn attention to the difficulty of comparing costs between different specialist providers with their differing mixes of inpatient and domiciliary care, their commitment to teaching, and their reliance on volunteer labour.

Providing more of a service, or even a new service is justifiable if it leads to a general rise in standards of care (for the greatest number), and has health or social benefit spin-offs. What the hospice movement has possibly not been able to demonstrate is whether 'better' always means 'more' (and more of the same) (Torrens 1985), and this is also the dilemma facing health care purchasers. Should resources be directed to hospices and specialist teams in the community and hospital settings for the purpose of facilitating health care pluralism and the maintenance of patient choice; or are the opportunity costs too high? (Should the money spent on hospices be better spent on resourcing and educating primary health care teams to take on almost all the palliative and terminal care required, or indeed, QALY for QALY would the money be better spent elsewhere in the health service?)

It is clearly important as to whether specialist palliative care services are deemed to be effective, and to begin there needs to be a definition of specialist palliative care and then a view as to what elements of palliative care can be assessed meaningfully in relation to the concept of effectiveness.

Defining specialist palliative care

In its broadest sense, palliative care is an approach rather than a discrete intervention. Caring, the palliative way, is to focus on the medical, nursing, spiritual, emotional and social needs of patients and their families, and seek to meet them through a variety of means. It is thus a style of caring: an acknowledgement of the need to approach patients 'holistically', and to be inventive in the range of solutions offered. The types of care using this approach can be grouped in various ways. There is a range of skills and competencies which are felt to be part of the repertoire of specialist practitioners in palliative care such as expert pain and symptom control, psychosocial support and bereavement counselling, and domiciliary supportive nursing. Equally, there is a range of settings in which such skills can be applied – inpatient, outpatient; domiciliary and continuing care settings – and a range of diseases for which the palliative care approach can be indicated (for example, cancer, the end-stages of major organ failure, and degenerative neurological conditions). The different permutations of palliative intervention with setting and illness type (including the vast heterogeneity of needs of cancer patients at different stages of their illnesses) has led to difficulties with defining what palliative care is and entails.

A distinction which has come to dominate discourse in this area is that between specialist and non-specialist palliative care (Doyle *et al.* 1993). Where practitioners are almost exclusively concerned with the needs and care of terminally ill patients, and also have formal qualifications in care of dying people/palliative medicine, then the service provided by such practitioners is tended to be labelled 'specialist palliative care' (NCHSPCS 1995c). If specialists actually provide something which non-specialists cannot or do not, then the label is probably justified. However, in the case of palliative care, it is not always clear what, in addition, specialists provide over non-specialists. Is it up-to-date knowledge of pharmacological and non-pharmacological advances in pain and symptom control? Is it counselling skills in breaking bad news, and effective communication? Is it practical advice on benefits and financial matters? Equally possible, could it be a matter of resources, such as *time* for unhurried consultations and nursing sessions, or *easily* accessible beds for respite and terminal care, or *effective* multidisciplinary teamworking?

Specialist palliative care services are generally provided in addition to mainstream services: the community nurse continues to visit a patient receiving specialist input, and the nurse may feel the burden of responsibility shared; the general practitioner (GP) will continue to prescribe medication and offer advice but may feel that extra help is more easily obtainable if the situation warrants a second opinion. In some circumstances the specialist services may effectively take over the primary care, particularly so if the patient chooses to use inpatient hospice facilities. However, the point here is that specialist palliative care does not have a 'pure' effect, and terminally ill patients who do *not* receive specialist palliative care services *may* receive care of an appropriate and acceptable standard from mainstream services; indeed, many practitioners working in the general health services have undertaken training in palliative care although they are not primarily identified as specialists in palliative care.

Effectiveness of palliative care

Effectiveness can be assessed using a variety of process and outcome indicators, but is generally accepted to be concerned with efficiency, impact and quality (Drummond and O'Brien 1993). Quantitative indicators of effectiveness include those which are essentially clinical (cure or remission rates, associated morbidity or mortality, etc.), those which are cost-related (the ratio of inputs to outputs or consequences, valued in particular ways) and those relating to impact on health status, well-being (both social and psychological well-being) and preference. Effectiveness can also be assessed by qualitative means, by eliciting the perceptions of the different stakeholders, and through an iterative process, comparing and contrasting different perceptions in relation to the experiences of service provision (Smith and Cantley 1985).

Applying these types of indicators to palliative care services necessitates clear definitions of the content of services, and yet – as the previous section illustrated – it appears that an astonishing variation in the pattern and mix of specialist and non-specialist, voluntary and statutory services has developed over the years. To be able to assert that specific services are effective requires a comparison between the service and the alternatives to the service (which may be other types of similar services or very limited interventions of any kind). Many of these basic comparative studies, taking into account outcomes, measures of performance and cost, have not been carried out for palliative care services. For example, there have not been recent studies which have studied the effectiveness of specialist palliative care advisory home nursing services in comparison to the community nursing services, nor the effectiveness of hospice care compared to care offered by community hospitals or other non-acute inpatient settings. While the impetus for developing palliative care services came from surveys that illustrated deficiencies in the care of terminally ill people in the community and hospital settings in the mid-1970s, it has been assumed that the patterns of services which developed to meet these needs actually developed in the most effective way. On the one hand, it would appear to be self-evident that palliative care services are effective under minimum criteria because patients use the services (and professionals refer patients to them) and there is enormous support for the continuation of the services (for example, the sheer volume of charitable and volunteer support for the independent hospice sector). On the other hand, relying on such sentiment as evidence of effectiveness is not without its perils in the current political climate of effectiveness, economy and efficiency. It also ignores the developments which have taken place in mainstream services in the meantime.

Considerable progress has been made in recent years in palliative care research to establish the tools for assessing performance of palliative care services, and for addressing the questions of standards and quality assurance. Various organizations have been working on the development of a minimum dataset for palliative care (across the variety of settings in which it is delivered) in order to produce performance indicators, not only for management purposes within each setting, but also to provide a comparative picture (for example, the National Council for Hospice and Specialist Palliative Care Services); a review of outcome measures in palliative care summarizes progress to date and lists the sources of the various instruments which have been used to measure outcome from the variety of perspectives (NCHSPCS 1995a); cost analysis in palliative care has proved more difficult to undertake although the attempts have been reviewed (King *et al.* 1993; Whynes, Chapter 2 in this volume); while organizational audit and quality assurance have become well researched (Higginson 1992).

Palliative care developed in the USA as rapidly as it did in the UK, but the effectiveness of services came under scrutiny much earlier, possibly because of the more overtly commercial nature of US health care financing systems. Both experimental and quasi-experimental approaches to evaluation were used which demonstrated some advantages of hospice care over conventional care. In the UK, there have been comparatively few attempts to compare hospice (or specialist) care with conventional care prospectively. There have been descriptive surveys of the inadequacies of conventional care (for example, Wilkes 1965; Haines and Booroff 1986; Herd 1990); a considerable amount of self-evaluation research in hospices and specialist palliative care teams (for example, Doyle 1991; Hinton 1994), and there have been the retrospective surveys of the circumstances surrounding terminal illness and death as reported by nearest carers (Cartwright and Seale 1990; Addington-Hall and McCarthy 1995). One major comparative study which has been collecting prospective data over recent years has yet to report its results (the York University Study). (Summaries of the findings of recent palliative care research is provided by Higginson 1995; Robbins 1996.) In the UK, it appears that the problems and issues involved in evaluating the effectiveness of palliative care are well understood, but technical difficulties deter research from taking place (quite apart from the difficulty of obtaining research funding), while the political issues surrounding the heavy involvement of the voluntary sector distort the research agenda further.

To summarize this section, it appears that the research record does not furnish the types of evidence that health care purchasers require for service planning according to the theoretical principles of health care commissioning at the present. Particularly, research on the most effective models of care across the different settings is not available.

Needs assessment

A framework of need

Defining what constitutes *need* as opposed to *demand* and *supply* has exercised many minds over the years. In the health and social services Bradshaw's taxonomy of need has been referred to as a beacon of practical thinking in the mire of confusion about relative and universal needs. Interestingly, 25 years on, Bradshaw himself was less certain of the utility of the word in relation to health needs: 'the concept of need has always been too imprecise, too complex, too contentious to be a useful target for policy' (1994: 45), and he suggests a distinction between need for health, and need for health services which can usefully be applied to the case of palliative care.

Needs assessment in palliative care can start from two angles. First, a needs assessment can begin by examining the care needs of terminally ill people, and asking what form of welfare and provision best meets those needs. Alternatively, a needs assessment can start with the assumption that palliative care services, as they are currently structured, constitute the best way of meeting the needs of terminally ill people. The question to be answered therefore is about the appropriate quantity of such services for a defined population. The difference between these is that the former begins with the person-based indications for health and social care (e.g. lack of home support, uncontrolled symptoms, the desire for spiritual discussion) while the latter starts with requirements for defined palliative care services (e.g. number of hospice beds or home care nurses per head of population). These alternative options are shown in Table 1.1, which maps out the relationship between the policy option of providing high quality care for terminally ill people, and the way in which the policy can become operationalized.

Pragmatically, few population-based health care needs assessments start with the assessment in the population of the need for health care; needs assessments have tended to be operationalized in relation to discrete services, on the assumption that these services are effective and appropriate. Needs assessments of palliative care have followed this model.

No health district in the UK would start off a needs assessment at present with a blank sheet in relation to palliative care services. Most districts have a variety of specialist palliative care services provided across the statutory and voluntary sectors, and in the different settings (Clark *et al.*

Table 1.1 The relationship between policy for care of terminally ill people and its operationalization

Aim	Objective	Operationalization of objectives	Criteria for judging objectives	Indicators for assessing criteria
High quality, responsive care for people with terminal illness	Routine provision of palliative care in all care settings	*Option 1* Specialist palliative care services separately funded within health care services	● Pain and symptom control ● Family support (pre and post bereavement) ● Psychosocial and spiritual support for patient ● Equitable access to services ● Cost-efficiency ● Public, patient and provider acceptability and accountability	Performance measures, costs and quality of life assessments relating to ● Inputs ● Processes ● Outputs ● Outcomes (impacts) reflecting the variety of participant perspectives
		Option 2 Palliative care provided within existing primary, secondary and tertiary care sectors		
		Option 3 No clear model. A combination of Options 1 and 2.		

1996). In turn this will tend to mean that future provision will be determined at least in part by the legacy from the past. This does not, however, mean that a fragmentation of funding and managerial accountability across the different sectors is an ideal way of providing what should be a routine, general access system of care. If maternity care were provided by a patchwork of voluntary, independent hospitals and charitably funded midwives, together with some provision in NHS facilities and GP services, rationalization and equity of access would become pressing issues. However, with palliative care, because the independent hospice movement has been so proactive, there is a widespread acceptance of the involvement of the voluntary sector in providing palliative care (especially terminal care) and a routinization and incorporation of its provider status.

In the UK, following the NHS and community care reforms of 1990, health authorities and social service departments have been charged with the task of providing needs led services. More attention is therefore focused on the process of needs assessment, and how this can be done in ways which feed into policy and planning. There are three main models of health care needs assessment which are currently used in health planning and commissioning (Stevens and Raftery 1994). One model starts with population based measures of disease (epidemiological approach); another model starts with variations in health care utilization and costs (comparative approach); and the other model starts with the preferences and demands (rather than needs) of the different interested parties in health service provision and uptake (corporate approach). The most robust approach is considered to be the epidemiological approach but this is not necessarily suited to a range of service level, broad based interventions. The comparative and corporate approaches represent more pragmatic, alternative strategies. A discussion of each of these models is presented, with illustration of the extent to which each has been used in the planning of palliative care services.

Epidemiologically based needs assessment

The epidemiological approach to needs assessment has been the model recommended by the Department of Health in the UK to district purchasers and GPs, for best informing health care planning and commissioning. This is a triadic model, with measures of prevalence and incidence at one corner, evidence concerning effectiveness and cost-effectiveness at another, and knowledge of existing services at the third. It is asserted that these three components form the basis of 'triangulation' whereby purchasers can determine the policy directions they wish to pursue (Stevens and Raftery 1994). Amassing the sort of evidence required for needs assessment represents a considerable task for district health authorities. Various recent initiatives have been funded by the Department of Health to make the task

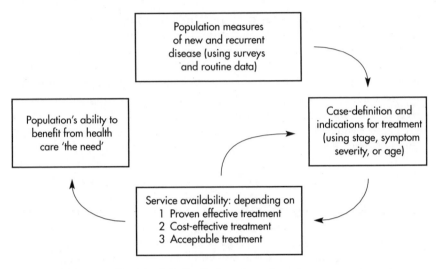

Figure 1.1   Stages of epidemiologically based needs assessment

easier, for example the 'DHA Health Care Needs Assessment' series, the 'Effectiveness Bulletins' produced by the NHS Centre for Reviews and Dissemination, providing expertise in reviewing research evidence through the Cochrane Collaboration, and the production of the Public Health Common Data Set.[1]

Figure 1.1 shows the way in which the three points of the epidemiologically based model relate to each other. The relationship between indications for treatment and service availability is clearly one likely to be in flux as new treatments are developed, possibly widening the clinical indications for treatment, and as research findings confirm or refute the effectiveness of treatments.

It is clear that the epidemiological approach to needs assessment works best when the prevalence and incidence of internationally classified diseases can be reliably measured in the population, and when there are clear clinical indications for widely agreed (and effective) interventions. There are not many diseases which fall into this category; those that do, tend to be sudden onset conditions, with relatively unambiguous or uncontested treatments (e.g. appendectomy for acute appendicitis). None the less, the epidemiological model is considered to be the most robust method informing the planning of health care for populations, and is attempted, with varying degrees of success for all major areas of health care provision. This approach is clearly based on definitions and standards set by the non-user; often academic researchers using expert clinical (medical) opinion, and represents a kind of 'top down' approach to needs assessment.

Given the emphasis placed on epidemiological approaches to needs assessment it is interesting to see how far they have been applied to the case of palliative care. Routine data (disease classification data and health service activity data) do not readily furnish rates of prevalence or incidence of patients requiring palliative care. Extensive use is made of malignant neoplasm rates since palliative care is closely associated with the care of patients with advanced cancer. However, these rates overestimate the number of cancer patients likely to benefit from *specialist* palliative care interventions (assuming that all patients who have an anticipated death – 50 per cent of all deaths – need palliative care).[2] They also underestimate the number of patients dying from other diseases who would also benefit from specialist palliative care services (end-stage major organ failure, neurological conditions, chronic respiratory disease, etc.).

Another source of prevalence data that has been used in the epidemiological approach is that provided by population surveys of various symptoms experienced during terminal illness (Higginson 1995). These data have mainly been obtained from retrospective surveys of reported prevalence by the nearest carer of a sample of deceased people. For example, extrapolating from the figures produced by Cartwright and Seale (1990) and Addington-Hall and McCarthy (1995), Higginson suggests that in a population of 1 million, each year 2400 people with cancer are likely to have pain which requires treatment. Similar extrapolations are performed with regard to other symptoms and levels of anxiety requiring support. Apart from the fact that these data are derived from carers rather than patients themselves, the difficulty with these extrapolations is that they may fairly represent the prevalence of symptoms in the population of terminally ill people, but they do not suggest what proportion require specialist palliative care services. Pain control can be achieved in many settings; indeed many primary health care teams now routinely set up and use syringe drivers for the administration of analgesia, and may also employ a practice based counsellor for psychosocial problems. It is therefore problematic to assume that instances of unrelieved symptoms recorded during long time periods (i.e. in the last year of life) are necessarily indications for specialist palliative care.

Comparative needs assessment

The comparative approach is concerned with levels of service utilization rather than patterns of disease, and starts with the premise that it is meaningful to compare local levels of activity against national averages. Studies of clinical practice variation over recent years have drawn attention to geographical and specialty disparities in health care utilization, implying that some populations are under-served, and some may be over-provided. Where a local level is found to be different from a regional or national average, then under this approach, attention is drawn to ways of bringing the level closer to the average. Comparison in this manner, cannot assume that the average level is necessarily the most appropriate level for the population taking into account other factors (such as demographic profile, socio-economic status and ethnic mix), but it can be used as a relatively rough 'league table' of health service utilization. This approach is based on the assumption that services basically 'muddle through'; they probably meet most of the need for them most of the time.

In relation to palliative care services this approach has been widely used. For example, statistics produced by the Hospice Information Service relating to numbers of specialist palliative care beds in each health district or region, and number of home care advisory nurses, or day care places are regularly used for descriptive and comparative purposes. Eve and Smith (1994) have also attempted to link the services available with throughput, i.e. the number of patients using the specialist services each year. Districts do vary considerably in the number of inpatient beds available, and also in the proportion of the patients using these services. In some districts it is possible that 50 per cent or more of people dying of cancer each year have some involvement with specialist palliative care services; in other districts the figure may be much lower.

There is of course a danger in using national average service or utilization levels for setting appropriate levels of provision within a district, since districts can vary considerably from each other. The provision of other non-acute inpatient facilities within a district (such as community hospitals) can have an influence on the demand for hospice beds, and so it is important to take into account the characteristics (or case-mix) of districts. An improvement on using national averages might be to perform a kind of cluster analysis where districts or even health care trust catchment areas could be grouped together in terms of common characteristics (such as number of acute care hospitals, whether the district/trust houses regional or supra-regional facilities, its urban/rural profile, etc.). These could then be compared in terms of number of hospice beds, inpatient hospital beds devoted to palliative care, number of specialist palliative care practitioners, and proportion of palliative care services supported by the voluntary sector.

Corporate needs assessment

Another approach to health care planning is to ask the various interested parties for their perceptions about the adequacy of services and any shortfalls in provision. A 'corporate' view is achieved by combining the views of those who provide and purchase health care services, as well as those who receive them, the public in general, politicians and the media. The corporate view is clearly a cultural construct, and is influenced by political and popular ideology, and will tend to reflect personal interests as well as specific group interests. Corporate needs assessment is one of a number of other strategies designed to engage users and stakeholders in the evaluation and quality assessment of health care services. Typically, how this is done involves questionnaire surveys, focus groups, interviews, and methods of achieving consensus through Delphi techniques, nominal groups and expert panels.

The corporate approach to needs assessment represents a 'bottom up' approach as opposed to the 'top down' approach typified by the epidemiologically based approach. This approach is based on ideas of citizenship, and the ideal that services should be organized around the needs and interests of ordinary people, and should be a source of empowerment.

This approach is increasingly being used in the health services as a way of engaging with users, and making services more accountable, although unlike the previous two models discussed above, a formal methodology has not been generally adopted. Conway *et al.* (1995) report a corporate needs assessment for the purchase of district nursing services which has parallels for the assessment of need for palliative care services. They observe that community nursing is unsuited to an epidemiological approach since patients' conditions are not amenable to either classification or quantification, and because community nurses work in variable ways across and between districts. Using a qualitative methodology, the researchers carried out a corporate needs assessment within an inner-city area, where the population of almost 1 million received nursing services from two community trusts and social services from three local authorities. Theoretical sampling was used to select nursing staff from areas which had differing socioeconomic profiles. Taped interviews were carried out with nine district nurses, and the transcripts were subsequently analysed for common themes. This type of qualitative work always exposes the complex and infinitely variable features of life and work as it is lived, and while rich and illuminating it can be difficult to draw conclusions. However, the authors drew attention to a series of needs which they recommended should inform future purchasing strategies. The most important needs were more effective teamwork, communication, and flexibility in working methods, and they suggested that service specifications should focus on changes at the interfaces of care (with social services and GPs), to enable more effective working.

Heslop (1995) reviewed the various ways in which a corporate needs assessment approach may be applied to palliative care which particularly incorporates the views of service users. She described the types of qualitative research methods which may be of use – interviews, surveys, focus groups, search conference and rapid appraisal – but pointed out the difficulties of using these methods with people who are receiving palliative care (either as patients or carers). All research methods which are applied to palliative care are challenged by the need for extreme sensitivity and consideration for the feelings of people who are facing death and bereavement.

While prospective work is possible with the users of palliative care, and is likely to provide a very important perspective on the acceptability of the different models of services, it represents a considerable task within each district (for example, the corporate needs assessment carried out in South Derbyshire: Clark *et al.* 1996). The value of corporate needs assessment is that it comments very directly on a local situation within a district, and although some findings are likely to be of general relevance, each district would really need to carry out its own research exercise. In addition to service user views, it would also be important to take account of the views of the different specialist and non-specialist providers of palliative care. Indeed, a forum of the different providers and purchasers of palliative care within a district can have the important function of regularly reporting back on issues regarding the provision of palliative care.

Models of needs assessment applied to palliative care

Clark and Malson (1995) suggest a framework for needs assessment in palliative care which incorporates aspects of each of the models outlined above: the use of population data, the collection of stakeholder perspectives, and the use of comparative data. Other approaches to needs assessment also bring together varying sources of information. For example, the 'needs audit' reported by Percy-Smith and Sanderson (1992), which attempted to understand local needs in Leeds, combined the use of existing data with information derived from a postal survey, in-depth interviews, focus groups and public meetings. Their framework for needs assessment is possibly robust enough to adopt for a range of health and social services, including palliative care. In essence, their framework includes the following steps:

1 Application of a conceptual framework (e.g. Doyal and Gough's theory of universal human need for critical autonomy and autonomy of agency, cited in Percy-Smith and Sanderson 1992).
2 Examination of people's own perceptions of their needs and comparison with views of purchasers, providers, and community representatives.
3 Examination of how far needs are currently being met.
4 The articulation of people's experience of services and their views of how they could be improved.
5 The attempt to reconcile differing perspectives and achieve a consensus on what the priorities for action should be.
6 The identification of strengths and weaknesses in the needs assessment model used.

(Percy-Smith and Sanderson 1992)

These frameworks are comprehensive and require a substantial amount of work. However, health districts have been charged with the task of assessing health care needs for their populations for a number of years, and from recent surveys it is clear that there has been some variation in approach to assessing needs for palliative care. From a survey of English health districts in 1994, it appeared that not only had some districts done much more work than others, but also much work still needed to be done, with the persistent cry for better quality data and information on effectiveness (Robbins and Frankel 1995). Help for health districts has come from a number of quarters: the National Council for Hospices and Specialist Palliative Care Services has produced a briefing pack for purchasers which includes information about specialist palliative care services and some guidance on assessing needs (NCHSPCS 1995b), information on outcome measures in palliative care (NCHSPCS 1995a), and the report of a project examining access to hospice and specialist palliative care services by members of black and ethnic minority communities (NCHSPCS 1995d); and the epidemiologically based needs assessment produced by Higginson (1995) within Series Two of the DHA needs assessment series also provide useful information for districts embarking on their own needs assessment for palliative care.

There appear to be two major areas which complicate needs assessment in palliative care and which will challenge the 'rational' planning processes of district health authorities and GP fund-holders:

- The balance of service and educational provision between the statutory and voluntary sectors (unless the boundaries between sectors become impossibly blurred).
- What a specialty of palliative care involves and how it integrates with, or superimposes itself on, other specialties, e.g. oncology, care of elderly people, renal medicine, neurology, respiratory medicine, cardiology and most importantly primary care.

These are major organizational issues which require some kind of resolution or decision before palliative care services, as they currently stand, can be neatly incorporated into the commissioning process.

Conclusion

This chapter has reviewed the concepts of needs assessment and effectiveness in relation to specialist palliative care services in order to ask the following questions. How applicable is the current approach of health care commissioning to the case of specialist care services? Is it possible to quantify the need for palliative care? By implication a number of other controversial areas have also been mentioned.

The National Health Service in the UK is becoming increasingly pluralistic, and in one sense the specialist palliative care sector is both a symptom and cause of this. About 25 per cent of all operations in the UK are now carried out in the private sector for those people with health insurance or who can afford to pay (Yates 1995). Around 5 per cent of all deaths each year in the UK occur in hospice beds (only 17 per cent of these are NHS hospice beds), with more than 50 per cent of these costs being met by the voluntary sector. The trends imply that smaller proportions of care are being paid for out of public taxation and government grants, and more is being paid for either directly out of pocket, or through insurance companies or charities. It is thus an increasingly complex situation in which health care purchasers are having to carry out needs assessment, with a challenging balance to maintain between what people want or expect as individual patients/clients/consumers/customers; what people want or expect as groups or communities; what people need as determined by professional groups; and what people should have in the view of politicians.

The palliative care sector has been born out of the voluntary hospice movement but this in itself has become a difficult legacy and makes needs assessment problematic. The world of gap-plugging by charities and volunteer labour in the welfare services does not sit comfortably with this mission of rational planning, and as long as palliative care is subsidized by the voluntary sector, it is less likely that the statutory services will provide routine specialist palliative care services. While government policy has positively encouraged a mixed economy of care in the personal social services, the same policy has not overtly been applied to health care provision (apart from the recent Private Finance Initiative for hospital building and refurbishment). It seems that almost by default, however, the mixed economy has arrived with palliative care.

The complexities of assessing the effectiveness of, and need for, palliative care which this chapter has described need to be turned into opportunities rather than be regarded as insuperable obstacles. It is important that palliative care research engages further with the wider agenda of social and health services research, to explore in depth the various methodological and epistemological issues relating to this area. This could have the effect of making the debate about effectiveness and needs assessment more sophisticated and self-reflective. In turn this may bring about a clearer mandate for the continuation and development of appropriate care for all people experiencing an anticipated death.

Notes

1 More information can be obtained from the following contact points.

   Cochrane Collaboration: Including the Cochrane database of systematic reviews; the database of abstracts of reviews of effectiveness; the Cochrane review methodology database.

Email	update@cochrane.co.uk	(UK)
	tstarr@powergrid.electriciti.com	(USA)
	david.badger@flinders.edu.au	(Aus)
Fax	+44 1865 516918	(UK)
	+1 619432 6650	(USA)
	+61 8276 3305 (attn David Badger)	(Aus)

Marketing and distribution of disks and CD-ROM by BMJ Publishing House, BMA House, Tavistock Square, London WC1H 9JR.

Effectiveness Bulletins: These are published under the title *Effective Health Care*, and are produced by a consortium of the Nuffield Institute for Health, University of Leeds, NHS Centre for Reviews and Dissemination, University of York and the Research Unit of the Royal College of Physicians. Available from Churchill Livingstone, London (fax +44 171 896 2145).

DHA Needs Assessment Series: Commissioned by the Department of Health, UK, Series One was published in 1994 in two volumes under the editorship of Andrew Stevens and James Raftery, Wessex Institute of Public Health Medicine (see publication details for Stevens below). Series One covered needs assessments for diabetes mellitus, renal disease, stroke, lower respiratory disease, coronary heart disease, colorectal cancer, cancer of the lung, total hip replacement, total knee replacement, cataract surgery, hernia repair, varicose vein treatments, prostatectomy for benign prostatic hyperplasia, mental illness, dementia, alcohol misuse, drug abuse, people with learning difficulties, community child health services, family planning, abortion and fertility services. Series Two was published in the autumn of 1996 and included a needs assessment for palliative care.

Public Health Common Data Set: Statistics relating to health regions/districts in the UK, combining Office of Population Censuses and Surveys (OPCS) data with various health activity data. These are commissioned by the Department of Health and available through the Stationery Office.

2 This assumption is derived from the National Council for Hospice and Specialist Palliative Care Services *A Statement of Definitions*: paragraph 4.1 'Half of all deaths in the UK are anticipated. It is this 50 per cent of patients who need palliative care. A significant minority need some – or all – of the skills and facilities provided by a specialist palliative care service' (1995c: 6).

References

Addington-Hall, J. and McCarthy, M. (1995) Regional Study of Care for the Dying: methods and sample characteristics. *Palliative Medicine*, 9: 27–35.

Allsop, J. (1995) *Health Policy and the NHS: Towards 2000*, 2nd edn. London: Longman.

Bradshaw, J. (1994) The conceptualization and measurement of need: a social policy perspective, in J. Popay and G. Williams (eds) *Researching the People's Health*. London: Routledge.

Cartwright, A. and Seale, C. (1990) *The Natural History of a Survey: An Account of the Methodological Issues Encountered in a Study of Life before Death.* King Edward's Hospital Fund for London.

Cheetham, J., Fuller, R., McIvor, G. and Petch, A. (1992) *Evaluating Social Work Effectiveness.* Buckingham: Open University Press.

Clark, D. (1993) Whither the hospices?, in D. Clark (ed.) *The Future for Palliative Care.* Buckingham: Open University Press.

Clark, D. and Malson, H. (1995) Key issues in palliative care needs assessment. *Progress in Palliative Care,* 3(2): 53–5.

Clark, D., Neale, B. and Heather, P. (1995a) Contracting for palliative care. *Social Science and Medicine,* 40(9): 1193–202.

Clark, D., Small, N. and Malson, H. (1995b) Hospices to fortune. *Health Service Journal,* 23 November: 30–1.

Clark, D., Heslop, J., Malson, H. and Craig, B. (1996) *As Much Help as Possible: Assessing Palliative Care Needs in Southern Derbyshire,* occasional paper no. 18. Sheffield: Trent Palliative Care Centre.

Conway, M., Armstrong, D. and Bickler, G. (1995) A corporate needs assessment for the purchase of district nursing: a qualitative approach. *Public Health,* 109: 337–45.

Coulter, A. (1991) Evaluating the outcomes of health care, in J. Gabe, M. Calnan and M. Bury (eds) *The Sociology of the Health Service.* London: Routledge.

Cox, I.G. (1995) General practice, primary care and the community focus for palliative care (letter). *Progress in Palliative Care,* 3(6): 214.

Doyle, D. (1991) A home care service for terminally ill patients in Edinburgh. *Health Bulletin,* 49: 14–23.

Doyle, D., Hanks, G.W.C. and MacDonald, N. (1993) Introduction, in D. Doyle, G.W.C. Hanks and N. MacDonald (eds) *Oxford Textbook of Palliative Medicine.* Oxford: Oxford University Press.

Drummond, M. and O'Brien, B. (1993) Clinical importance, statistical significance and the assessment of economic and quality-of-life outcomes. *Health Economics,* 2: 205–12.

Eve, A. and Smith, A.M. (1994) Palliative care services in Britain and Ireland – update 1991. *Palliative Medicine,* 8: 19–27.

Fitzpatrick, R. and Boulton, M. (1994) Qualitative methods for assessing health care. *Quality in Health Care,* 3: 107–13.

Goddard, M. (1989) The role of economics in the evaluation of hospice care. *Health Policy,* 13: 19–34.

Goddard, M. (1993) The importance of assessing the effectiveness of care: the case of hospices. *Journal of Social Policy,* 22: 1–17.

Haines, A. and Booroff, A. (1986) Terminal care at home: perspective from general practice. *British Medical Journal,* 292: 1051–3.

Herd, E.B. (1990) Terminal care in a semi-rural area. *British Journal of General Practice,* 40: 248–51.

Heslop, J. (1995) Palliative care needs assessment: incorporating the views of service users. *Progress in Palliative Care,* 3(4): 135–7.

Higginson, I. (1992) *Quality, Standards, Organisational and Clinical Audit for Hospice and Palliative Care Services.* London: National Council for Hospice and Specialist Palliative Care Services.

Higginson, I. (1995) *DHA Project: Epidemiologically-Based Needs Assessment. Series 2: Palliative and Terminal Care.* London: Department of Health.

Hinton, J. (1994) Can home care maintain an acceptable quality of life for patients with terminal cancer and their relatives? *Palliative Medicine,* 8: 183–96.

Johnston, G. and Abraham, C. (1995) The WHO objectives for palliative care: to what extent are we achieving them? *Palliative Medicine,* 9: 123–37.

King, M., Lapsley, I., Llewellyn, S., Tierney, A., Anderson, J. and Sladden, S. (1993) Purchasing palliative care: availability and cost implications. *Health Bulletin,* 51: 370–84.

Klein, R. (1996) The NHS and the new scientism: solution or delusion? *Quarterly Journal of Medicine,* 89: 85–7.

Lunt, B. and Hillier, R. (1981) Terminal care: present services and future priorities. *British Medical Journal,* 283: 595–8.

NCHSPCS (1995a) *Outcome Measures in Palliative Care.* London: National Council for Hospice and Specialist Palliative Care Services.

NCHSPCS (1995b) *Information for Purchasers.* London: National Council for Hospice and Specialist Palliative Care Services.

NCHSPCS (1995c) *Specialist Palliative Care: A Statement of Definitions.* London: National Council for Hospice and Specialist Palliative Care Services.

NCHSPCS (1995d) *Opening Doors: Improving the Access to Hospice and Specialist Palliative Care Services by Members of the Black and Ethnic Minority Communities.* London: National Council for Hospice and Specialist Palliative Care Services.

Ong, B.N. (1993) *The Practice of Health Services Research.* London: Chapman & Hall.

Øvretveit, J. (1995) *Purchasing for Health.* Buckingham: Open University Press.

Percy-Smith, J. and Sanderson I. (1992) *Understanding Local Needs.* London: Institute for Public Policy Research.

Robbins, M. (1996) *Evaluating Palliative Care.* Oxford: Oxford University Press.

Robbins, M. and Frankel, S. (1995) Palliative care services: what needs assessment? *Palliative Medicine,* 9(4): 287–94.

Sackett, D.L. and Rosenberg, M.C. (1995) On the need for evidence-based medicine. *Journal of Public Health Medicine,* 17: 330–4.

Smith, G. and Cantley, C. (1985) *Assessing Health Care: A Study in Organisational Evaluation.* Milton Keynes: Open University Press.

Standing Medical Advisory Committee and Standing Nursing and Midwifery Advisory Committee (1992) *The Principles and Provision of Palliative Care.* London: HMSO.

Stevens, A. and Raftery, J. (eds) (1994) *Health Care Needs Assessment: The Epidemiologically Based Needs Assessment Reviews, Volumes 1 and 2.* Oxford: Radcliffe Medical Press.

Torrens, P.R. (1985) Hospice care: what have we learned? *Annual Review of Public Health,* 6: 65–83.

Wilkes, E. (1965) Terminal cancer at home. *Lancet,* i: 799–801.

Yates, J. (1995) Serving two masters, *Dispatches.* Report for Channel 4 television.

2 Costs of palliative care

DAVID WHYNES

In December 1948, just four months after the launch of the UK's National Health Service (NHS), the Minister of Health announced to his colleagues in government that the budget allocation for the first year of operation was being revised upwards by some 28 per cent. He ascribed the need for revision to the unanticipated high levels of both demand and health care costs once the service had been initiated (Klein 1995). In this respect, the UK received an abrupt and early warning of a trend since observable in all industrialized countries, namely, the tendency of health care expenditures to rise over time. In 1960, the countries of Europe allocated, on average, 3.9 per cent of their annual gross domestic products (GDPs) to health care yet, by 1992, this proportion had more than doubled to reach 8.3 per cent. The relative change for the world's largest spender on health care – the USA – was even more extreme; the share of health care in that economy rose from 5.3 to 13.8 per cent of GDP over the same period (Office of Health Economics 1995).

Since the 1980s, the observation that medical expenditures are absorbing ever-increasing proportions of national output has placed the costs of care at the top of the health policy agenda. As a result, cost-containment strategies have been implemented in the public health sectors of most industrialized countries. These range from limitations on forms of treatment, the introduction of co-payment and modifications in the structure of physicians' remuneration to, in some cases, the radical overhaul of the entire health care system (Organization for Economic Cooperation and Development 1990). Irrespective of the particular form chosen, all cost-control strategies are essentially operating in one of two ways. Put simply, reducing the growth of health care expenditure means either constraining the growth of demand or limiting the rise in the cost of treatment. In turn, the former resorts either to rationing, by modifying eligibility to benefit criteria, or to increasing the price of health care to the consumer, while, for its part, constraining the growth of costs is essentially concerned with the pursuit of efficiency in provision.

Irrespective of the cost-containment strategy adopted, it has become increasingly difficult for health care providers in any industrialized country to contemplate initiating courses of treatment in the expectation of achieving therapeutic benefits, without also considering the costs of care incurred by those treatments. In some countries, this need to balance costs and outcomes in determining spending priorities has been made explicit, one well-known example being the Oregon experiment in Medicare resource rationing in the USA (Dixon and Welch 1991; Kitzhaber 1993). In similar vein, the 1990 reforms of the health services in the UK were prefaced with the observation: 'If the NHS is to provide the best service it can for its patients, it must make the best use of resources available to it. The quest for value for money must be an essential element in its work' (Department of Health 1989: 7). Clearly, if the value-for-money criterion is to apply at all, it is to apply equally to all possible treatments, and this would therefore include palliative care.

The issue of cost is especially prominent in the case of palliative care for one very simple reason. By its very nature, palliative care is typically a prelude to patient death. Death, however, is extremely demanding of health care resources, as detailed studies of the US Medicare system – public health insurance for elderly people – have shown. In 1978, 5.9 per cent of Medicare enrolees died, yet they accounted for 27.9 per cent of all Medicare expenditures in that year (Lubitz and Prihoda 1984). A replication of this calculation for 1988 yielded broadly similar proportions of 5.1 and 27.2 per cent, respectively. About 40 per cent of all Medicare costs in the last year of life accrued in the 30 days prior to death (Lubitz and Riley 1993). It is, of course, obvious that not all of these 'high costs of dying' (Ginzberg 1980) can be attributed to palliative care alone. A proportion must be ascribed to bona fide attempts at curative treatment which, with the benefit of hindsight, evidently failed. This fact notwithstanding, it is clear that the provision of palliative care must make *some* contribution to the relatively high health care cost associated with the final period of patients' lives.

Costs and palliation modalities

To the economist, any medical procedure is a production process, whereby inputs (such as drugs, labour, specialist equipment and so forth) are employed to generate an outcome (for example, improved survival or quality of life benefits). Typically, the procedure will not be defined as a unique technology or modality, i.e. there will be more than one clinically acceptable way of producing the desired result (Whynes 1995). For example, heart disease might be amenable to either surgical or medical management in either a normal hospital ward or an intensive care unit, with recovery taking place either in hospital or the patient's own home (Wennberg 1990). It is the range of the inputs employed, and their intensity of use, which determines the precise cost and outcome of treatment for each possible therapeutic modality. In the specific case of palliative care, we might follow the World Health Organization (WHO) in taking the outcome to encompass a death which is neither hastened nor postponed, where there is relief from pain and other symptoms, and where the spiritual, psychological and social support of both patient and family are attended to (World Health Organization 1990). Differing palliation modalities offer the possibility of differences in both cost and outcome, and perhaps the most obvious variation to consider initially is the institutional care setting.

The institutional setting of palliative care is closely associated with the place of death. In the earlier part of the twentieth century, prior to the development of comprehensive public health services, the majority of people in industrialized countries would have died in private homes, with the comfort of whatever palliation their families or charity might provide. In the USA, a trend towards dying in hospital and other institutions appears to have emerged in the interwar period and the proportion of all deaths occurring in institutions has been roughly stable, at around two-thirds, since the 1960s (Scitovsky 1984). Figure 2.1 presents more recent data for England and Wales, which indicate that the proportion of deaths occurring in institutions is continuing to grow in these countries, from 63 per cent of the total in 1974 to 74 per cent in 1992. Since the early to mid-1980s, institutions outside the NHS, which include those operated by the voluntary and private sectors, have evidently come to play a more significant role. An equivalent growth in institutional care also appears to be occurring in Canada (Wodinsky 1992).

The institutional setting in which palliative care is delivered is a key determinant of overall care costs, as the results of recent studies have demonstrated. Perhaps the most obvious investigation to take as an example is the US National Hospice Study, which ran between 1978 and 1985 (Greer et al. 1986; Mor et al. 1988b). The initiation of this study was a direct result of the rapid growth of the hospice movement in the USA which, in turn, was leading to pressure for the inclusion of hospice benefits within Medicare. The study compared both costs and outcomes of conventional care (CC), as administered in hospitals, with those of hospice, either hospital-based (HB) or centred around home care (HC). In total, 40 hospice and 14 CC sites were the subject of detailed investigation. Total costs per patient per week over the last year of life were estimated for nearly 6000 patients drawn from the three modalities. Overall, the cost of CC for the year amounted to $14,800 on average, the totals for HB and HC being estimated at $12,700 and $10,800, respectively. Thus the HB and HC

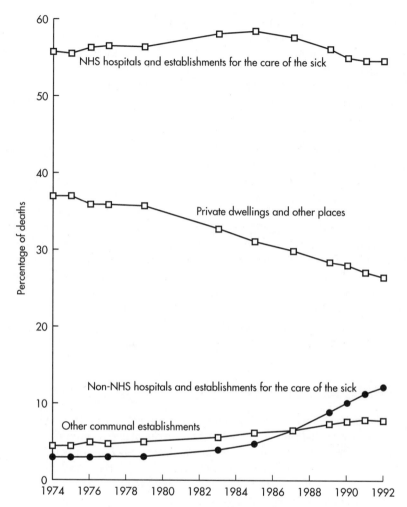

Figure 2.1   Place of death, England and Wales, 1974–92
Source: OPCS Mortality Statistics, Series DH1, nos. 1–27

modalities represented cost savings for the year over CC of 14 and 27 per cent, respectively. It should be noted that, up until the final two months, the weekly costs of CC were actually marginally lower than those of the hospice modalities. The cost-saving effect of hospice thus occurs thereafter and the effect is especially pronounced during the last 30 day: weekly costs for this time period were estimated at $551, $607 and $1482 for HC, HB and CC, respectively. In all settings, weekly costs rose as death approached, although the rise in CC costs was obviously the most pronounced.

The findings with respect to comparative costs can be interpreted quite simply. Although the three modalities comprise quite different input combinations, the principal factor distinguishing them in terms of total cost over a given period of time is the differential length of hospital inpatient stay. Hospital days, which are characterized by the more intensive use of medical treatment and physicians' labour, inevitably emerge as being considerably more expensive than outpatient and home care visits, or days in nursing homes or in other non-hospital institutions. Thus, in limiting the extent of required stay in hospital, the HC modality (and, to a lesser extent, the HB) appears significantly cheaper than CC. This dominant influence of hospital inpatient stay on the costs of palliative care modalities has also been observed in other hospice and home care evaluations (Bloom and Kissick 1980; Brooks and Smyth-Staruch 1984; Gray *et al.* 1987; Beck-Friis *et al.* 1991), while a study of terminal care for AIDS patients in the Netherlands has similarly concluded that hospital inpatient care is by far the more expensive palliation option, in comparison with a mixture of home care and hospital outpatient consultations (Postma *et al.* 1995). Concluding from these findings, it would appear that the overall cost of dying in the USA is likely to have stabilized, give the observed constancy in the proportion of patients dying in institutions. As the proportion of UK patients dying in institutions shows, as yet, no signs of having stabilized (Figure 2.1), we must predict further rises in the cost of dying in the UK case.

Issues in cost measurement

In broad terms, these research findings with respect to palliative care replicate those for most other forms of medical treatment, in finding that home care is typically cheaper than institutional care and, among institutions, hospitals are the most expensive. Let us explore further why this should be the case. Although it is certainly possible that relative efficiency effects might exist, one suspects that a very large proportion of the perceived cost differences between modalities can actually be explained by the possibility that 'like is not being compared with like' (Whynes 1993).

At present, there exists no agreed protocol for the delivery of palliative care to patients with end-stage disease. If patients under one modality actually receive more care inputs than under another, then the costs of the former are likely to be higher. In the National Hospice Study, for example, it was found that CC patients were far more likely to have received physician-supervised intensive medical interventions (such as chemotherapy and surgery), diagnostic tests and transfusions prior to death. The higher intensity of treatment clearly represents a factor in explaining the higher costs of hospital care (Mor *et al.* 1988b). Against the trend, one US study actually determined that hospice care was no cheaper than hospital care, although it should be noted that the hospice service being considered was actually operating with a higher staffing ratio than the hospital service with which comparisons were being made (Kane *et al.* 1984).

When cost comparisons between modalities are being made, it is generally the case that only formal costs (that is, cases where real money, as it were, changes hands) are considered. In the case of palliative care, this exposes the cost estimates to bias. First, the hospice movement in both the UK and the USA has always maintained a strong voluntary element in its labour force. The National Hospice Study detected a wide range of paid staff to volunteers in its sample, from 1:1 to as high as 1:5 (Mor *et al.* 1988b). Volunteers were typically engaged in counselling and companionship, but also undertook tasks such as patient transport, cleaning and administration. A contemporary study of 40 UK hospices determined that the number of volunteers per hospice varied between 50 and 350, undertaking much the same tasks as those in the US study (Hill and Oliver 1988). From the point of view of cost estimation, it is clear that, if volunteers are undertaking work which would otherwise have to be undertaken by paid staff, then the costs of hospice will appear artificially low, particularly when compared with, for example, a non-charitable hospital using only paid staff. Similar remarks can be made in cases where hospices are in receipt of charitable donations, which enables them to subsidize their services in a manner not available to institutions dependent on full-cost care contracts (Clark *et al.* 1995).

Second, in comparison with all forms of institutional care, home care typically displays lower costs. However, the bias here arises because, in this case, a large part of the care burden falls upon informal carers whose efforts are not usually costed in the formal sense. Outpatient chemotherapy, for example, typically appears cheaper than the equivalent treatment administered on an inpatient basis because the 'hotel' costs are borne, not by the institution, but by the patients themselves, or by their family and other carers (Friedlander and Tattersall 1982; Ferris *et al.* 1991). In one US study, 20 out of 140 patients receiving outpatient chemotherapy spent more than 50 per cent of their incomes on non-medical expenses associated with attendance (Houts *et al.* 1984). One Swedish comparison of terminal cancer care explicitly recognized that the cost economies of home, as opposed to hospital, care essentially result from the willingness of the patient's family to shoulder the care burden. 'A helpful next-of-kin in most instances is a prerequisite' and home care for a 'dying, multi-symptomatic cancer patient without aiding relatives would presumably require much more nursing, and thus entail higher costs' (Beck-Friis *et al.* 1991: 263).

One final problem in comparing the costs of palliative modalities arises from the fact that patients are not homogeneous. As with most branches of medicine, it is reasonable to argue that, the more complicated the case, then the more probable is an eventual referral to hospital. From the cost point of view, a form of adverse selection operates, with hospitals attracting those cases likely to require the largest amount of expenditure on palliation and potential remedial treatment. In addition, the National Hospice Study identified a considerable degree of selection bias, in the sense that the hospice sites tended both to recruit physicians and to attract patients for whom intensive interventions were unattractive (Greer *et al.* 1986). When adjusted for patient mix, for example, the perceived cost advantages of hospital-based hospice over conventional care during the final weeks of life largely disappeared (Kidder 1988). More recently, it is emerging that the patient mix within US hospices is changing, due to circumstances beyond the hospices' control. With the increased provision of hospice services in the USA, and in an effort to control their own costs, US hospitals have begun a movement towards 'quicker and sicker' discharge of their elderly patients. Modern hospices are now observed to provide more acute care and more skilled nursing. Therefore, not only are US hospices moving towards the medical model of palliation which the hospice movement once sought to replace, but also their cost structures are coming to mirror those of conventional hospital care (Estes and Swan 1993).

Bearing all these caveats in mind, it emerges that costing palliation modalities is problematic, even when, ostensibly, the same types of institutions are being compared. By way of example, a UK study of 11 hospices estimated a mean cost per bed day of £132, within a range of £58 to £260 (King *et al.* 1993). Factors such as those identified above – the use of volunteers, patient mix, differential inputs, passing on costs to informal carers – accounted for the variation. Although earlier studies had indicated the presence of scale economies in hospice care (Goddard 1989), it is interesting to note that the two hospices at the extremes of the cost range were of the same size.

The scope for economies in palliative care

In a general environment of cost-containment, no single area of health care can hope to escape scrutiny with a view to seeking economies. Accordingly, what scope exists for achieving reductions in the cost of palliative or terminal treatments? The literature identifies three broad sets of possibilities, namely, the increased use of advance directives, efficiency gains in institutional settings and the reduction of 'futile care'. Each of these will be considered in turn.

Advance directives

The use of advance directives (ADs) in the USA has arisen from the belief in the need to empower patients in relation to their choice over the manner of their eventual deaths. The AD permits the patient to specify in advance his or her desired modality of terminal care and is activated at the onset of pre-specified clinical circumstances. While the ostensible objective of ADs is to permit the patient, rather than the physician, to control the manner of the former's demise, it has been widely assumed that the use of ADs will produce an economic spin-off benefit. ADs should tend to be cost-reducing, on the grounds that, given the choice, patients are likely to prefer less intensive and aggressive terminal care than that routinely offered by the medical profession (Lo *et al.* 1986).

Although one of the earliest randomized controlled trials of terminal care produced no evidence of differences in terminal care costs between patients with and without ADs, the population considered was highly selected, no adjustment for diagnostic mix was made and ADs were typically written very close to the point of death (Schneiderman *et al.* 1992). More recent comparisons, which overcome the problems just noted, have indeed demonstrated the expected result of significantly higher terminal hospitalization charges for non-AD patients. In one, the cost differential was of the order of 60 per cent overall, falling to 35 per cent after adjustment for age, sex and diagnosis (Weeks *et al.* 1994). In another, total hospital charges for AD patients were found to amount to less than one-third of those for non-AD decedants (Chambers *et al.* 1994). Actual cost savings could be even higher if AD patients elected to die in non-institutional settings.

Efficiency gains

Efficiency gains in institutional settings may take one of two forms. First, on the basis of the evidence considered earlier, cost savings might well result from the transfer of palliative care from a hospital to a hospice or home care setting. However, it should be borne in mind that, in certain cases, financial cost savings may be found to result simply from the reclassification of expenditures; they do not therefore represent true economies. From a health authority point of view, for example, discharging hospital patients to informal carers reduces institutional expenditures but imposes burdens on families and social services. Even if economies are obtainable overall, they would not be as large as the reduction in the health authority budget would suggest. In many countries, the achievement of economies is hindered by the rigid structure of public and private sector bureaucracies, implying considerable difficulty in transferring savings across budgetary headings (Wodinsky 1992).

Second, there is a growing volume of trial evidence related to the cost-effectiveness of particular palliation regimens in given settings. For example, shorter courses of continuous chemotherapy or radiotherapy for breast cancer may yield results at least as good as prolonged courses of intermittent therapy, and at considerably less unit cost (Hancock 1992). Audit procedures can ensure that care providers routinely use only the most cost-effective regimens (Rubens 1990). From the point of view of any given institution, relatively simple changes in management structure might give rise to economies in operation, for example, the simplification of admission procedures and the increased usage of volunteers (Baker 1992).

Futile care

That which constitutes 'futile care' is controversial, although an intuitive definition would be the offering of medical resources in the absence of any reasonable expectation of therapeutic benefit. It is evident that, for any patient, attempting to treat 'incurable disease unto death is patently unacceptable' (Munro and Sebag-Montefiore 1992: 309). Not only is it likely that such medical intervention will impose quality of life costs on the patients, who are thereby denied the use of their final days as they wish, but resources are clearly being expended to achieve a therapeutic effect with virtually no positive probability of any success, at the expense of other patients whose expected gains may be far higher. The paradigmatic case of futile care is usually taken to be cardiopulmonary resuscitation for patients dying of cancer (Tomlinson and Brody 1990). A further potential candidate is chemotherapy for unresectable non-small-cell lung cancer, which appears not to enhance survival prospects or quality of life nor to palliate pain (Ihde 1992).

More intriguing, however, are findings such as those from a Swedish randomized trial of palliative chemotherapy in advanced gastrointestinal cancer (Glimelius et al. 1995). Chemotherapy plus best supporting care, while being more expensive than best supporting care alone, produced net survival gains, although death was the inevitable end-point for all patients. Overall, the average costs of medical care per day for both groups were statistically indistinguishable. From such a result we can derive two, potentially conflicting, implications as regards the acceptability of using the enhanced modality. On the one hand, it can be argued that if best supporting care is considered not futile (on the basis of an assessment of cost per life day), then the enhanced modality must be so considered also. On the other, the use of the enhanced modality to postpone death is difficult to square with our working WHO definition of the acceptable outcome of palliative care.

It should be noted that each of these three issues is symptomatic of a conflict which lies at the heart of the palliative care debate. Certainly in the USA, there appears to exist a widespread view among the public that it is the medical profession which is responsible for 'cruelly and needlessly prolonging the lives of the dying' (Gillick 1994: 2134), thereby inflating the costs of terminal care. Various motives have been ascribed, including avarice (US physicians, unlike hospitals, are paid per patient day rather than per episode), a passion for using technology and a fear of malpractice litigation, resulting in the use of any and all treatments offering the slightest possibility of improving the patient's condition. Certainly, the first- and last-mentioned represent strong economic incentives to continue treatment.

Assuming it were to be possible to implement all of these cost-reducing measures simultaneously, how much cost could be saved? According to a study of the USA based upon the most recent published cost estimates, if each dying citizen were to execute an advance directive, chose hospice care and refuse intensive hospital inpatient treatment, the expected saving on the last year of life might amount to around 27 per cent of health care costs for that year (Emanuel and Emanuel 1994). This would represent 3.3 per cent of US health care spending and 6.1 per cent of the entire Medicare budget. This scenario is, of course, optimistic for several reasons. First, the use of ADs is infrequent at present and, even if the practice were to increase slowly over time, it would still be many years before sizeable cost savings would accrue via this route. Second, the published cost advantages of hospice and home care might well be overstated, owing to selection bias among patients, uncosted informal support structures and the increasing trend for hospices to become more like hospitals. Finally, cases where the legitimate discontinuation of futile care might be contemplated certainly exist yet, as discontinuation is likely to take place close to the actual point of death in any case, potential savings are unlikely to be large. The sum involved – perhaps $30 billion to $40 billion per annum at present – represents a considerable absolute saving on health care spending although, to put matters into perspective, it is considerably smaller than the annual loss occasioned by administrative inefficiencies (Woolhandler and Himmelstein 1991).

Costs and ethics

From the foregoing discussion, the sources of the costs of palliative care, and thus the sources of economy in these costs, are relatively easy to identify. Any modality which employs fewer resources than the alternatives, or which employs a given resource less intensively or over a shorter period of time, will emerge as being cheaper. Even in a world of cost containment, however, the pursuit of low cost *per se* is not the proper goal. Our choice of appropriate modalities of care for dying people is governed by ethical considerations although, and this is a central point, ethical positions themselves entail costs. In this respect, we need to consider three basic propositions.

First, do we accept that there will exist a point in a patient's life when death will ensue irrespective of medical intervention and that, beyond this point, it is right and proper to let nature take its course? If we answer 'No' to this question, then we must encourage our physicians to administer *all* forms of therapy which would offer even the most remote chance of prolonging the patient's life. This will inevitably entail a very high cost for each patient, because the range of therapeutic options is likely to be very wide. Moreover, and assuming that resources in any health care system are finite, we are thereby denying inputs to other patients who might well benefit more positively. If we answer 'Yes' to the question, then we require that our medical profession establishes the existence of an acceptable cut-off point, such that it can say: 'This patient is now dying and it is proper that attempts at remedial treatment will henceforth cease'. Unless our physicians can be placed in a protected position, this is a very difficult decision for them to reach, given professional pride and the risk of malpractice litigation. Unfortunately, placing physicians in such a protected position carries with it a further set of problems, in that, in some degree, protection insulates them against accountability.

Second, assuming that some cut-off point has indeed been established, what is the proper palliation modality for the dying patient? Patients who are permanently and heavily sedated, and oblivious to their surroundings, are likely to be far cheaper to treat than those in whom consciousness is maintained and who retain an involvement with their environment. Just as with treatment, of course, there is no limit to the extent to which environmental stimulation can be provided (pleasant surroundings, supervised activities, etc.) and thus, again, no limit on cost. Assuming the latter option is preferred on the grounds of quality of life, do we accept that the quality of life during the dying process should be equal for all? One critic of the UK hospice movement, for example, has argued that incorporation of hospice into the National Health Service would overcome the substantial inequity in death which currently prevails: 'Why should only the minority who die of malignancies – and precious few even of them – be singled out for de luxe dying' in the independent hospices, 'agreeable secluded little places to die amid leafy glades' (Douglas 1992: 579). Naturally, this equity argument surrounding death is bound up with that related to treatments in public and private medicine more generally. It appears to require that, just as societies are establishing acceptable protocols for curative treatments, we need to establish a 'standard of dying'.

Third, how significant are patient preferences to be in the treatment and palliation decisions? We have already seen that, in the UK, the proportion of deaths occurring in institutions continues to rise, in spite of evidence that there exists a strong preference for dying at home (Townsend *et al.* 1990). That which prevents this happening is generally the lack of financial and social support for the familial carers of the dying patient. Dying at home would inevitably require an increase in social services costs. Although it is more than probable that these increased costs could be more than recouped by savings in the hospital budget, the financial autonomy of local and central government departments makes such overall resource savings extremely difficult to engineer. A potentially powerful cost-reducer driven by patient preference – voluntary euthanasia – is technically out-lawed throughout the industrialized world, although official tolerance of physician-assisted suicide is increasing in countries such as the USA and the Netherlands. Even so, few observers expect that even a legalized pro-cess would do more than serve a very small minority of terminally ill people whose suffering is so severe that normal measures of comfort are of no avail (Gillick 1994). This having been said, economic forces behind legal-ized euthanasia create a difficult moral scenario. For example, informal carers or, for that matter, institutions, would face an economic incentive to encourage dying patients to opt for euthanasia in order to escape care costs. To speculate further, would it be appropriate to offer a dying patient a financial inducement (payable, presumably, to the beneficiaries of his or her will) to opt for euthanasia, paid out of the health care resources saved as a result of earlier death?

Conclusion

In the UK at least, research and development activities in palliative care appear to be far less well advanced than in the cases of curative or pre-ventive medicine. Serious economic evaluation in the field is only just beginning (Normand 1996) and a sizeable minority of UK health authorit-ies appear neither to have conducted a needs assessment for palliative care nor to have an overall strategy in this respect (Clark et al. 1995). There are plausible reasons for explaining this comparative neglect. First, out-comes of palliative care are essentially qualitative and thus appear far less tangible than those of curative treatments, where significant survival or life-year gains are likely to be observable. Economists find appraisals of intangibles difficult to conduct, in the absence of an agreed valuation of the quality of life in relation to quantity. Second, it is quite possible, in a world of increasing cost-containment, that health care agencies feel the need to concern themselves primarily with the health of the living rather than comfort for the dying. Third, and as we have already seen, cost and resource use structures are particularly complex for palliative care, typ-ically involving inputs from the public health care sector, social services, charities, informal carers and others. Being complex, resource use is dif-ficult to disentangle and the provision of palliative care is distressingly simple to pass off as another agency's problem.

At the root of the whole argument over the costs of palliative care is a simple economic question – how much are we, the public, willing to pay to ensure that terminally ill patients die in a proper manner? Recent survey evidence suggests that there are grounds for believing that the answer, for the UK at least, may be more than had been previously thought. In the first prioritization exercise based on a large random sample of a national population (n = 2000), 'special care and pain relief for people who are dying' was ranked second only to 'treatments for children with life-threatening diseases', and above well-established curative interventions such as hip replacements, psychiatric services, long stay hospitals for elderly people and surgery for life-threatening diseases in adults (Bowling 1996). Palliative care would appear to be an excellent example of a health care issue where the wishes of the users are at variance with the policies of the providers.

References

Baker, M. (1992) Cost-effective management of the hospital-based hospice program. *Journal of Nursing Administration*, 22: 40–5.

Beck-Friis, B., Norberg, H. and Strang, P. (1991) Cost analysis and ethical aspects of hospital-based home-care for terminal cancer patients. *Scandinavian Journal of Primary Health Care*, 9: 259–64.

Bloom, B.S. and Kissick, P.D. (1980) Home and hospital cost of terminal illness. *Medical Care*, 18: 560–4.

Bowling, A. (1996) Health care rationing: the public's debate. *British Medical Journal*, 312: 670–4.

Brooks, C.H. and Smyth-Staruch, K. (1984) Hospice home care cost savings to third-party insurers. *Medical Care*, 22: 691–703.

Chambers, C.V., Diamond, J.J., Perkel, R.L. and Lasch, L.A. (1994) Relationship of advance care directives to hospital charges in a Medicare population. *Archives of Internal Medicine*, 154: 541–7.

Clark, D., Small, N. and Malson, H. (1995) Hospices to fortune. *Health Service Journal*, 23 November: 30–1.

Department of Health (1989) *Working for Patients*, Cm 555. London: HMSO.

Dixon, J. and Welch, H.G. (1991) Priority setting: lessons from Oregon. *Lancet*, 377: 891–4.

Douglas, C. (1992) For all the saints. *British Medical Journal*, 304: 579.

Emanuel, E.J. and Emanuel, L.L. (1994) The economics of dying: the illusion of cost savings at the end of life. *New England Journal of Medicine*, 330: 540–4.

Estes, C.L. and Swan, J.H. (1993) *The Long Term Care Crisis*, Newbury Park, CA: Sage.

Ferris, F.D., Wodinsky, H.B., Kerr, I.G., Sone, M., Hume, S. and Coons, C. (1991) A cost-minimization study of cancer patients requiring a narcotic infusion in hospital and at home. *Journal of Clinical Epidemiology*, 44: 313–27.

Friedlander, M.L. and Tattersall, M.H.N. (1982) Counting the costs of cancer therapy, *European Journal of Cancer and Clinical Oncology*, 18: 1237–41.

Gillick, M. (1994) The high costs of dying: a way out. *Archives of Internal Medicine*, 154: 2134–7.

Ginzberg, E. (1980) The high cost of dying. *Inquiry*, 17: 293–5.

Glimelius, B., Hoffman, K., Graf, W., Haglund, U., Nyren, O., Pahlman, L. and Sjoden, P.-O. (1995) Cost-effectiveness of palliative chemotherapy in advanced gastrointestinal cancer. *Annals of Oncology*, 6: 267–74.

Goddard, M. (1989) The role of economics in the evaluation of hospice care. *Health Policy*. 13: 19–34.

Gray, D., MacAdam, D. and Boldy, D. (1987) A comparative cost analysis of terminal cancer care in home hospice patients and controls. *Journal of Chronic Diseases*, 40: 801–10.

Greer, D.S., Mor, V., Morris, J.N., Sherwood, S., Kidder, D. and Birnbaum, H. (1986) An alternative in terminal care: results of the National Hospice Study. *Journal of Chronic Diseases*, 39: 9–26.

Hancock, B.W. (1992) Quality and cost in the palliative care of cancer. *British Journal of Cancer*, 65: 141–2.

Hill, F. and Oliver, C. (1988) Hospice: an update on the cost of patient care. *Health Trends*, 20: 83–6.

Houts, P.S., Lipton, A., Harvey, H.A., Martin, B., Simmonds, M.A., Dixon, R.H., Longo, S., Andrews, T., Gordon, R.A., Meloy, J. and Hoffman, S.L. (1984) Nonmedical costs to patients and their families associated with outpatient chemotherapy. *Cancer*, 53: 2388–92.

Ihde, D.C. (1992) Chemotherapy of lung cancer. *New England Journal of Medicine*, 327: 1434–41.

Kane, R.L., Wales, J., Bernstein, L., Leibowitz, A. and Kaplan, S. (1984) A randomised controlled trial of hospice care. *Lancet*, i: 890–4.

Kidder, D. (1988) Hospice services and cost savings in the last weeks of life, in V. Mor, D.S. Greer and R. Kastenbaum (eds) *The Hospice Experiment*. Baltimore, MD: Johns Hopkins University Press.

King, M., Lapsley, I., Llewellyn, S., Tierney, A., Anderson, J. and Sladden, S. (1993) Purchasing palliative care: availability and cost implications. *Health Bulletin*, 51: 370–84.

Kitzhaber, J.A. (1993) Prioritising health services in an era of limits: the Oregon experience. *British Medical Journal*, 307: 373–7.

Klein, R. (1995) *The New Politics of the National Health Service*, 3rd edn. London: Longman.

Lo, B., McLeod, G. and Saika, G. (1986) Patient attitudes to discussing life-sustaining treatment. *Archives of Internal Medicine*, 146: 1613–15.

Lubitz, J.D. and Prihoda, R. (1984) The use and costs of Medicare services in the last 2 years of life. *Health Care Financing Review*, 5: 117–31.

Lubitz, J.D. and Riley, G.F. (1993) Trends in Medicare payments in the last year of life. *New England Journal of Medicine*, 328: 1092–6.

Mor, V., Greer, D.S. and Goldberg, R. (1988a) The medical and social service interventions of hospice and nonhospice patients, in V. Mor, D.S. Greer and R. Kastenbaum (eds) *The Hospice Experiment*. Baltimore, MD: Johns Hopkins University Press.

Mor, V., Greer, D.S. and Kastenbaum, R. (eds) (1988b) *The Hospice Experiment*. Baltimore, MD: Johns Hopkins University Press.

Munro, A.J. and Sebag-Montefiore, D. (1992) Opportunity cost: a neglected aspect of cancer treatment. *British Journal of Cancer*, 65: 309–10.

Normand, C. (1996) Economics and evaluation of palliative care. *Palliative Medicine*, 10: 3–4.

Office of Health Economics (1995) *Compendium of Health Statistics*, 9th edn. London: OHE.

Organization for Economic Cooperation and Development (1990) *Health Care Systems in Transition*. Paris: OECD.

Postma, M.J., Jager, J.C., Dijkgraaf, M.G.W., Borleffs, J.C.C., Tolley, K. and Leidl, R.M. (1995) AIDS scenarios for the Netherlands: the economic impact of hospitals. *Health Policy*, 31: 127–50.

Rubens, R.D. (1990) Auditing palliative cancer chemotherapy. *European Journal of Cancer*, 26: 1023–5.

Schneiderman, L., Kronick, R., Kaplan, R., Anderson, J. and Lager, R. (1992) Effects of offering advance directives on medical treatments and costs. *Annals of Internal Medicine*, 117: 599–606.

Scitovsky, A.A. (1984) 'The high cost of dying': what do the data show?, *Milbank Memorial Fund Quarterly*, 62: 591–608.

Tomlinson, T. and Brody, H. (1990) Futility and the ethics of resuscitation. *Journal of the American Medical Association*, 264: 1276–80.

Townsend, J., Frank, A.O., Fermont, D., Karran, O., Walgrove, A. and Piper, M. (1990) Terminal cancer care and patients' preference for place of death: a prospective study. *British Medical Journal*, 301: 415–17.

Weeks, W.B., Kofoed, L.L., Wallace, A.E. and Welch, G. (1994) Advance directives and the cost of terminal hospitalisation. *Archives of Internal Medicine*, 154: 2077–83.

Wennberg, J.E. (1990) On the need for outcomes research and the prospects for the evaluative clinical sciences, in T.F. Andersen and G. Mooney (eds) *The Challenges of Medical Practice Variations*. London: Macmillan.

Whynes, D.K. (1993) Counting the true costs of palliative care. *Progress in Palliative Care*, 1: 47–50.

Whynes, D.K. (1995) The cost-effectiveness of cancer therapy: the health economist's view. *Proceedings of the Royal College of Physicians of Edinburgh*, 25: 67–75.

Wodinsky, H.B. (1992) The costs of caring for cancer patients. *Journal of Palliative Care*, 8: 24–7.

Woolhandler, S. and Himmelstein, D.U. (1991) The deteriorating administrative efficiency of the US health care system. *New England Journal of Medicine*, 324: 1253–8.

World Health Organization (1990) *Cancer Pain Relief and Palliative Care*, Technical Report Series 804. Geneva: WHO.

3 | Resource allocation and palliative care

☐ CALLIOPE FARSIDES AND EVE GARRARD

Due largely to the influence of the American bioethicists Beauchamp and Childress (1994) ethical issues in health care are often thought to fall under four main moral principles: the principle of beneficence, the principle of non-maleficence, the principle of respect for autonomy, and the principle of justice. Although the dominance of their approach has been the subject of some criticism (Holm 1995), their four principles are undoubtedly a useful organizing tool (Gillon 1995). The idea behind the approach is relatively straightforward and uncontroversial. Basically it is claimed that theirs is a 'common-morality theory' which 'takes its basic premises directly from the morality shared in common by the members of a society – that is unphilosophical common sense and tradition' (Beauchamp and Childress 1994: 100). On the basis of these premises they offer their four principles, a consideration of which will help to analyse specific bioethical problems.

Traditionally the main focus has been on the first three principles. This is not surprising given the common assumption that the minimal moral duty placed on any individual is that they should not cause harm to others, and the commonly held belief that health care professionals have a special duty to do good for others. The emphasis on autonomy is more culturally determined, with some theorists arguing that Anglo-American bioethics affords undue primacy to the principle of autonomy for broadly ideological reasons (Holm 1995). Putting aside this criticism, it is still clear that by focusing on issues of autonomy, beneficence and non-maleficence one is more likely to concentrate the gaze upon the relations between individual carers and patients. This emphasis is reflected in traditional ethical codes which tend to be framed in terms of an individual professional's duty to an individual patient.

While it is important to acknowledge that there are considerable numbers of complex ethical issues arising out of such relationships, it is also important to appreciate that these relationships exist within a much wider context, and that this context will determine the existence of further issues. One obvious consequence of acknowledging the importance of the broader context and its influence on individual relationships between carers and clients is that the principle of justice is elevated to a status more equal to the other three.

Justice is by definition a social concern, referring as it does to the distribution of goods between individuals or groups. In the context of health care provision the goods in question vary widely in their form (time, money, skill to name but a few), but have the shared purpose of promoting health, curing disease or, as in the palliative care context, relieving suffering. Ethical problems arise because in all but a few contexts these goods are in short supply, and decisions have to be made about how to best allocate them.

Thus the main issue arising under the principle of justice is the allocation of scarce resources. The issue can be approached at a number of levels. First, there are decisions to be made about how much money the health care system should be given in relation to other institutions and practices placing demands on the public purse. Once this has been decided the amount allocated has to be divided between different specialisms and care sectors and across different geographical boundaries. Finally, once particular care providers have secured their resources they have to decide how best to use them in treating their patients.

All these decisions are ethically sensitive. In order to decide at a macro level how much money should be allocated to the health care service one has to compare its value (in the fullest sense of the word) to that of a range of other important services such as education and defence. One must also decide the extent to which individuals will be held responsible for funding their own health care needs (either directly or indirectly) and how much the state is prepared to subsidise them. In fact there may be little room for flexibility if the state is committed to a low taxation, low expenditure model.

At the intermediate level, where money is distributed within the health care system, claims based on need and responsiveness to public demand will have to withstand pressure imposed by long established patterns of territoriality. And the unfashionable and unglamorous will have to clamour for recognition alongside the technological and exciting specialisms. The worry is that the institutionally powerful or the emotively appealing disciplines may not be the most worthy of funding on dispassionate grounds even though they win out in any competition for resources.

At the micro level one will eventually get to the point of discussing which patients should and should not be treated where it is not possible to treat everybody. This is immediately more difficult than discussing how to treat a particular individual whose treatment is secured, even if we have to acknowledge that resource considerations could prevent us from exploring all possible avenues for the patients we do treat. In the first case by denying treatment or care one is harming an individual in a quite significant manner. If the procedure required is lifesaving, one is allowing the patient to die. Blanket non-treatment decisions motivated by resourcing considerations will result in an individual receiving less than optimal care and might even put the patient's life at risk. If a patient receives some level of care but certain procedures are not offered because they are too expensive, for example, the person is once again harmed in the sense of not being given the best possible care available, but theirs and others' basic needs may have been met.

In either type of case it is difficult for professionals who define their activities in terms of a duty of care to engage in discussions of who should and should not be helped, and how much should be done for those in their care. None the less, ethicists believe that it is important to allocate resources on the basis of a principle or formula which can be ethically defended, and, protected by their relative detachment, they have become involved in devising theories and ethically auditing those offered by health economists and policy makers. The purpose of such theories is twofold. First, to help to allocate resources between various disciplines and sectors of health care. Second, to allow us to make rational choices between individual patients.

A variety of theories have emerged, but the majority seem to share some basic assumptions. Most obviously they share the assumption that the provision of health care is directed primarily at the goal of prolonging life and effecting cures. It would be misleading to claim that no attention is given to improving quality of life in the absence of cure, but qualitative considerations are always considered alongside more quantitative issues. This point can be illustrated by considering one of the most widely publicized theories of resource allocation, the QALY theory (Bell and Mendus 1988; Cubbon 1991).

QALYs and palliative care

The purpose of a QALY calculation is to establish the effect of offering a certain treatment or intervention in terms of three factors. First, the effect on the degree of pain or distress suffered by the patient; second, the degree of incapacitation; third, the number of extra years the patient may reasonably look forward to after the treatment. If an intervention leaves a patient virtually pain free, mobile and with a long life expectancy it will secure a high QALY rating. If a treatment can secure the patient only a few months or weeks of life during which the patient will be in pain and bed-bound the QALY rating will be very low. Given the underlying assumption that it is desirable to relieve pain and suffering and prolong life, treatments with a high QALY rating will be valued over those with a low one. However, there is a further factor to be taken into account, which is cost. By considering the cost of the procedure one can come up with a price per QALY, which in turn allows one to compare different treatments in terms of their value for money.

This is thought to be the major advantage of the QALY approach: that it affords policy makers a rational means by which to compare quite different forms of interventions. For example, when deciding whether to allocate resources to a new state of the art coronary care unit which will perform heart transplants and other pioneering procedures, one could look at the cost per QALY of the treatments proposed. These values could then be compared to those attached to less glamorous projects such as an expansion of the hip replacement programme or the development of district nursing services.

There are a number of potential problems with this approach, some of which are beyond the remit of this chapter (Harris 1985; Rawls 1989). However, in the present context it is important to acknowledge that adopting such an approach to resource allocation questions would have serious implications for a number of medical specialisms. It is immediately apparent that those who choose to adopt the QALY approach will have little reason to provide significant resourcing for palliative care services. Since it is relatively expensive, even a very substantial improvement in the quality of someone's life will be outweighed by the relatively short time for which the benefit could be enjoyed. Furthermore, in absolute terms the quality of life achievable through intervention often compares unfavourably with the quality of life ensured by other forms of care offered to patients with acute or chronic conditions.

There are several reasons why we should be concerned by this outcome. But the first point to stress is that palliative care should not be defended through simply territorial interests. It is a natural tendency to favour one's own specialism and to wish to promote the interest of one's own patients. However, if one is committed to securing a just allocation one has to provide a defence of one's own specialism which clearly demonstrates the basis of its claim for support.

Perhaps one could begin such a defence by claiming that we generally share strong moral intuitions that there is more to health care than the extension of life. As well as the length of a life, we are concerned about the *quality* of a life, in ways that are not captured by the very quantitative and 'functional' approach of QALYs. By functional we mean that the QALY approach tends to judge incapacitation in very physical terms, and assumes that there can be very little quality of life to enjoy once a patient is bedridden and unable to participate in normal daily activities.

Within palliative care many patients will be severely incapacitated in a physical sense, but this does not exclude the possibility of significantly improving their quality of life not only through pain relief and symptom control, but also by providing support aimed at minimizing the effects of their incapacitation.

Such interventions are assumed to be valuable even if their results can be enjoyed for only a relatively short time. And, where non-treatment decisions are made they would more probably be based on a belief that the treatment was too burdensome given the benefit it offered and the time-span involved.

However, there is a more fundamental reason why it is difficult for the QALY calculation to capture the value of interventions in a palliative care setting. Given that palliative care ultimately focuses on the terminal phase of a patient's life, those offering such care will be concerned not only with the manner in which patients live, but also in the way in which they die. As individuals we are concerned about the manner in which we take leave of our lives. Indeed at the end of life, the quality issue seems largely to trump the quantity issue; for many people at least, appropriate care will not necessarily entail prolonging or even maintaining life (Dworkin 1993).

So within palliative care, of necessity we move from a model of care which emphasizes curative outcomes, to a more holistic model which assumes that medical and nursing care is also relevant to the dying process. This creates immediate problems in terms of evaluating care. However, there is still a responsibility to do so in order to decide whether particular interventions have a justified claim on resources, and whether palliative care as a specialism can compete effectively with, for example, orthopaedic surgery or cardiology.

While it is possible to consider whether patients enjoy a longer amount of time at a higher quality of life than they could have expected without treatment, it is more difficult to present the claim that they 'died a better death' in a manner which sits happily with the broadly economic terminology of the QALY approach.

However, the fact that it is more difficult to evaluate interventions in these terms is not a reason to abandon attempts to do so. Qualitative research could be useful in this instance, for example interviewing patients, carers and professionals and asking them to reflect on the extent to which caring interventions facilitated an individual experiencing a good death. By analysing the interview data it should be possible to make claims about which types of interventions appear to be effective.

So the claim made here is that irrespective of its low scoring in QALY terms palliative care interventions can be shown to be of value (Crisp et al. 1996). As such there is a clear justification for funding them. The problem is that the purpose of palliative care is in important respects different to that which underpins the traditional medical model of care, and which in turn informs many theories of resource allocation. However, if we accept that it is important to manage dying and not abandon the patient once a cure is infeasible, these differences should not prevent palliative care competing effectively with other disciplines for funding. However, this macro-allocation justification still leaves open the intermediate allocation question of how palliative care resources should be distributed between the various components of palliative care.

Intermediate level allocation

Commonly understood, the goals of palliative care are threefold: pain control; symptom control; and psychological support (World Health Organization 1990: 11). Given the commitment to the four moral principles we started with, there will always be a strong case, deriving from beneficence, for putting resources into pain control. Some philosophers distil the whole of morality down to an obligation to minimize pain and maximize pleasure, ensuring that any intervention with these effects will be given top priority (Singer 1994: 306–12). Few would deny that resources spent on keeping people pain free and controlling the distressing symptoms of disease count as money well spent. It is also relatively straightforward to argue with hindsight that the psychological support offered to a patient did or did not benefit them. It is less clear in advance, however, who will benefit and to what extent. Similarly it might be less clear which psychological problems are linked directly to the individual's illness and thus in a strict sense the responsibility of the palliative care team, and those which are not.

Where resources are limited, prioritizing decisions have to be taken. The following question then arises – should one offer complete care tailored to individual patients' needs until the budget runs out, thus leaving some untreated? Or should one abandon the goal of a Rolls Royce service for a limited number, and aim instead at universal access to effective pain control at least, plus further support if the budget allows? These were the sorts of questions recently debated in the US state of Oregon where it was decided that it is more important to offer basic health care to all those who cannot fund their own care, than to offer the full range of services to the (necessarily) limited number of people who previously qualified for aid.

In countries where palliative care services are only just developing the priority tends to be the introduction of effective pain control (see Stjernsward, Chapter 13 in this volume). Where resources are really short anything else might be considered a luxury. One might choose to argue that in the absence of sufficient resources it is better to relieve the physical suffering of a large number of people, than to attempt to relieve the physical and mental anguish of a far smaller group. This is not to leave nurses and doctors free from the responsibility of acknowledging the psychological suffering of patients and responding appropriately. Rather it is to limit the availability of specialized professional interventions designed to deal with specifically psychological problems.

The interesting question to ask in response to this observation is whether this practice of giving less priority to psychological support is an unacceptable remnant of the medical model of care and its preoccupation with organic disease, or whether there might be some justification for placing a higher priority on different forms of intervention.

Discounting the possibility of prejudice against this form of intervention one would probably be forced to say that the issue is one of efficacy. To justify the use of scarce resources in one way rather than another one has to show that there is a good chance of effecting a significant improvement, or at the very least that the intervention will prevent further suffering. In any one case it is much more difficult to know in advance either the extent to which we can actually alleviate a psychological problem, or the cost, in terms of time, staff resources and funds, of providing the support. Furthermore, it will often be difficult to tell which aspects of patients' psychological needs are actually directly produced by, or are even related to, their illness. Those who work with terminally ill patients know that patients bring their problems with them, and sometimes the fact that they are dying is the least of those problems.

The conclusion may at first appear unacceptably harsh: if we cannot predict with sufficient accuracy the benefits to any one patient of concentrated psychological intervention, we have less of a justification for funding such care over more proven interventions such as pain relief or (physical) symptom control. Therefore it might be preferable to save money by assigning less psychological support to patients so long as that money is used to provide more basic care to a larger number of patients.

Some might say that by placing less of an emphasis on the need for psychological support services one is increasing the burden of terminal illness on those least equipped to cope, and this in turn might undermine the treatment being given for their physical symptoms. It would of course be wrong to suggest that there is a fixed hierarchy of importance within the various aspects of palliative care. To do so would be to transport remnants of the medical model into a context where it does not necessarily fit. It is a positive feature of the palliative care philosophy that patients are viewed holistically and care is offered across a number of dimensions. However, if the choice is between relieving the physical pain and suffering of a significantly larger number of people or addressing all the problems of a smaller number of people one might be prepared to say that the ideal type model should remain intact, but in the real world treating more patients will relieve more suffering.

None the less, the objection which claims that failure to fully treat psychological symptoms will in fact undermine the treatment of physical suffering, must be met. The claim may well be true; but even if it is, it does not tell against the model of palliative care provision being presented here. Holistic connections between the psychological and the physical cannot be a reason for focusing resources on the treatment of psychological symptoms in those who are already receiving good physical palliation. For any suffering they might have to undergo in the absence of psychological support from their carers is *already* being undergone by those not lucky enough to be receiving specialist palliative care, and there are far, far more of them. Those outside the circle of care will *also* be undergoing more physical suffering, so it is difficult to see what could justify allocating resources away from them, and towards the treatment of the psychological distress of those who are already receiving excellent treatment for their physical symptoms.

Failure to acknowledge the weight of these essentially egalitarian considerations may stem from an inappropriate prioritizing of the interests of 'our patients', i.e. those who already come within the circle of care. But full acknowledgement of the principle of justice requires us to take into account the needs of *all* patients, potential and actual. Here is an example of a situation in which our tendency to emphasize the principles of beneficence, non-maleficence, and respect for autonomy has diverted our attention from the equally important demands of the principle of justice.

It is worth noting here that a Rolls Royce service is psychologically satisfying for *carers*, who do not normally see those who remain untreated because there are no further resources, and who quite understandably resist the idea of 'dropping their standards'. But carer-satisfaction, of course, is not the primary aim here. However, carers would need to know that by providing a 'basic model' of care they were not sacrificing quality to the extent that they were offering an *unsatisfactory* level of care, albeit to larger numbers of people.

On a reassuring note, it is at least possible that within some contexts of care institutional philosophy may compensate for non-provision of a personalized high-cost service. However there are bound to be people who lose out as a result of this method of allocation but on *any* method there are always people who lose out, and maybe these could not be adequately helped by any realistic provision of resource. None the less it is important to face the implications of taking this approach.

If resources are concentrated on pain relief and symptom control rather than psychological support, for some patients, there will be no relief of (mental) suffering, possibly for two reasons: first, we cannot remove the fact of their illness or offer them a cure and that may be the source of their mental anguish; second, we are unwilling to direct resources towards relieving the mental anguish. Having admitted this, we should surely accept some responsibility for what follows, both in terms of acknowledging the suffering of the patient and in terms of responding sympathetically to demands and behaviours their condition might generate.

Ethical judgements and the issue of euthanasia

When judging the provision of palliative care, we should not be seduced into flying the standards appropriate to more curative models of health care. In fact there might be relatively intangible benefits meted out to patients by the atmosphere and philosophy of care of the institution within which they are being treated. The hospice philosophy which has been adopted and adapted throughout the palliative care sector is essentially supportive of patients' psychological needs, but there is a tendency towards illiberalism when considering ideas which at present seem incompatible with that philosophy. As public debate on the issue of euthanasia grows, it would be wrong to assume that patients, however grateful for the benefits of the hospice philosophy, are necessarily hostile to views which are currently opposed to it. There is a need for tolerance, which often demands that we pay attention to views we currently consider not only misguided but also morally wrong.

It is possible that individuals who are not directly treated for the psychological sequelae of their physical disease will decide that for them life is no longer worth living. If we suspect that such a demand is the result of a treatable psychological disturbance such as depression, we surely have a responsibility to treat it. Thus part of the basic package of care might include some level of psychological support. However, some people would reach a similar conclusion and this would not indicate that they were depressed. In fact some terminally ill people will decide they want their life to end sooner rather than later irrespective of the care offered. In these cases spending money on psychological support might be wasteful.

Consider for example people who have previously made a clearly stated advance directive, and now while still competent feel that the point is approaching at which they wish to refuse any further life-prolonging interventions. Or people whose life has been full of activity and whose existence is defined in terms of creativity and productiveness. They may well feel that a certain type of life is not worth living, and a particular type of death is a preferable option. In such cases an offer of psychological counselling would probably be perceived as a denial of their autonomy, and an undermining of their notion of the good. In these cases the provision of care is almost irrelevant to individuals' evaluation of their life and desire for death, and a request for euthanasia should not be interpreted as a failure of care or a demand for more (Farsides 1996).

However, where we have to admit that non-availability of care at a certain level contributes to the patient's desire to die sooner rather than later, we have to accept a degree of responsibility for the patient's level of distress, and acknowledge that an unsympathetic response to any request that desire might generate would amount to a further substantial harm to the patient. In the interests of a fair allocation of available resources particular patients may well be harmed by the non-availability of a care at the level appropriate to their needs. This is of course regrettable and a first response would probably be to demand more resources, but such a demand must take into account the opportunity costs for other disciplines if more money were to be directed at palliative care.

What seems to follow from this? At the very least, it follows that we must be prepared to treat the patient's request for euthanasia with some measure of sympathy and respect. This is the case in both situations described. If patients have chosen to value death over life in the absence of any pathological disturbance or distress, to deny the validity of their position is to undermine their autonomy. At the very least we must tolerate the expression of their wishes and discuss them in a non-judgemental manner. In the second case we have to accept that in another context we might be able to 'solve the problem' and prevent the demand being made. However, having decided to withhold care we must accept the possibility that this will generate a request for euthanasia and respond appropriately.

This must amount to allowing euthanasia at least to be discussed by the patient, and hence it must be on the agenda between patient and carer. If it is a matter for open discussion between patient and carer, then it must be a matter for open discussion between different groups of carers. For the sake of the patients, we cannot afford for this to be a completely prohibited topic of discussion within the palliative care movement. The fact that active euthanasia is illegal, perhaps rightly so, does not preclude the possibility of there being some few cases where passive euthanasia should at least be discussed as a possible option. Nor should it mean that a conspiracy of silence exists such that patients know not to mention the word, even though they have come to think that for them an act of euthanasia would secure a fitting end to their life.

Perhaps this is an unexpected conclusion to a chapter which began by discussing resource allocation, but it is hoped that the connection is clear on reflection. The principle of justice demands that we look at the interests of patients as a whole and seek to adjudicate their claims in the fairest possible way. At present palliative care services tend to work in such a way as to offer a very high level of care to the relatively few people who can access the service. To broaden the constituency of people receiving expert care may well necessitate pruning the service in ways which will (through omission) cause significant harm to a small number of individuals. This harm may in turn lead those individuals to prefer to die, a preference which might find expression through a request for euthanasia. Such requests must not be silenced but rather be met with compassion and understanding. In so doing one offers care to the patient even if prevailing moral standards and the law of the land mean that their request will never be acted upon.

References

Beauchamp, T. and Childress, J. (1994) *Principles of Biomedical Ethics*, 4th edn. Oxford: Oxford University Press.

Bell, J.M. and Mendus, S. (1988) *Philosophy and Medical Welfare*. Cambridge: Cambridge University Press.

Crisp, R., Hope, T. and Ebbs, D. (1996) The Asbury draft policy on ethical use of resources. *British Medical Journal*, 312: 1528–31.

Cubbon, J. (1991) The principle of QUALY maximisation as the basis for allocating health care resources. *Journal of Medical Ethics*, 17: 181–4.

Dworkin, R. (1993) *Life's Dominion*. New York: HarperCollins.

Farsides, C. (1996) Euthanasia: failure or autonomy? *International Journal of Palliative Nursing*, 2(2): 102–5.

Gillon, R. (1995) Defending 'the four principles approach' to biomedical ethics. *Journal of Medical Ethics*, 21: 323–4.

Harris, J. (1985) *The Value of Life*. London: Routledge.

Holm, S. (1995) Not just autonomy: the principles of American biomedical ethics. *Journal of Medical Ethics*, 21: 332–8.

Rawls, J. (1989) Castigating QUALYS. *Journal of Medical Ethics*, 15: 143–7.

Singer, P. (1994) *Ethics*. Oxford: Oxford University Press.

World Health Organization (1990) *Cancer Pain Relief and Palliative Care*, Technical Report Series 804. Geneva: WHO.

Half full or half empty?
The impact of health reform on palliative care services in the UK

DAVID CLARK, HELEN MALSON,
NEIL SMALL, KAREN MALLETT,
BREN NEALE AND PAULINE HEATHER

It is well known that the hospice movement in the UK had robustly independent beginnings. Its early founders drew inspiration from the work of religious orders which cared for dying people as well as from altruistic traditions which fostered charitable giving and voluntary work. When these were harnessed to new insights in pain and symptom control and developing psychological understanding of bereavement and loss, then the prospects for an alternative, and apparently more *holistic* system of care began to emerge (Saunders 1993). It was a system which, as James and Field (1992: 1363) put it, was 'unashamedly reformist' in character and which in the beginning had to occupy a territory outside the mainstream of health care provision. The first hospices in the UK were therefore independent charitable organizations. These were sometimes established with material or financial support from the National Health Service. Beyond this, however, they were easily distinguishable from the NHS in certain fundamental ways, such as in their model of care, in organizational culture and in their method of financing. While the early hospices had often sought to stand outside the constraints of health care planners and their associated bureaucracies, the maturation of the movement was to bring about a growing interdependence with the wider structures of health care delivery. This interrelationship between the hospice movement and the mainstream health care system is central to any full understanding of the history and development of hospices and specialist palliative care services in the UK. It is also relevant to understanding the problems of palliative care services

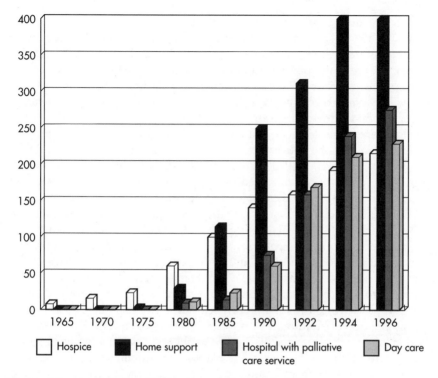

Figure 4.1 Growth of palliative care services in the UK
Source: The Hospice Information Service 1996

elsewhere, particularly those operating within policy environments which share similar problems and difficulties, such as those outlined in several other chapters (Robbins, Chapter 1; Whynes, Chapter 2; Gómez-Batiste *et al.*, Chapter 10 in this volume).

The development of palliative care services in the UK has been distinguished by two striking characteristics (see Figure 4.1). First, there has been a remarkable increase in the number of inpatient hospices, from less than a handful in the mid-1960s, to over 200 thirty years later. In 1996 three-quarters of these were independent, not-for-profit organizations. Second, there has been enormous diversification in activity. In addition to the inpatient hospices, dramatic expansion has also taken place in other modes of care. As Figure 4.1 also reveals, palliative care in the UK is now delivered through an expanding number of day care centres, through domiciliary services and through specialist hospital support teams as well as through inpatient care. Since day care and domiciliary services in particular are often linked to hospices, so a complex matrix of care has developed between independent and NHS providers. Smith and Eve (1996) estimate that these services provided care for some 53,000 inpatient admissions in 1993. This expansion and diversification has been driven in various ways.

Undoubtedly an important source of momentum has been the lobbying power of the hospice movement itself. Much expansion has been made possible by harnessing community support through local fund-raising and by placing pressure upon health authorities to give backing to new hospice services. By the late 1980s government recognition was added to this through a system of funding which gave special support to the independent hospices, in a move to create a 50:50 sharing of costs (Clark 1993). Furthermore, since 1987, health authorities have been required to prepare specific plans for the delivery of palliative care in their local areas. All of this has in turn been fuelled by the aspirations of health professionals and provider organizations convinced of the importance of palliative care and eager to promote service development. The resultant growth in activity has of course created certain concerns on the part of policy makers and planners.

By the late 1980s the Wilkes report had already cautioned against the too rapid expansion of inpatient hospices at the expense of developments in hospital and community-based care for dying people (Wilkes 1980). In the intervening years there have been fears that palliative care services continue to arise haphazardly and in response not so much to need as to emotive pleas from local champions. Critics argue that this has created a pot-pourri of services, not always properly matched to local circumstances (too many hospices in some places, not enough in others) and one in which the culture of charitable giving has played too prominent a part. This de luxe dying for a minority (Douglas 1992) is pointed to as the profound weakness of a system which has lacked the regulatory influence of either strategic planning or market forces. Protagonists of course counter these points with powerful arguments of their own. If the job had been left to the planners it would have never been started; hospices enjoy massive community support; they have become respected institutions within British culture, receiving wide endorsement across political parties and from leading figures in the establishment. Moreover, because they experience high levels of charitable subvention, they are available at relatively little cost to the taxpayer, coupled to the fact that their services are free at the point of delivery.

This is therefore a complex and unfolding history. We shall argue here that it is a history which must be linked increasingly to wider changes in the health care policy context. For while hospices achieved much at first by bracketing themselves from questions of health policy and finance, their success, particularly when linked to the growing range of developing palliative care services, raises important questions of a strategic nature and poses the problem of how and by whom they are to be paid for over time. In this chapter we shall outline some of the major changes that have taken place in the organization of the UK's National Health Service since the early 1990s. These have been so fundamental in character that their impact on hospice and palliative care services has been inescapable. Drawing on studies conducted within the UK over that time we shall make some assessment of the relationship of palliative care services to more general matters of health reform. We conclude that while hospices have had significant success in adapting to a new and unfamiliar environment, considerable progress has still to be made if the UK is to make any claim to the availability of a comprehensive and accessible range of specialist palliative care services.

Principles of health reform in the UK

Ever since the Second World War, governments of various political persuasions and in many countries have been grappling with issues of cost-containment in health care. Particularly in recent years the rhetoric of policy has tended to focus on issues of *efficiency* of operation and *effectiveness* of impact. This rhetoric of course is shaped by the financial concerns of accountants and tempered by the electoral worries of politicians – for health care is always a sensitive issue with the voting public. In the UK in the 1980s however, as also in the USA, these combined with a far stronger ideological drive, shaped by the concerns of the new right, to liberate health, social security and social care from the shadow of an allegedly overweaning nanny state and to expose welfare to the rigours of a marketized system. This project focused on 'bottom line' economics and cost-containment coupled with ideological principles which privileged individual choice and responsibility and even repudiated the notion of 'society' itself (Small 1989). Although such macro changes may seem remote from the day to day concerns of hospice providers, it is unquestionable that their subsequent translation into policy is having a direct bearing on the development of palliative care services.

Effectiveness in health care is an objective which is being pursued in many countries through the goals associated with evidence-based medicine. This approach is one which challenges custom and practice, local tradition or anecdotal justification in favour of a strategy for health care which is scientifically grounded in the results of research, where the gold standard is the result of properly conducted randomized controlled trials. Clearly, such an objective will impact only in the medium to longer term as it demands deep-seated changes in the delivery of medical education and in the conduct of day to day clinical practice. Efficiency, however, is a goal which can be tackled within a much shorter timescale, reflecting the day to day concerns of policy making and politics. Accordingly, we have seen far more examples of this aspect of health 'reform' in the course of the 1980s, for it is predicated on the reorganization of systems and structures and the creation of new financial arrangements within which health care is delivered.

Table 4.1 Key aspects of health reform in the UK

- Separation of purchasing and providing functions
- Promotion of mixed economy of care
- Development of primary-care-led services
- Further development of community care
- Creation of 'quasi-markets'
- Establishment of health commissions
- Introduction of GP purchasing

It was a conservative government led by the then Prime Minister Margaret Thatcher which brought forward wide-ranging proposals for health reform in a 1989 white paper entitled *Working for Patients* (Department of Health 1989). The key principles of the changes that were to follow are set out in Table 4.1. A central feature of the drive for both cost-containment and effectiveness was a major structural alteration in which the functions of providing health care were separated out from those of purchasing it. Large and complex district health authorities which both planned and delivered care were altered root and branch. The new cadre of purchasers, subsequently known as health commissions, which arose out of the ashes of the former district health authorities and family health service authorities, were to be more slender organizations charged with procuring health care for their local populations. The *providers* of care, on the other hand, were to become separate organizations, NHS trusts which would contract with the purchaser to deliver certain services. Purchasers were encouraged to look to a mixed economy of care, wherein providers would include the newly formed trusts, together with charitable/not-for-profit organizations, as well as private health care businesses. Such a 'market', it was argued, would stimulate efficiency, competition and promote the adoption of business values in what was perceived to be a bureaucratic and poorly administered NHS. It would be further stirred by the power to be given to general practitioners (GPs) to purchase care directly from tertiary providers, seeking the best 'deal' for individual patients. The creation of GP fundholding in this way was to give a spur to a primary-care-led NHS in which care in the community was deemed preferable to institutional care.

Following extensive review of the policy literature (Neale *et al.* 1994; Clark *et al.* 1995), we argued that the key to understanding the implications of the NHS reforms for palliative care lay in the concept of the *purchasing cycle* (see Figure 4.2). In this theoretical model could be determined the mechanisms whereby the new market for health care was to unfold. As a *model*, the purchasing cycle contains an underlying rationality. Crucially, it begins with a conviction that health care must be procured in relation to the identified needs of given populations. Health needs assessment (Clark and Malson 1995, 1996) should be the vehicle for this.

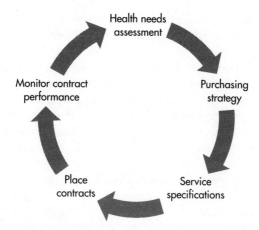

Figure 4.2 The purchasing cycle

Having developed a detailed demographic, epidemiological and qualitative understanding of local need, purchasers must then formulate a clear strategy for meeting it. The purchasing strategy will encompass the values and goals underpinning purchasing intentions. It will also be the foundation upon which can be laid detailed service specifications – i.e. statements about the volume, character and quality of services which will be necessary in order to fulfil the needs that have been identified. At this stage the purchaser can place contracts with providers (possibly after a process of competitive tendering). With contracting comes monitoring and performance review in order to assess the extent to which the contracted services have been successful in meeting the needs identified at the start of the process. From here the cycle recommences and knowledge gained through contract monitoring and quality assurance can be fed back to promote a more refined understanding of need.

These principles, we have suggested, should be central to the entire process of health reform which has been taking place within the British system if there is to be any resulting benefit to patients. Accordingly, they provide the key framework in which palliative care services must function. Understandably, they were to create worries within UK hospices. To what extent would purchasers prioritize palliative care services? Would hospices find a position within the new 'contract culture'? How might health needs assessment affect services which had developed out of historical precedent, local demand and in response to persuasive lobbying? Above all, would the new market culture lead to cost-cutting and disinvestment from hospice and palliative care services?

It is well known that the major alterations brought about in the UK as a result of the so-called 'reforms' represent a massive, untested experiment, for which there were no pilot or demonstration projects. Our purpose has therefore been one of conducting real-time studies in an attempt to monitor the impact of the NHS reforms upon palliative care services and to feed back our findings to both purchasers and providers as they themselves grappled to implement the new system. In doing this we quickly found a mismatch between the carefully weighed public statements to be found in the policy guidance and the altogether messier realities of life within the health system itself. Most striking was the fact that, with the formal introduction of the new system in 1991, attention focused not on the 'rational' starting point for the purchasing cycle (health needs assessment), but rather upon the contracting process itself. The reasons for this are clear. At this stage the primary imperative was to kick start the new system and formalize the emerging market arrangements through the contracting procedure. Despite such inconsistencies, we have chosen, for clarity of presentation to structure our observations here around the formal elements of the purchasing cycle and to make comment upon the extent to which it was taking effect by 1995, four years after introduction. Our evidence is drawn from two separate empirical studies, one conducted among purchasers in the Trent region of England in 1993–4 and the other conducted with hospices across the whole of the UK in 1994–5.[1] These are coupled with wide-ranging and more general observations of the palliative care scene in the UK. Of course, such research is very much focused upon a moving target of organizations and individuals within them grappling with major changes. To this must be added difficulties associated with making sense of issues which may relate to the maturation of the hospice movement itself, rather than to specific policy changes. Above all there are dangers in reifying 'the reforms' and in objectifying a series of complex, fragmented and often contradictory processes into a unified and integrated whole. These generate in turn a number of practical difficulties for researchers and may be responsible for a degree of caution among respondents who carry heavy responsibilities to make the new system work. Nevertheless, we hope that our work provides some helpful commentary on the unfolding health policy framework in the UK as it affects palliative care directly.

Needs assessment

As we have argued, health needs assessment should be the cornerstone of the purchasing system, providing accurate information upon which to build a strategy. Purchasers see the relevance of this, particularly where palliative care services to date have developed in a relatively *ad-hoc* and uncoordinated way. In these circumstances health needs assessment may shed vital light on the question of whether current services are correctly conceived and formulated. At the same time there are problems in this, for example a stark mismatch between identified need and current provision could raise

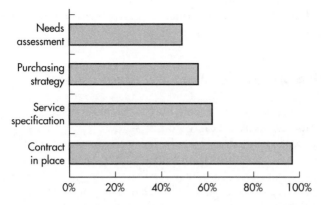

Figure 4.3 Proportion of purchasers in the UK which have developed

the possibility of either decommissioning an existing service or of development of new services, according to the evidence. Furthermore, a properly conducted needs assessment, incorporating epidemiological data, stakeholder and user views, together with some comparison with other districts, is likely to be seen as a costly and unaffordable exercise. One Trent purchaser told us 'it's unlikely we'll fund a need assessment – it would deplete all the funds we are currently able to put into purchasing a service.' Of course such concerns are reinforced by some of the definitional problems involved in conducting a palliative care needs assessment: how is the population to be defined; what constitutes a need for palliative care; and what model of palliative care is being used as a starting point? This could be hampered in turn simply by lack of knowledge of existing provision of palliative care, particularly in general hospital and community settings.

In a national survey of purchasers conducted in 1994, Robbins and Frankel (1995) found that 49 per cent claimed to have conducted some form of palliative care needs assessment. A year later, our own national survey of hospices and inpatient palliative care units showed that, by the account of the providers, the same proportion (49 per cent) of main purchasers were thought to have undertaken needs assessments for palliative care (Figure 4.3). Providers of specialist palliative care saw needs assessment as very important in 73 per cent of cases and 28 per cent of those replying had actually gone so far as to request their main purchaser to undertake some work of this kind, even though such a decision would be the responsibility of the purchaser rather than the provider. Needs assessments in less than half of purchasing authorities may be seen as a rather disappointing figure, particularly in relation to its 'cornerstone' place in the purchasing cycle. However, some examples from our study showed positive outcomes following such work. For example comments on one questionnaire included the following: 'The needs assessment carried out has formed the basis for development of services at the hospice and is fundamental to the business plan.'

Purchasing strategy and service specifications

Where the functions of health care purchasers and providers are separated, then the importance of a clear vision of services for the locality, incorporated into a purchasing strategy, becomes vital. In the context of palliative care, as we have seen, health authorities have been required to produce such strategies since 1987, a date preceding the introduction of the internal market by several years. It was therefore disappointing in our 1995 survey to find that only 56 per cent of purchasers appeared to have produced strategies for palliative care; 35 per cent of hospices responding to our survey stated that their main purchaser had not produced a strategy for palliative care, and 9 per cent of hospices did not know one way or the other. Evidence also exists for insufficient involvement of specialist providers in the strategic planning process. Only 32 per cent of hospices considered themselves to be fully involved in this area, with just under 50 per cent reporting partial involvement and a worrying one-fifth (21 per cent) stating that they were not at all involved. Where palliative care purchasing strategies did exist however, the overwhelming majority commented positively on their value.

Of the UK hospices we surveyed in 1995 a higher proportion of purchasers (61 per cent) had produced service specifications for palliative care than had developed strategies (56 per cent). It is likely that this reflects pressures on purchasers to push ahead with contracting as the highest priority within the purchasing cycle. Yet despite such pressures, over 25 per cent of hospices stated that their purchasers had no service specifications for palliative care and 13 per cent did not know. Moreover, there could be an element of cynicism about such procedures. One hospice matron we interviewed put it this way:

> Specifications are sort of motherhood and apple pie phrases like 'it will be done in accordance with normally accepted standards for this kind of work', you know, which means as long as you don't put your foot in it nobody's going to object. If you do something wrong you can get jumped on from a great height. Nobody can argue with it, but it really doesn't say anything. Again, everybody is just feeling their way towards how do you specify these things.

A particular point which emerged when talking to purchasers in the Trent region related to the extent and nature of generic care for terminally ill people, in other words ways in which palliative care could be delivered more effectively in the mainstream settings of home, nursing home and hospital. This is likely to represent a substantial proportion of overall provision, but remains very difficult to gauge. Palliation may be mentioned increasingly in generic contracts as a component of specific roles (mainly nursing), but is rarely specified in any detail. It therefore remains a hidden commodity, still to be accounted for in the planning, budgeting, procurement and monitoring processes, and provided at the discretion of individuals.

Contracts

One purpose of the special ring-fenced government monies allocated to hospices in the early 1990s was said to be to assist in the process of preparation for the world of contracts (Clark 1993). This would involve a transition from the relative freedom associated with receiving a health authority's grant-in-aid, to the potentially more restrictive contractual situation which implies detailed agreements, targets and monitoring. Indeed in our study in the Trent region of England in 1993–4 there was strong evidence that purchasers would seek to use the contracting process as a mechanism for reining in apparently recalcitrant hospices which had hitherto enjoyed high levels of autonomy and self-determination. There was also a sense that market mechanisms might provide some regulation of hospice developments where strategic planning had so palpably failed. Fears therefore existed among some hospices that such measures, by eroding their perceived independence in the eyes of the public, might also lead to a diminution in levels of public giving or the willingness of individuals to offer their services on a voluntary basis. While contracts for services should operate on the basis of mutual trust, there was clearly the potential for them to be used as a mechanism for control unless purchasers and providers opened up a constructive dialogue and reached some understanding of each other's perspectives. This, then, was a scenario of inherent risk, with two clear options for hospices. On the one hand, they could ignore the contract culture, and rely entirely on charitable giving, endowments, and the use of voluntary staff to conduct their activities. In this way it might be possible to remain unfettered by contractual chains, but the associated uncertainties would be high. On the other hand, hospices could get into a contractual relationship with one or more purchasers and seek to build the assurance at least of a medium-term source of income, albeit with potential restrictions.

It was therefore with some degree of eagerness that we awaited the results of our 1995 national survey in which we sought to assess what portion of inpatient hospices and specialist palliative care units had entered into contractual relationships with health care purchasers. To our considerable surprise we found that only 3 out of 128 hospices replying to our questionnaire did not have a contract with a purchaser (Figure 4.3). A single contract or service agreement was the most common arrangement (59 per cent); however 16 per cent had contracts with two purchasers, 9 per cent each had three or four contracts; 4 per cent had five; and a single unit, exhibiting very high levels of entrepreneurial adaptation, had a total of six contracts. This last arrangement could of course bring problems and one respondent we interviewed remarked that a large number of small contracts can generate a significant administrative burden. Overall, however, such figures suggest to us a significant level of adjustment to the new funding arrangements among a sample of hospices, three-quarters of which were in the voluntary sector.

There was, however, another and also significant finding on the question of contracts, this time of a more critical nature. We have already referred to government commitment to an equally shared funding mechanism for independent hospices, whereby monies raised from charitable sources would be matched by state resources. On the evidence of our survey, this remains a fairly distant aspiration. Among the independent hospices who replied to our questionnaire, mean income from NHS contracts/service agreements amounted to just 38 per cent of the total. Even among NHS hospices, which would be expected to be fully funded, mean income from contracts was just 91 per cent of the total. Over two-thirds of hospices had three year contracts with their purchasers, with the remainder mainly having contracts of one year's duration. This mismatch between policy rhetoric and contractual reality is a source of continuing grievance among hospices, and helps to explain why their services represent such a favourable option for purchasers.

Contract monitoring

The process of monitoring contracts provides the detailed context in which the purchasing 'lever' (Department of Health 1994) can exert influence. Through careful scrutiny of performance against the contract, and in particular through attention to quality assurance procedures, it becomes possible to assess the extent to which local needs are being met by current services. The UK NHS reforms of the early 1990s therefore placed considerable emphasis upon clinical audit as a route to achieving a more efficient and effective health service. As Higginson (1993) has shown, palliative care has not been slow in rising to the challenge of this and a great deal of interest in audit has been displayed by palliative care practitioners.

Our research has again given some insight into the development of contract monitoring, quality assurance and audit work in a context where both purchasers and providers have been on a steep learning curve, grappling to adopt new ways of thinking about the delivery and assessment of health services. In our 1993–4 study in the Trent region, the following comment from a purchaser captures some of the issues:

> We feel we're buying activity from the providers. It doesn't give sufficient information. We would like to move towards purchasing outcomes of care. The problem is how? Within community services we may purchase a programme of care with input from different disciplines, rather than the number of contacts with patients. That's what we're aiming for. We haven't given thought to how we can purchase palliative care more meaningfully.

We found at this time therefore that contracts were still rather general in tone, reflecting historic agreements with providers and lacking great specificity. In the 1994–5 national study, further light was shed on this. Among the hospices and palliative care units responding, contracts included the following elements in descending order: types of service (81 per cent); quality dimensions (74 per cent); volumes of services (62 per cent); educational provision (37 per cent); equal opportunities issues (34 per cent); and skill mix (17 per cent). This lack of detailed specification may well be true of NHS contracts generally (Flynn *et al.* 1995), but the low figure for education is surprising given its central place within hospice philosophy. Overall, there was also considerable variation in the way that our respondents *evaluated* their main contract. Nearly half thought it good (48 per cent), with one-fifth classing it as very good (21 per cent). Nevertheless, almost one-third classified it as poor or very poor.

By the time of our 1994–5 study contract monitoring was almost universal and there was general agreement that the introduction of contracting had led to an increase in audit activity. The *effects* of increased audit were viewed positively, with nine out of ten hospices regarding it as beneficial. However, our more qualitative data revealed some disappointment on the part of palliative care providers who had become enthused by audit work. There were common signs for example that purchasers often had a rather simplistic understanding of the work of palliative care, that they had a rather formulaic approach to quality assurance and that they might not be capitalizing on the results of the audit activity now taking place.

Conclusions: how full is this glass?

The hospice movement in the UK is rightly recognized as a source of many important developments. Its approach to care has won widespread public support and professional endorsement and has fuelled developments in the wider field of palliative care which go well beyond the work of the individual hospice units. As in the USA however (Magno 1992; Miller and Mike 1995), just as critical mass has been reached and a position of influence

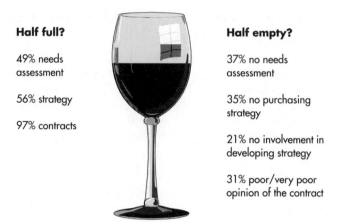

Half full?

49% needs
assessment

56% strategy

97% contracts

Half empty?

37% no needs
assessment

35% no purchasing
strategy

21% no involvement in
developing strategy

31% poor/very poor
opinion of the contract

Figure 4.4   How full is the glass? Palliative care and the UK health reforms by 1995

established, hospices have faced in the 1990s a series of problems relating to wider questions of health policy, and in particular funding mechanisms. To what extent have these endangered hospice developments? Can they be seen as an opportunity rather than a threat? After several years of observing the developing hospice scene in the UK, we are still unable to give an unequivocal answer to such questions. Perhaps one will never be possible. What can be made of the current situation, however, and what does it have to tell us about future scenarios?

Our conclusions are summarized in Figure 4.4. Whether we regard the glass as half full or half empty depends on our vantage point, our degree of optimism and our level of concern about the future.

To view the situation positively makes it possible to say that some good things have occurred. Contracts are now the norm for most hospice providers, securing some level of funding stability. Over half of all purchasers appear to have strategies for the delivery of palliative care and a half of purchasers have conducted needs assessments to underpin these. From this perspective hospices might be seen as having adapted successfully to the conditions of an internal market for health care. Indeed, there is considerable evidence to suggest that hospice providers have made important contributions to strategic planning, needs assessment, and quality assurance activity. Some hospices are therefore able to report good relations with their purchasers, based on mutual understanding and a shared vision for palliative care. There was also evidence in some cases of closer links with other NHS providers of palliative care.

Conversely, our findings could be read as indicating only patchy evidence that the 'purchasing cycle' is working to the benefit of palliative care. For example, 37 per cent of purchasers appear not to have conducted a needs assessment. Moreover, one-third of purchasers may have no strategy for palliative care and one-fifth of hospices report no involvement in strategy development. Almost one-third of hospices have a poor or very poor opinion of their contracts.

Overall, perhaps, a sense of optimism prevails. When asked how they view the prospects for their future development an overwhelmingly buoyant viewpoint emerges, with 56 per cent seeing it as very positive and 39 per cent as quite positive. A triumph of hope over experience, or a measured consideration of the prospects? For us the jury is still out. The UK has undergone massive alteration to its health care system in the 1990s. Hospices and specialist palliative care units, the majority heavily reliant upon charitable subvention, have made a remarkable adaptation to changing times. Within a very short period they appear to have become comfortable with the vagaries of marketized health care. Such adaptation will represent at least one crucial aspect of their survival and development into the twenty-first century.

Note

1 Full details of the Trent palliative care purchasing study can be found in Neale *et al.* (1994). The broad aim of this study was to examine the process of palliative care procurement in each of the then eleven District Health Authorities within the Trent region of England, from a purchaser perspective. Data collection took place in the autumn and winter of 1993–4. Two principal methods of data collection were used: interviews with key individuals involved in palliative care purchasing in each district, and analysis of district policy documents, minutes of meetings, service specifications, contracts and financial data.

The national study of the impact of the NHS reforms on UK hospice and specialist palliative care services was kindly supported by the Nuffield Health and Social Services Fund. Full details of the methodology and study can be found in Malson *et al.* (1996). The study was conducted in 1994–5 and had three key components: first, a postal questionnaire to all inpatient hospices and palliative care units in the UK (n = 203) in which 128 replies were received, giving a response rate of 63 per cent; second, detailed case studies of a representative sample of 12 hospices, using interviews and documentary analysis, and third, interviews with national experts.

References

Clark, D. (1993) *Partners in Care? Hospices and Health Authorities*. Aldershot: Avebury.

Clark, D. and Malson, H. (1995) Key issues in palliative care need assessment. *Progress in Palliative Care*, 3(2): 53–5.

Clark, D. and Malson, H. (1996) Needs assessment in cancer care, in B. Hancock (ed.) *Cancer Care in the Community*. Oxford: Radcliffe Medical Press.

Clark, D., Neale, B. and Heather, P. (1995) Contracting for palliative care. *Social Science and Medicine*, 80(9): 1193–201.

Department of Health (1989) *Working for Patients*, Cm 555. London: HMSO.

Department of Health (1994) *Purchasing for Health*. London: Department of Health.

Douglas, C. (1992) For all the saints. *British Medical Journal*, 304: 579.

Flynn, R., Pickard, S. and Williams, G. (1995) Contracts and the quasi-market in community health services. *Journal of Social Policy*, 24(4): 529–50.

Higginson, I. (1993) *Clinical Audit in Palliative Care*. Oxford: Radcliffe Medical Press.

Hospice Information Service, The (1996) *Hospice Facts and Figures, Fact Sheet 7*. London: The Hospice Information Service.

James, N. and Field, D. (1992) The routinisation of hospice: charisma and bureaucratisation. *Social Science and Medicine*, 34(12): 1363–75.

Magno, J. (1992) USA hospice care in the 1990s. *Palliative Medicine*, 6: 158–65.

Malson, H., Clark, D., Small, N. and Mallett, K. (1996) Impact of National Health Service reforms on palliative care services in the UK. *European Journal of Palliative Care*, 3(2): 68–71.

Miller, P.J. and Mike, P.B. (1995) The Medicare hospice benefit: ten years of federal policy for the terminally ill. *Death Studies*, 19: 531–42.

Neale, B., Clark, D. and Heather, P. (1994) *Palliative Care and the Purchasers: A Study of Recent Developments in the Trent Region*, occasional paper no. 13. Sheffield: Trent Palliative Care Centre.

Robbins, M. and Frankel, S. (1995) Palliative care services: what needs assessment? *Palliative Medicine*, 9(4): 287–94.

Saunders, C. (1993) Foreword, in D. Doyle, G.W.C. Hanks and N. MacDonald (eds) *Oxford Textbook of Palliative Medicine*. Oxford: Oxford University Press.

Small, N. (1989) *Politics and Planning in the National Health Service*. Buckingham: Open University Press.

Smith, A.E. and Eve, A. (1996) Survey of hospice and palliative care in-patient units in the UK and Ireland, 1993. *Palliative Medicine*, 10: 13–21.

Wilkes, E. (1980) *Report of the Working Group on Terminal Care*. London: Department of Health and Social Security.

PART II

Service developments

Introduction to Part II

The first part of this book has examined questions of policy, ethics and evidence as important aspects integral to shaping palliative care in the future. In Part II, the contributors address the current development of a wide range of different specialist palliative care services. The majority of our contributors here, in a variety of contexts, have been at the forefront of the development of palliative care services since the early 1980s, when the hospice movement in the UK first started to have a greater impact worldwide. In addition to describing the establishment of various services across the world, several authors reflect on issues such as equity, culture, historical context and their impact on developing programmes. Palliative care services have tended to include one or more of the following components: inpatient hospice unit, a home care service, or a consulting service/palliative care team in the hospital. Reference is made to all these models of care in the following chapters.

Jo Hockley begins this part of the book (Chapter 5) by capturing the evolution of the hospice approach from a global perspective. The development of the hospice unit is probably what is most significant about the growth of specialist palliative care services in the UK and therefore related aspects of admission, funding, children's hospices, day hospice, and respite 'at home' teams are addressed. Clearly there are challenges ahead for the future of the hospice unit. Many wonder whether the hospice movement in the UK might not be a victim of its own success: in what ways can it continue to develop its contribution as palliative care begins to be delivered in a wide range of settings? It is important that those working in specialist hospice units continue to promote the multidisciplinary model with its emphasis on education and research. New and innovative aspects of caring for dying patients and their families need to be thought through and then channelled into the wider health care system in order to heighten continually the profile of palliative care.

There is always a danger that a specialist service may 'deskill' those who care for dying people as part of their wider duties, especially in the acute setting and the community. This must certainly be guarded against. Hospices are not going to be able to care for all those who are dying, so the dissemination of the principles and ideals of hospice care must continue to filter to other specialities. The greater knowledge that we now have in the care of dying patients must be made widely available.

Although Chapter 5 gives an overview of the core hospice services that developed worldwide during the early 1980s, authors from various countries, including Spain, eastern Europe, India, Australia, Sweden and Italy, contribute chapters which highlight not only the global character of specialist palliative care services, but also the different aspects of development, service orientation, and government interest and support that occur in individual contexts.

Roger Hunt and Ian Maddocks, in Chapter 6 on historical aspects and equity issues relating to palliative care in South Australia, highlight the question of governmental responsibility for funding. Because of societal pressure for hospice palliative care services during the earlier part of the hospice movement, many programmes were set up voluntarily. Now that the specialty has become an integral part of health care and medical training in many countries, governments are being asked to take greater financial responsibility. There has been a positive response from many governments but Hunt and Maddocks state that much of the response of government funding in Australia is sponsored more by a sense of easing the 'acute' bed situation rather than underlying concern for the care of dying people. One aspect of the hospice movement is a concern to educate society as a whole about death and dying. Funding hospices to ease the acute situation runs the risk of creating an enlarged 'side-room syndrome' while conveniently hiding dying people from the wider society. With government funding comes the responsibility of integrating services within mainstream healthcare settings, so that patients dying from non-malignant diseases can benefit from expertise developed within the hospice/palliative care services. Otherwise it could be argued that patients dying from cancer are more privileged than those dying from other diseases.

In India, it would appear from Gilly Burn's personal account (Chapter 7) that there are few appropriate facilities. The main hospice units in Bombay, Delhi and Goa seem isolated from the 80 per cent of India's population who live in rural areas. Issues of inequality here relate not to the funding of palliative care for cancer patients versus non-malignant disease as it might be in Australia or other affluent countries, but more to the inappropriate use of resources at a much higher level of the system. Apparently, one cancer centre's resources were spent sending their doctors to the USA to learn about stereotatic radiotherapy when the same centre had no oral morphine tablets and no professional with in-depth knowledge of palliative care. New technology is important and should never be denied to developing countries but it is vital that limited resources are matched appropriately to the need. India accounts for one-sixth of the world's population, with 80 per cent of cancer patients presenting with their disease in the incurable stage of their illness. Rural community programmes exist for preventive care, hygiene and public health. It would seem appropriate, as Gilly Burn suggests, that an already established network could be used to promote palliative care more effectively.

The extended family life and sense of community which can be found in eastern and developing countries can contrast with the individualistic and materialistic society of so-called developed countries. In some cases one of the major benefits may be that the sick person is cared for by the family and able to die at home. Giorgio di Mola stresses the point in Chapter 8 on 'home care' that home is where the majority of people feel comfortable and most truly themselves. Several of the authors in Part II, including di Mola, put forward the idea that home is where people want to die and yet results of studies show that, although length of stay at home during the palliative stage of illness is increasing, often people end up dying in institutions. Why this happens is difficult to determine. Circumstances in the home, inadequacy of family support, distressing symptoms, and sudden deterioration without warning are all aspects that can prevent a dying patient from remaining at home. It may also reflect on the expertise of the specialist key worker. Opening up a conversation about dying can be very threatening all round; yet so often if this has not been done the greater fear of feeling out of control and unsure of what is happening can precipitate an admission to hospital, which might appear a more 'safe' environment. Home is certainly where a lot of government and hospital administrators want people to die because it appears the cheaper option. However, di Mola argues that to provide appropriate and skilled support, not just from the perspective of specialist palliative care, then good generic care is often still a considerable expense.

Barbro Beck-Friis (Chapter 9) details a cameo on the home care services set up since the mid-1970s within a single district in Sweden. In the county of Ostergotland the government has funded Hospital Based Home Care Teams (HBHCTs) to help give 24-hour care for dying patients in their own homes. Although Giorgio di Mola sees the home as a low-tech environment as far as health care is concerned, Beck-Friis details how the HBHC teams will perform reasonably high-tech procedures within the home setting, for example, paracentesis or blood transfusions. The commitment over the years to developing what is clearly a most respected service, albeit in a small area of Sweden, is considerable.

Commitment and clear professional leadership are just two of the characteristics that Xavier Gómez-Batiste and colleagues (Chapter 10) insist play an important part in setting up specialist palliative care services. A five year plan to establish a mixture of different services in Catalonia was backed by the World Health Organization in 1990. Over a three year period 51 teams (9 inpatient units, 8 support teams in hospitals and 34 teams in the community) were established. The government in Catalonia is certainly committed to listening to an expert in the field of palliative care and to taking on board suggestions for rational planning. This chapter, besides reiterating the importance of needs assessment, is also committed to the importance of evaluation and cost-effectiveness of the care implemented. The authors stress the importance of having a definition of specific services and standards before starting out, in order to prevent the confusion between palliative care, pain services, oncology and more long-term care. In many ways this may sound somewhat ruthless, and yet in setting out a new specialist service which may well be over and above a generic service that already exists, it is vital for both professionals and the public to see how it fits in to existing provision. Where there is no generic service in the home, like in Sweden, then perhaps one can take on a broader remit.

In eastern Europe, Jacek Luczak from Poland describes in Chapter 11 an enthusiasm for palliative care services that has been unsurpassed by the lay public in many other countries. Despite the impediment of a political and economic system in the 1980s that excluded care of the dying, hundreds of people, both lay as well as those with medical and nursing qualifications, helped in the promotion of an informal voluntary hospice movement. Many nurses and doctors gave of their time after a day's work to care voluntarily on a hospice programme. It is this sort of commitment that so often will push forward the boundaries of care for dying people. Clearly the WHO has played a major part more recently in targeting various countries of the former 'eastern bloc' over cancer pain policies and in particular, the introduction of morphine preparations which were almost non-existent prior to the early 1990s. Much of the development of specialist palliative care in eastern Europe has been recorded in various hospice bulletins with a limited circulation. Professor Luczak has now brought together here a detailed description of how the various countries are trying to promote their palliative care programmes in the wake of political reform and major socio-economic transformations.

Turning to South East Asia, we see once again similar problems facing the development of palliative care services, albeit manifesting themselves in different ways. Epidemiological and demographic trends both indicate high levels of need for palliative care in local populations, and some services have begun to develop. In Chapter 12, however, Ian Maddocks's personal view of the prospects for palliative care in Asia identifies several areas for attention and guards against apparently easy options based on the transplantation of western models. First, the cultural and religious context must be addressed. Western concepts of good works and autonomy do not apply in Asia. Palliative care must develop in relation to the appropriate context of ethics and cultural norms. Professional considerations of various kinds can serve to limit the development of palliative care, for example: a preference in Asia for curative treatments; a confidence in hospital care; physical restrictions on home care as well as a lack of insurance cover for home care or professionals able to deliver it. Other barriers, more political in character, include governments' unease about and resistance to the prescribing of opioids. Finally, in a context where the educational needs for palliative care in Asia are expanding, Maddocks warns of the dangers of this particular 'market' becoming dominated by western providers who are insufficiently aware of the context in which they seek to teach.

These themes of service development, of cultural variation and of professional, organizational and political resistances are at the heart of the final chapter in Part II, contributed by Jan Stjernsward just as he came to the end of a 16 year period as chief of the World Health Organization's cancer unit. Chapter 13 summarizes the WHO cancer control strategy, highlighting the importance of palliative care within it. Stjernsward focuses upon the priority of cancer pain as a global public health problem and shows what can be achieved through a strategy which aims to build consensus on key issues and establish rational policies for implementing existing knowledge. The success of the strategy is revealed through the establishment of a global network of support and evidence of development projects and initiatives even in some of the poorest countries of the world. This chapter should be read by anyone with an interest in palliative care in the developing countries, but it also provides considerable material for reflection on the future of palliative care in other, more materially favoured, parts of the world.

New themes and key questions in Part II

The development of services

- The WHO Cancer Pain and Palliative Care Programme has set out a broad range of principles which can be applied to the development of palliative care services in all contexts. There is concern that shrinkage in the activities of WHO may impede further progress in the development of palliative care services in the poorer countries.
- Political support, integration within wider matters of health policy, and the role of local 'champions' are all vital to new palliative care service developments, whether at the national, regional or local level.

- Increasingly, service development must take place in the absence of new resources. The redirection of some resources from oncology and the redeployment of resources from mainstream care must be looked to as a possible strategy, supported by careful appraisal of options, evaluation and review.
- In emphasizing an overtly quantifiable and medical problem (e.g. pain) as the primary focus of development for new palliative care services, attention must be paid to the danger of overlooking the wider cultural and psychosocial aspects of need. These will vary from setting to setting and it is important that new services reflect these local factors and do not seek merely to replicate or impose models of care which appear to have been successful elsewhere.

Service organization and place of care

- Although, in many cultures, there is a preference for death to take place at home, the proportion of deaths taking place in hospital remains relatively unchanged. Why should this be?
- In the poorest countries, community based palliative care is the only feasible option. How can such services be developed comprehensively and how can family members and other informal carers be more empowered and better informed?
- In the affluent nations, death in a nursing home is becoming more common. How can liaison with hospice and hospital be improved and what systematic approach would best meet the palliative care educational needs of staff in nursing homes?
- Is 'high-tech' palliative care at home a viable option? Is it likely further to extend the medicalization of death?
- Complacency over the quality of care given in hospices must be guarded against and hospices must examine closely the legitimacy of their claims to be 'centres of excellence'. What is the appropriate role for hospices as the wider specialty of palliative care begins to consolidate?
- Hospital-based home care teams have arisen in relation to a lack of comprehensive day and night care for dying patients at home. The respect they have gained has resulted in demand for their services among patients returning home after surgery. Clearly this has been important in the dissemination of good multidisciplinary practice, but there may be a danger of losing the focus on palliative care.

International collaboration and cooperation

- Lack of national policies for palliative care, lack of oral morphine and restrictions on opioid prescribing, together with poor educational opportunities, all continue to hamper the development of palliative care in some places. Frequently these problems are compounded by inadequate public health infrastructures, poor administrative systems and underlying poverty.

- Cooperation and partnership between palliative care organizations around the world have a vital part to play in continuing development. This can take place at many levels – international associations, professional bodies or local providers.
- Is the question of euthanasia currently only relevant in the more affluent countries of the world which are characterized by chronic illness, ageing populations and high-cost health care systems?
- In what ways can the new information technologies be harnessed to the clinical and educational needs of palliative care, particularly in the international context?
- The way in which a society cares for its dying people is said to be a measure of its overall value and worth. Is such a concept widely applicable, and if so what does it tell us about the potential for palliative care to contribute to much wider processes of social improvement?

5 The evolution of the hospice approach

JO HOCKLEY

Since the mid-1960s the hospice movement in the UK has had a considerable impact on the care of dying people. Although compassion for destitute and dying people has been the mission of many in differing nations (Saunders 1984), it was Dame Cicely Saunders's work with the establishment of St Christopher's Hospice, as the first teaching and research-based hospice unit in 1967, that fired the imagination of many health professionals across the world. Such a movement laid the foundation for the concept of hospice care to be recognized as a specialty, namely 'palliative medicine', by the Royal College of Physicians (London) in 1987.

The image of a hospice being a place of rest and nurture for those wearied at the end of life's journey is mirrored by the fact that the hospice movement itself has been 'journeying'. It has not remained static. Its emphasis on an holistic approach to patient care, the family as the focus of care, and the importance of multidisciplinary collaboration on a day to day basis, is a philosophy that can be adapted to different settings and indeed cultures. In the UK, the knowledge and skill developed in the hospice units has had a ripple effect into the community via home care teams and day hospice, and now full circle back into the acute hospital setting (Hockley 1996). Globally, differing countries and continents have begun to adapt aspects of the hospice philosophy that are most acceptable to their specific contexts and cultures.

To what extent is the hospice movement a victim of its own success in the UK? What is the life expectancy in terms of an established hospice unit? What innovative ideas can maintain its impact and interest in society as a whole? How will the freestanding hospice survive in the twenty-first century? What is the worldwide impact of hospices? How, precisely, does hospice philosophy adapt to differing cultures?

This chapter will consider issues facing the direction of hospices in the UK, the core development of hospices worldwide, and their global development. It will look at where hospice care might be on its journey and whether, as some might suggest, a further 'crossroads' is being reached (Scott 1981; Clark 1994).

Hospices in the UK

Besides emphasizing the proper control of pain and other symptoms, one of the important aspects of the hospice movement in the UK has been to re-encourage a more holistic approach of care within the science of medicine. For hundreds of years the mind, the soul and the body were seen as an integral part of illness. However, with the gradual emphasis on the science of illness and technological advances, in the main the wholeness of patient care and the needs of the family lost their focus. The hospice movement has not only helped to redress the balance but also stressed the importance of the multidisciplinary team, working together with the patient and family at the centre of care. It has highlighted the necessity of controlling pain and other symptoms; the need to face the fear of dying and to consider ways of exploring that fear, both with patients and their families, as well as with staff. The 'time' given to patients and families to talk and to 'be with' has been given priority, and the nurse–patient ratio adjusted accordingly.

The admission criteria to hospice units has always been an important issue. If a hospice unit is to benefit as many patients and families as possible, it is important that beds are not 'blocked' by long-stay patients (i.e. patients with a number of years to live). Generally a patient coming to a hospice would be expected to have less than three months to live. The most common length of stay of a hospice patient in the UK is 12–14 days (Eve and Smith 1996) but some patients may be cared for in a hospice for a number of weeks. Kirkham and Davies (1992) found that in their 20-bedded hospice 12 per cent of patients occupied their beds for 28 days or more. Research has shown that patients in a hospice can experience an adverse effect when subjected to a number of patients dying around them (Honeybun et al. 1992).

The number of beds in a hospice unit will automatically limit the length of stay. A small hospice of 8–12 beds will obviously require different policies about length of stay compared to a hospice with 30 beds or 60 beds (Regnard 1989). St Christopher's Hospice and St Joseph's Hospice (both situated in London with 62 beds and 63 beds respectively) are the largest hospice units in the UK. They can therefore comfortably accommodate a situation when a patient suddenly reaches a plateau in the end-stage of an illness. Kirkham and Davies (1992), however, state that if clinical activity of hospice units is to be a useful indicator at a national level, statistics recording number of patients referred, number of new admissions, discharges, readmissions and inpatient deaths, mean length of stay and mean midnight bed occupancy should be collected uniformly by all hospice units, so that 'throughput is then taken as the total annual number of new and subsequent admissions divided by the number of beds' (Kirkham and Davies 1992: 53).

Admission to a hospice is secured either by a senior nurse or doctor from the hospice visiting and assessing the patient at home or in the hospital, or by the referring team completing a hospice admission form. Such a form can range from a simple overview of the medical situation to that of a detailed document requiring medical, nursing and social aspects of care. If there is some ambiguity about the request then further contact (either by phone or a visit) can be made by the hospice doctor or nurse prior to admission. Most hospices will see an urgent community referral as a priority over and above that of a patient already in a hospital bed. The largest percentage of admissions to hospice units in the UK comes from home (Eve and Smith 1996).

Much of society unfortunately still has the idea that hospice units are just places where you go to die. Recent figures, however, show that 45 per cent (Eve and Smith 1996) of admissions to a hospice unit are discharged. Obviously these patients will remain under the care of the hospice unit but it does not mean that the only patient exit out of a hospice unit is 'feet first'.

Funding of hospice units in UK

In 1996 there were 217 inpatient hospice units in the UK and Republic of Ireland with a total of 3215 beds (Hospice Information Service 1996). Funding for hospice units up until recently has been on an *ad-hoc* basis. A few units have been totally self-funded using fund-raising initiatives and charities to help support them, other units have been part funded by the government, and still others fully funded and run as NHS hospice units. In the mid-1980s the government, in acknowledgement of the success of the hospice movement with its enormous support from the public, decided to fund the work 50:50. This meant that for every £1 raised by hospice fund-raisers, the government would match it 'pound for pound'. More recently a special allocation of Department of Health monies has been available to independent hospices (Clark 1993). This figure has increased more than fivefold, from £8 million in 1990 to £43 million in 1993. Unfortunately controversy has occurred between the independent hospices for whom these monies were made available and NHS-funded hospices. It appeared that those health authorities that had taken the initiative and built their own NHS-funded hospices lost out and were thereby penalized. However, in the current climate of purchaser/provider and the new market-place economy, hospices have to enter the world of contracting with health authorities or budget-holding general practices (see Clark and colleagues, Chapter 4 in this volume).

The challenge in the future is the availability of hospice care for all terminally ill patients (SMAC/SNMAC 1992). At present 3 per cent of hospice admissions are represented by patients suffering from diseases other than cancer such as motor neurone disease and AIDS. This rises to 6 per cent of admissions if specialist hospices dedicated only to AIDS/HIV are included (Eve and Smith 1996). To admit all patients who are dying can-not be the way forward otherwise hospice units would simply become enlarged hospital 'side-rooms'. There is a difference between those people living with a disease that cannot be cured and those for whom a prognosis clarifies that they are actually *dying* from a disease that cannot be cured (Biswas 1993). This is the necessary clarification that distinguishes those patients with advanced non-malignant disease and those with advanced cancer, AIDS, or motor neurone disease. Hospice units have set the stand-ard for the cancer patient, those suffering from HIV/AIDS and motor neurone disease, where in each case the disease process and prognosis is reasonably predictable. The challenge is to know how to extend the prin-ciples effectively. To disseminate the philosophy and ideals of care, to share knowledge of symptom control with the differing specialties and the prim-ary care teams is therefore paramount. The care of elderly people is per-haps a reasonable example of where hospice principles can be taught and are being transferred into a differing setting. Another example is that of the children's hospice units.

Children's hospices

By 1996 there were eleven operational hospice units for children with terminal illness in the UK (St Christopher's Information Service), beginning with the establishment of Helen House, Oxford, in 1982. Many of the admissions into children's hospice units are for respite care for children with a wide range of complex and often rare life-limiting illnesses rather than for cancer. Children's hospices grew out of the vision for adult units but have a slightly different emphasis. Many are non-institutional with no resident doctor. The care is family driven (Worswick 1994) with a greater emphasis on 'respite'. Interestingly during 1993 there were 2434 admis-sions to a total of 45 beds in five hospices but only 38 deaths (Eve and Smith 1996). Some adult units admit children on occasions, but only 12 units (7 per cent) had actually done so in 1993. Six of these units employed paediatric nurses to care for the children.

Day hospice

One of the main developments of hospice in the UK since the mid-1980s has been the establishment of day hospice units (Fisher and McDaid 1996). These units are often attached to well-established hospices but occasionally stand alone, sometimes alongside a hospital or GP unit, in order to support a home care team. In 1996 there were 232 day hospice units in the UK and Republic of Ireland (Hospice Information Service 1996). Criteria for admission to a day care programme vary but would generally include the hospice philosophy that a person has a progressive, far advanced disease. However, practical issues are also important:

- *Patient's physical ability*: all patients need to be able to get down the stairs and into the car of a volunteer driver.
- *Balance of support from other resources*: day care must not become the only resource so that when patients are no longer able to attend because of physical disability they are not devoid of all their support.
- *Balance of a patient's individual needs and that of the rest of the group attending the day hospice*: often a patient will be limited to two sessions a week at the hospice but in special circumstances this is reviewed.

Much of what can or cannot be achieved in day care depends on appropriate leadership, and a mix of professional skills (for example, those of the occupational therapist, physiotherapist, or art therapist) together with the skills of volunteers. For many patients facing advanced disease the energy required for 'doing' has often waned. However, the literature reports that the understanding and skill of people in day hospice can enable patients to enjoy a creativity that they thought they had lost, to be able to continue to participate in life and have a degree of normality albeit in the context of advanced disease (Gibson 1995). In many ways such rehabilitation in palliative care from a day hospice perspective re-emphasizes hospice philosophy:

> The skilled help given to enable a person and their family to re-adjust to a situation that is unlikely to remain static for more than a few weeks at a time, because of progressive, far-advanced disease. Such help involves not only the expert control of distressing physical symptoms, but the exploration of strengths/coping strategies in relation to the patient's emotional/psychological/spiritual health. The outcome of such assistance alongside specialist therapies is designed to positively effect the quality of life making the time lived worthwhile.
>
> (Hockley and Mowatt 1996: 14)

The concept of respite care in the home that is being developed by a number of hospice home care teams may well be the way forward to at least help patients dying of non-malignant disease to die at home.

'Respite Care at Home' teams

In many ways the concept of 'respite care' is not new, but with greater emphasis on community care the emphasis is on respite in the patient's home. Johnson *et al.* (1988) first described a Relative Support Scheme set up in 1984 by St Luke's Hospice in Sheffield. Outcomes of this scheme showed that 60 per cent of the 227 patients who used the scheme died at home. In 1992 the hospice home care team of The Ellenor Foundation in south London, set up a 'Respite Care at Home' team service providing support and care for the carer in the home and seeking to enable patients to remain in their own homes for as long as possible, and to die at home if that is their wish. There are now 68 units offering home respite care (Hospice Information Service 1996) although the extent and quality of cover is not reported.

There are a number of reasons why such a service is thought to be appropriate:

- lack of the extended family to help and support;
- as the main carer devotes time to the person who is dying, other family members especially children may be losing out on the attention of a parent;
- the patient may need constant caring, repositioning in bed;
- a prolonged dying period can often leave carers, especially if they are elderly, feeling emotionally drained;
- many families are afraid of death and are comforted with the presence of a team member in their home.

Contrary to beliefs, families or the carer using such a scheme were not looking for a team member to be present in the house for a 24-hour period. The carers were more likely to ask for a 4–7 hour block; in this way they felt strengthened in their caring but their privacy was not invaded (Stone and Blade 1994). It is impossible to predict the need of a respite nursing service within a home care team. Many families are able to manage to care for their loved one at home with the help of a hospice home care team and the normal local community services. This makes it difficult to calculate how many nurses are needed to cover the respite care service. A 'respite nurse bank' specific to the hospice home care team is probably the most flexible and cost-effective way of organizing such care. Nurses are paid by the hour, and at the end of each visit the respite nurse will report to the hospice home care nurse. There is no sickness or holiday entitlement. All nurses on the respite bank team are trained in hospice care and attend team meetings every six weeks. Clear criteria need to be given for request of such a service so that it is used as a specialist input to augment statutory services in order that a patient can die at home. An evaluation into the effectiveness of such a service is currently being considered with the respite care team at St Christopher's Hospice, London (Dale 1995).

Core development worldwide

The responsibility of any new specialty is to enhance growth and share its expertise with others. With growth comes the responsibilities not just to challenge health care professionals but to join the debate of governmental policies. Palliative care is a recognized specialty in the UK, Canada and Australia (Jackson 1993).

Canada

Canada was perhaps the first country outside the UK that actively pursued the concept of hospice. In the early 1970s consideration was given within the health care system to alternative models of hospice care other than the freestanding unit. Health professionals at Winnipeg and Montreal both adopted the concept of a Palliative Care Unit within the acute hospital setting. The word 'palliative' was used to describe the care of the dying person rather than 'hospice care'. Already the interpretation of hospice as a philosophy of care was being extended and not restricted to bricks and mortar. Between 1981 and 1986 there was a 200 per cent increase in the number of different palliative care programmes in Canada (Scott 1992). By 1990, however, despite the existence of 346 different programmes, some were floundering (O'Donnell 1992). As a result, an Expert Panel on Palliative Care was formed to put forward certain recommendations concerning the allocation of monies, the establishment of regional palliative care centres, home care projects, a compulsory and tested palliative care curriculum for all health care professionals, a stronger focus on the control of suffering, and reimbursement to families for lost income. It was around this time that the Ottawa-Carleton Regional Palliative Care Association set up five committees to help coordinate a specific aspect of palliative care within the region and to prevent duplication or fragmentation of services (O'Donnell 1992).

United States of America

In many ways the development of hospice care in the USA might be described as a 'bottom-up' approach. The federal government has responded as a result of demand from society but a universal complaint of the USA hospice movement has been the lack of involvement of the medical profession in the delivery of hospice care (Magno 1992). Although there has been considerable action from professional groups with the establishment of freestanding hospice units, much of the interest has come through home care teams using a considerable number of volunteers.

In the early and mid-1980s major innovative research was carried out looking at the evaluation of conventional terminal care in hospital, free-standing hospice and hospice home care (Wales *et al.* 1983; Greer *et al.* 1986). Since then governments have been lobbied and funding made available through Medicare for patients with a prognosis of six months or less to live. However, a further Medicare proviso stated that continuity between the home and the inpatient unit had to be maintained and that patients were allowed only 20 per cent hospice inpatient care out of the total care provided, which added considerable pressure to hospice facilities (Magno 1992), forcing many hospices not to apply for Medicare funding. Both the lack of medical input and the problems of funding have held back the establishment of hospice care as a specialty in its own right. The Academy of Hospice Physicians, established in 1985, and renamed the American Academy of Hospice and Palliative Medicine in 1996, is none the less pushing not only for the effective introduction of palliative medicine into the curricula of medical schools (see Ingham and Coyle, Chapter 16 in this volume) but for hospice/palliative medicine to be recognized as a subspecialty of medicine in order that more physicians with an interest in this field can make it their career (Magno 1992). In 1990 a National Hospice Census reported 1529 operational hospice programmes, with 41 per cent being community-based, 30 per cent hospital-based, 23 per cent home health-agency based and 5 per cent being other organization-based (National Hospice Organization 1990).

Australia and New Zealand

Australia and New Zealand have developed hospice care principles along similar lines to that of the UK. However, a greater proportion of the population in Australia and New Zealand probably has private insurance. Hospice units with their home care teams, palliative care units within the acute hospital, and hospice home care teams have been establishing themselves since the mid-1980s. Like many of the western countries, research for parliamentary select committees into aspects of death and dying (Ashby and Wakefield 1993) is invited and supported. This is often as a result of the knock-on effect of the support and development of hospice care in a country where it is widely practised and established (see Hunt and Maddocks, Chapter 6 in this volume).

Western Europe

The development of hospices in western Europe has had an increasing impact on nearly every country although each has had to contend with differing problems. In **Germany** where the concept of hospice is often misinterpreted and misunderstood, any integration of the different services is hampered by the ways in which health care is financed and by the fact that no authoritative body has met together to work out a strategy (Albrecht 1990). Groups have arisen in most major towns but a considerable amount of palliative care is carried out within the general acute setting rather than in freestanding hospice units.

It must be said that where nursing has a major voice as a professional body in a country, care for the dying patient and the family appear to have more of a chance of establishing an identity alongside medical colleagues. **France, Belgium, Norway and Sweden** are all countries which are making an impact in hospice/palliative care – although again the emphasis is on specialized palliative care consultation teams in the acute hospitals and in the community rather than on freestanding hospice units. In Norway 80 per cent of deaths occur in institutions. The government has recently recommended the establishment of palliative care units at university hospitals in the five health regions of the country (Schjolberg 1995). The three main cities of **Finland** each has a hospice and it is the dissemination of knowledge from these hospice units that is their main function besides clinical input into patient and family care. Because many of the families live far away, Scandinavian hospices have special facilities for families to stay over.

In the **Netherlands** with the widespread public attention given to issues of euthanasia, many have thought that hospice care would never be fully recognized. Much of the care of dying patients has been within the acute oncology wards, nursing homes for elderly people, or in small 'hospice at home' houses where the major part of the care was organized and fulfilled by volunteers. However, in 1992 Dr Zylicz pioneered the work of the first multidisciplinary hospice unit in Arnhem and has a vision of two or three 'centres of excellence' in order to train specialists in palliative care (Zylicz 1993). In **Denmark** most hospice work is connected to the Danish Church. The first of two hospices opened in 1992.

Clearly, lobbying health departments to look at the needs of dying people is an important way of establishing a top-down approach for hospice care. In conjunction with the Cancer and Palliative Care Unit of the World Health Organization, Dr Gómez-Batiste (1994) set out a five-year plan for palliative care in **Catalonia, Spain** (see Gómez-Batiste and colleagues, Chapter 10 in this volume). He states that within three years there has been swift expansion of resources, training and education, and the prescription of morphine has been made much easier. In **Italy**, although there are highly esteemed units in Milan and Rome, there is little concrete backing from the Servizio Sanitario Nazionale (Italian National Health Service: see Toscani and Mancini 1989).

The European Association of Palliative Care is now well established and has played a major role in drawing together health care professionals of all the main disciplines. Bi-annual conferences are held in different European countries, thereby bringing professionals together and making the dissemination of research, clinical expertise, and the knowledge of services more accessible. Cultures vary across western Europe but hospice practice has been adapted to meet differing needs and circumstances. None the less there are still pockets in western Europe, especially in the Mediterranean islands (Gibraltar, Malta, Cyprus), where hospice work is in its infancy.

A detailed picture of hospice development in eastern Europe appears in Chapter 11 in this volume; it has been written by Professor Jacek Luczak, who has worked to develop hospice/palliative care in Poland and other countries of eastern Europe.

Global perspective

Africa

The core development of the hospice movement in Canada, USA, Australia, New Zealand and western Europe details the number of hospice units, home care programmes, education initiatives and government lobbying being undertaken. It is, however, important to see hospice development in a global perspective which takes account of countries in the developing world. As early as 1980, hospices in **South Africa** and **Zimbabwe** were being established. In the wake of industrialization in Africa the need for hospice has grown as the extended family becomes more fragmented with family members seeking work in the large towns (van Heerden 1981). In South Africa the hospice movement has been able to build bridges between communities – even crossing the bridge of racial prejudice. There are some 12 hospice units throughout South Africa. The work has continued to develop in the form of home care teams and day care units with home care teams rising from 13 to 16 in the period 1995–6. Exciting work of hospice outreach caring for terminally ill people in the townships continues in South Africa. Although a considerable amount of hospice care is being taught in South Africa, much of the rest of Africa remains isolated from hospice knowledge. The major input in Zimbabwe is through home care services. In **Kenya** a second satellite team has been set up outside Nairobi reaching into the homes of families in the countryside.

Latin America

It is probably true to say that no other health care movement has had such a ripple effect throughout the world as that of the hospice movement. Hospice/palliative care is more than just good pain and symptom control. It is about caring for the whole person in the context of the family as the unit of care. Despite obstacles of poverty, racial injustice and persecution, many individuals have valiantly pulled together to provide a service, often for no monetary reward, for dying people and their families. The work in eastern Europe (see Łuczak, Chapter 11 in this volume) is an amazing example of this but since 1988 considerable development of palliative care has occurred in some of the Latin American countries. Bruera (1992) details initiatives in **Argentina, Brazil** and **Colombia**. Eighteen palliative care programmes are now established in different Argentine cities. Some of these services are based on the San Nicolas model of trained volunteers providing an outpatient and home care service; others have moved into the teaching hospitals. In Brazil, after starting a palliative care consultation team in one of the regional cancer hospitals, a hospice unit is to be opened which will act as headquarters for a regional programme. Colombia boasts the first freestanding 52-bedded hospice unit in Latin America. However 'widespread poverty . . . lack of communication between patient and families and the health care staff in issues such as the diagnosis of cancer and prognosis makes it necessary to use different standards for the assessment and management of these patients' (Bruera 1992: 184).

Asia

Much of the work in Asia is still in its infancy and patchy. Fellow colleagues in **China** (Kerr 1993) and **India** (see Burn, Chapter 7 in this volume) in particular still grapple with the enormity of the task – where the suffering of terminally ill people is largely a result of inefficient governmental bureaucracy, and underdevelopment and endemic poverty (Thomas et al. 1995). However, hospice care programmes in **Japan** (Suzuki et al. 1993), **Hong Kong, Singapore** (Goh 1994), and the **Philippines** are well established both from a clinical and governmental viewpoint (see also Maddocks, Chapter 12 in this volume).

Challenges for the future: 'hospice crossroads'

One of the strengths of the hospice movement has been the commitment and collaboration of the differing health professionals involved in the care of dying people. As hinted in the introduction and then seen in the global development of hospice care, the movement has not stood still. A journey has taken place. But where are we on that journey? Has it come to an end, or are we at a major junction as we face the twenty-first century? Ever since the beginning of Dame Cicely Saunders's work in establishing St Christopher's Hospice, people along the way (Mount 1973; Scott 1981, 1992; Clark 1994) have challenged those involved in the care of the dying to re-evaluate their work, to stop, to 'take stock' of the direction and to examine carefully the task ahead. Are we at a junction where hospice care is being challenged? Or at a crossroads where the diversity of a developing specialty can encompass new ideas without abandoning what clearly has been a revolution in the care of dying people?

There have always been obstacles and difficulties even at the beginning of the hospice movement, and the present economic climate is no easy task to have to face in the light of the explosion of palliative care needs that are likely to take place into the twenty-first century. In Canada, Scott (1992) challenges those in palliative care about the difficult choices and the competing forces within their health care budgets. None the less, he feels that it is important to take stock of the obstacles that confront palliative care as a whole and palliative medicine as a specialty: 'the STOP sign offers us the opportunity to look around and shift direction to avoid obstacles. As palliative care approaches the year 2000, a wide variety of choices, obstacles, and opportunities will have an impact on its development' (Scott 1992: 6).

Multidisciplinary model

In looking to the future one must consider the past and take on board what has been helpful to continue and what has hindered growth. There is no doubt that caring for the dying has always been done. It may not have been so organized but that is not to say people did not care before – they did but emphases were different. What about leadership of hospice units? It was Dame Cicely Saunders's background as a nurse and then a social worker that inspired her with the thought of better care for dying people. She went on to train as a doctor simply because she was told that the medical profession otherwise would not take her seriously. The multidisciplinary role model was so much a part of Dame Cicely's work – she could so easily identify with the different roles – she knew what it was to contribute to the care of the dying from the different specialities in which she had worked. She saw the strength in bringing these roles together in multidisciplinary working. Surely therefore the best units/teams are those which are led from a multidisciplinary standpoint. It is important that this multidisciplinary strength is not undermined by the fact that palliative medicine has now become a specialty. The clear danger is that all that has been built up over the years could be undermined if the multidisciplinary emphasis is to be watered down because of overly strong medical or nursing direction. Although palliative medicine has now been recognized as a specialty in its own right, there is a danger that doctors coming into hospice/palliative care will lose sight of the vision of the multidisciplinary approach in decision making and leadership.

Lack of accountability

One of the dangers of the freestanding hospice unit is the lack of accountability. Yes, to a degree there is accountability to the families of patients in the unit. However, unlike that of the hospital palliative care team, and even when working alongside general practitioners in the community, there is no other specialty involved in the care of the patient to which accountability is required. In this context, the hospice unit can become isolated in its caring if there is not a continual flow of new ideas and challenges. The analogy of the Dead Sea where no fish survive, and only the River Jordan flows into it without any outflow of water is an interesting one. If a unit is to remain healthy there needs to be the stimulation of movement. The most obvious is the movement of staff – new doctors and nurses coming into the specialty with the freshness and stimulation of having worked in a different environment.

Support and stress of hospice work

A review of the literature looking at stress among hospice/palliative care staff (Vachon 1995) shows that through education programmes and support, stress in hospice care is less of a problem than it was in the early 1980s. The satisfaction then in caring for dying people and their families in an atmosphere of good symptom control and multidisciplinary care may well be supportive in itself. Hospice work is none the less demanding and in many ways caring for dying people is rather an unnatural occupation. Although considerable research has been done on coping styles, personal value systems, and work stressors, there is little reference to energy levels of hospice nurses directly involved in full-time, day to day physical care of dying patients. Some would argue that full-time health professionals directly involved in the physical care of dying people should not remain in their positions for more than five years. The benefit, if nothing else, would be the further dissemination of hospice principles into other areas of care. There is certainly a need for proper appraisal of staff, support and education in order to enhance staff morale and coping mechanisms.

Hospice units have the clear advantage of attracting health professionals from other disciplines if they can continue to support their staff and make them feel valued. The lack of resources and care for staff in the NHS and the inability of many nurses to fulfil their desire to care for patients because of staff shortages is taking much of the satisfaction out of nursing. Since the mid-1980s in the UK there has been an alarming drop in the number of nurses qualifying. In 1997/98 only 9000 nurses will qualify compared to 14,000 in 1995/96 and 37,000 in 1983 (Hancock 1996). In the future if nurse–patient ratios are maintained in hospice units, nurse satisfaction and appreciation of the work they do may well attract staff.

Flexibility

Hospice care has been built on a patient/family focused system of care which differs from the more rigid systems of nursing tasks, and medical ward rounds of the acute hospital setting of the mid-1960s. The flexibility necessary for instituting this focus has been a hallmark of the hospice movement. However, with the development of hospices there is sadly the risk of creating new, but equally rigid systems. With the emergence of palliative care in other settings and services 'growing up' in nearby health authorities, hospice units need to be open to new ideas.

> Like all good movements the impact of the hospice movement does not depend on bricks and mortar but on the interest its ideas generate and the changes in practical care which these have brought about.
>
> (Young 1981: 2)

Twinning of hospice units in other countries

Twinning of hospices has become an interesting concept set up by the British Association of Hospices Abroad in 1994. In many ways the twinning of hospices sounds rather an inept idea, more usually associated with local community groups than a medical specialty. There is no doubt, however, that this identification of practice in a different country can be mutually enhancing. Countries with well-established hospice programmes have much to relearn about the enthusiasm and commitment of people fired for the first time with a vision for the dying. Not only is it important to promote good practice, teaching and research in countries of the developing hospice world but also exchanges of personnel can enhance both places of work.

Conclusion

In this chapter certain patterns emerge as a global view of hospice care has been captured. In countries where hospice/palliative care is well established there is a need for regional networking. Palliative care is still a reasonably new specialty and we need to collaborate and not duplicate local initiatives. The organization of regional committees in education, research and policy making (O'Donnell 1992; A. Daley, personal communication, 1995) could help prevent repetition and help to strengthen the voice of palliative care at a regional level. It is important for these regional committees to be representative of all the different hospice/palliative care services whether funded independently, for non-profit making, NHS or private plan as well as all the different specialist disciplines.

In countries where hospice/palliative care services are emerging, then there is a responsibility to nurture and to advise. The twinning of hospice units and teams in different and developing countries enables a sharing of ideas, knowledge and experience. The WHO has had a great deal of influence on the development of the global networking in palliative care (Stjernsward *et al.* 1996; see also Stjernsward, Chapter 13 in this volume). People have been introduced and encouraged to work together on projects to help those countries where people are struggling with the day to day problems of poor health and poverty on top of a terminal illness.

We are at a difficult time of economic 'belt tightening' just when hospice/palliative care appears to be at an exciting stage of development, both clinically and educationally. It is important not to be distracted from the ultimate goal, of palliative care for all, but to work steadily and wisely forward. In many instances it will be necessary to stop and take stock, to wait and collaborate with colleagues in the differing disciplines and services; at other times it will need a boldness to confront the obstacles that persist with gentle firmness in the knowledge that our work is to better influence the care for dying people and their families.

References

Albrecht, E. (1990) Palliative care in West Germany. *Palliative Medicine*, 4(4): 321–5.

Ashby, M. and Wakefield, M. (1993) Attitudes to some aspects of death and dying, living wills and substituted health care decision-making in South Australia: public opinion survey for a parliamentary select committee. *Palliative Medicine*, 7(4): 273–82.

Biswas, B. (1993) The medicalization of dying, in D. Clark (ed.) *The Future for Palliative Care*. Buckingham: Open University Press.

Bruera, E. (1992) Palliative care programme in Latin America. *Palliative Medicine*, 6(3): 182–4.

Clark, D. (1993) Wither the hospices?, in D. Clark (ed.) *The Future for Palliative Care*. Buckingham: Open University Press.

Clark, D. (1994) At the crossroads: which direction for the hospices? (editorial). *Palliative Medicine*, 8(1): 1–3.

Dale, M. (1995) The Respite Care Team. *Hospice Bulletin*, 2(1). Issued by the Hospice Information Service, St Christopher's Hospice, Lawrie Park Road, London SE26 6DZ.

Eve, A. and Smith, A.E. (1996) Survey of hospice and palliative care inpatient units in the UK and Ireland. *Palliative Medicine*, 10(1): 13–21.

Fisher, R. and McDaid, P. (1996) *Palliative Day Care*. London: Edward Arnold.

Gibson, A. (1995) Creativity in hospice: a celebration of achievement. *Occupational Therapy News*, June.

Gómez-Batiste, X. (1994) Catalonia's five-year plan: preliminary results. *European Journal of Palliative Care*, 1(2): 98–101.

Goh, C.R. (1994) The Hospice Way (keynote address). *Proceedings of National Hospice Conference, Penang, 5 Nov 1993*. Penang: National Cancer Society of Malaysia.

Greer, D., Mor, V., Morris, J. *et al.* (1986) An alternative in terminal care: results of the national hospice study. *Journal of Chronic Disease*, 39(1): 9–26.

Hancock, C. (1996) News, *Nursing Standard*, 10(31): 5.

van Heerden, J.A. (1981) Africa, in C. Saunders, D.H. Summers and N. Teller (eds) *Hospice: The Living Idea*. London: Edward Arnold.

Hockley, J. (1996) The development of a palliative care team at the Western General Hospital, Edinburgh. *Supportive Care in Cancer*, 4(2): 77–81.

Hockley, J. and Mowatt, M. (1996) Rehabilitation, in R. Fisher and P. McDaid (eds) *Palliative Day Care*. London: Edward Arnold.

Honeybun, J., Johnston, M. and Tookman, A. (1992) The impact of a death on fellow hospice patients. *British Journal of Medical Psychology*, 65: 67–72.

Hospice Information Service (1996) *Information on children's hospices in the UK*. Obtainable from Study Centre, St Christopher's Hospice, Lawrie Park Road, London SE26 6DZ.

Jackson, A. (1993) Overview of spread of palliation: starting a new service outside Europe and North America, in C. Saunders and N. Sykes (eds) *The Management of Terminal Malignant Disease*. London: Edward Arnold.

Johnson, I.S., Cockburn, M. and Pegler, J. (1988) The Marie Curie/St Luke's Relative Support Scheme: a home care service for relatives of the terminally ill. *Journal of Advanced Nursing*, 13: 565–70.

Kerr, D. (1993) Terminal care in China. *American Journal of Hospice and Palliative Care*, July/August: 18–26.

Kirkham, S. and Davies, M. (1992) Bed occupancy, patient throughput and size of independent hospice units in the UK. *Palliative Medicine*, 6(1): 47–53.

Magno, J. (1992) USA hospice care in the 1990s. *Palliative Medicine*, 6(2): 158–65.

Mount, B.M. (1973/4) Death: a part of life. *Crux*, ii(3): 7.

National Hospice Organization (1990) Census: Statistical Snapshot 1989, *Hospice News*. Arlington, VA: National Hospice Organization.

O'Donnell, N. (1992) A regional approach to palliative care services. *Journal of Palliative Care*, 8(1): 43–6.

Regnard, C. (1989) Acute versus chronic palliative care? (editorial). *Palliative Medicine*, 3(2).

Saunders, C. (1984) *The Management of Terminal Illness*. London: Edward Arnold.

Schjolberg, T. (1995) Development of palliative care in Norway: an overview. *International Journal of Palliative Nursing*, 1(1): 53–6.

Scott, J.F. (1981) Canada: hospice care in Canada, in C. Saunders, D.H. Summers and N. Teller (eds) *Hospice: The Living Idea*. London: Edward Arnold.

Scott, J.F. (1992) Palliative Care 2000: what's stopping us? *Journal of Palliative Care*, 8(1): 5–8.

SMAC/SNMAC (Standing Medical Advisory Committee and Standing Nursing and Midwifery Advisory Committee) (1992) *The Principles and Provision of Palliative Care*. London: HMSO.

Stjernsward, J., Colleau, S.M. and Ventafridda, V. (1996) The World Health Organisation cancer pain and palliative care program: past, present and future, *Journal of Pain and Symptom Management*, August, 12(2): 65–72.

Stone, C. and Blade, S. (1994) *Respite Care Team 'Setting Up' Pack.* Available from The Ellenor Foundation, Livingstone Community Hospital, Dartford, Kent DA1 1SA.

Suzuki, S., Kirschling, J.M. and Inoue, I. (1993) Hospice care in Japan. *American Journal of Hospice and Palliative Care,* July/August: 35–40.

Thomas, M., Mathai, D., Cherian, A.M. *et al.* (1995) Promoting rational drug use in India. *World Health Forum,* 16: 33–5.

Toscani, F. and Mancini, C. (1989) Inadequacies of care in far advanced cancer patients: a comparison between home and hospital in Italy. *Palliative Medicine,* 4(1): 31–6.

Vachon, M. (1995) Staff stress in hospice/palliative care: a review. *Palliative Medicine,* 9(2): 91–113.

Wales, J., Kane, R., Robbins, S. *et al.* (1983) UCLA Hospice Evaluation Study. *Medical Care,* 21(7): 734–44.

Worswick, J. (1994) Helen House: a model of children's hospice care. *European Journal of Palliative Care,* 2(1): 17–20.

Young, G. (1981) quoted in Preface, in C. Saunders, D.H. Summers and N. Teller (eds) *Hospice: The Living Idea.* London: Edward Arnold.

Zylicz, Z. (1993) Hospice in Holland: the story behind the blank spot. *American Journal of Hospice and Palliative Care,* July/August: 30–4.

Terminal care in South Australia: historical aspects and equity issues

ROGER W. HUNT AND IAN MADDOCKS

Palliative care has become established as a medical and nursing specialty within many countries, notably in the English-speaking communities of the British Isles, North America and Australia, but increasingly in Europe and the wealthier cities of Asia. A palliative care programme has commonly comprised one or more of these components:

- a dedicated in-patient care facility, a 'hospice';
- a consulting service in a hospital;
- a home care service.

In Australia the availability of these three components within the one integrated programme of care has been generally accepted as an ideal to be effected wherever practicable, with the one multidisciplinary team having access to and opportunity for clinical oversight of patients with terminal illness wherever they are receiving care (Maddocks 1990).

As a new discipline, palliative care was required to jostle for recognition within the competing demands for public funding, inpatient beds, community resources and teaching time within the public and academic institutions of medicine. But its ethos of compassionate and effective care offered during the sad and stressful time of terminal illness captured the public imagination in many centres, and encouraged not only generous community fund-raising outside of official or commercial initiatives, but also the ready recruitment of many volunteers ready to contribute a wide range of professional and personal skills. The evangel of hospice, proclaimed with eloquence by charismatic individuals demonstrating a persistent and passionate advocacy for the dying, triggered a paradigm shift in interest and perception sufficiently persuasive to warrant the name 'Hospice Movement'.

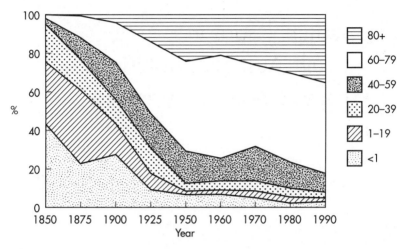

Figure 6.1 Proportion of deaths in each age-group, South Australia, 1850 to 1990

Quite rapidly many of the individual projects begun in this wave of enthusiasm consolidated, and won a recognized place within established medicine. The result has been an increasing acceptance of the palliative care 'specialist' within both medicine and nursing, the establishment of recognized paid positions within hospital work forces, and increasing, if often reluctant, government support for the maintenance of dedicated inpatient facilities and multidisciplinary outreach teams.

Inevitably, these developments have been patchy and often responsive to local demand rather than being planned as components of a comprehensive regional health care plan. Palliative care is therefore faced with major questions concerning its clinical and geographical fields of operation. Is this a service with a broad responsibility for care of dying people, or is it to be limited – whether on the basis of geography, site of care, diagnosis, age, ability to pay or clinical need?

This chapter seeks to explore this basic question by considering the development of palliative care in South Australia. South Australia centres on Adelaide, a city with just over 1 million people, but has also a vast country region, sparsely settled, with a population of 400,000.

The historical context

Age at death and cause of death

In the early decades after its first settlement by British colonists in 1836, death in South Australia affected primarily infants and young children. In 1850, three in every four deaths occurred in persons younger than 20 years (Figure 6.1). The proportion of deaths in persons over 60 years progressively

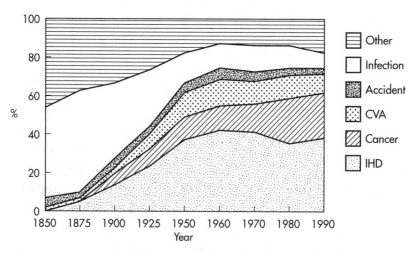

Figure 6.2   Cause of death by year, South Australia, 1850–1990

increased, and by 1990, 92 per cent of deaths were of persons older than 40 years (Hunt 1996).

A shift in the cause of death accompanied the change in age at death (Figure 6.2). Improved living conditions, especially improved nutrition and hygiene, and developments in bioscience and medicine, notably immunization programmes, aseptic procedures and antibiotics, led to a progressive reduction in mortality from infectious diseases like infant gastroenteritis, influenza, poliomyelitis, diphtheria, rheumatic fever and tuberculosis. Most people now die at an old age from a degenerative disease like cancer, ischaemic heart disease (IHD) or cerebro-vascular accident (CVA) (Hunt 1996).

During the last third of the twentieth century, mortality from ischaemic heart disease and cerebro-vascular accidents has declined, and cancer has become the leading cause, now accounting for about 26 per cent of all deaths in Australia.

Site of death

The proportion of deaths at home in South Australia decreased steadily from 92 per cent in 1875 to 21 per cent in 1990, and there was a corresponding increase in institutional deaths (Figure 6.3). Hospital and nursing home beds increased in number, sickness or extreme frailty more often led to institutional admission and, for terminal illness, continued through to death (Hunt 1996).

In common with experience in other western countries, however, the terminal phase of illness was not being managed well. When, for example, in a case of advanced cancer, the treatments available came to be recognized as futile, there was a risk of clinical negativism ('there is nothing

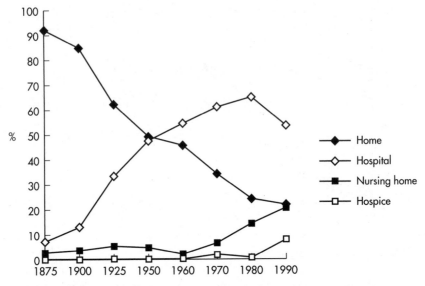

Figure 6.3 Proportion of deaths at each place by year, South Australia, 1875 to 1990

more we can do'), and the probability of isolation from simple comforts and familiar faces in the sterile gloom of a hospital side-room. Hospital terminal care was often inappropriate, depersonalized, and costly. Against this background, the concept of hospice care found strong support in South Australia.

Hospice development in Australia

Australia's hospice initiatives followed the examples set in the UK and North America. 'Forerunner' hospices, established by religious organizations, had long been offering nursing care for dying persons (but had little medical supervision compared to the modern 'hospice'). In the 1980s there was a rapid growth of new services throughout Australia, inspired by initiatives like St Christopher's Hospice in London, and the outreach programmes served by Britain's Macmillian nurses (Harris and Findlay-Jones 1987). Recognition that existing attitudes and practices failed to meet the needs of dying persons grew rapidly. The hospice concept offered a tangible new direction, a specific alternative to conventional hospital care of dying patients.

Associations formed in all states of Australia to promote hospice care and to lobby government for funds. In the 1988–9 federal budget, funds were allocated specifically for palliative care, primarily because it was hoped that better alternative arrangements for the care of dying persons would reduce the burden of care in hospitals and allow reduction in hospital expenditure.

The suggestion that palliative care services would reduce the number of hospital bed days occupied by terminally ill patients is also found in budget statements for subsequent years. The efficient use of hospitals, rather than a recognition of the real needs of dying patients and their families, appeared to be the prime motivation for funding palliative care.

Nevertheless, governments and their instrumentalities have recognized gradually the value assigned to hospice and palliative care services by the Australian public. The ways in which this recognition by government has been manifested vary. Dedicated funds for palliative care have continued to be distributed to the states by the national (Commonwealth) government. The South Australian Health Commission (1992) published a hospice care policy which states:

> The Government is responsible for ensuring the provision of comprehensive hospice/palliative care services to all South Australians. This can be achieved through the direct provision of services or in co-operation with other established health care providers.
> (South Australian Health Commission 1992: 2)

Acceptance by government of such responsibility was driven by a growing confidence and cooperation among non-government bodies interested in palliative care. In 1989, the South Australian government had established a Hospice Care Coordinating Committee, comprised of representatives of bodies delivering palliative care services. The committee met regularly with government representatives to review needs, and to suggest ways of achieving equitable and efficient services for the whole state.

The first academic chair in palliative care was established at Flinders University of South Australia in 1988, and quickly established postgraduate awards in palliative care, available also by distance study. The example was apparently persuasive, and by 1996 there were four Australian chairs in palliative care. In most Australian universities, palliative care topics now appear in undergraduate and postgraduate curricula.

The first national conferences on hospice and palliative care was held in Adelaide in 1990. The national body formed on that occasion, the Australian Association for Hospice and Palliative Care (AAHPC, a federation of state associations), quickly became a focus for dialogue with government, and a powerful advocate for changes which would improve services for terminally ill persons. The association publishes a National Directory of Hospice Services in Australia which listed 122 hospice and palliative care services in 1990; 166 in 1995.

The Australian and New Zealand Society of Palliative Medicine (ANZSPM) was established in 1993 and by 1996 included over 160 medical graduate members. In 1995, the society initiated dialogue with Royal

Australasian College of Physicians which aimed to lead to the formation of a Faculty of Palliative Medicine within the college, an opportunity for practitioners from diverse backgrounds, such as family medicine, psychiatry, oncology or anaesthesia, to obtain appropriate preparation and achieve specialist recognition in palliative care.

The impact of palliative care services

In spite of the obvious popularity and acceptance of palliative care services, few systematic data about their impact are available. Early evaluations of services have been largely descriptive (Bird *et al.* 1990).

The AAHPC, with government support, in 1996 began to formulate accreditation standards for the wide range of rural and metropolitan services. Work is also being undertaken to standardize data collection, and provide consistent reports of clinical activity across the nation, while the first results of innovative case-mix and costing studies were becoming available in 1996.

There have also been legislative changes to support palliative care practice, including the South Australian Natural Death Act 1983 and the Victorian Medical Treatment Act 1988. The Consent to Medical Treatment and Palliative Care Act 1995, believed to be the first parliamentary legislation to include the words 'palliative care' in its title, places emphasis on the wishes of terminally ill patients, whether expressed directly or, if the patient is incompetent, via an advance directive or a medical agent. This Act also provides civil and criminal protection for clinicians who properly administer palliative treatment with the intention to relieve pain and distress, even if death is hastened. Moves to legalize voluntary euthanasia received support from the Northern Territory's Rights of the Terminally Ill Act, proclaimed in 1996. Although strongly opposed by both the AAHPC and the ANZSPM such an initiative possibly draws on the philosophy espoused by palliative care, which emphasizes patient autonomy and quality of life in the terminal phase (Hunt 1994).

Although there is little evidence that palliative care services in Australia have increased the proportion of individuals who die at home, they may increase the proportion of the terminal phase which is managed in the home. The transfer of terminally ill patients between sites is indicated by a sample of cancer patients who were tracked over their final weeks of life. Up until the final three weeks of life 50 per cent or more of patients were at home (Figure 6.4). As functional status declined and death approached, the proportion who remained at home decreased steadily and in-patient care in a hospital or hospice unit became more likely (Hunt 1996).

The major initial effect of hospice development in South Australia has been the displacement of terminally ill cancer patients from hospitals to

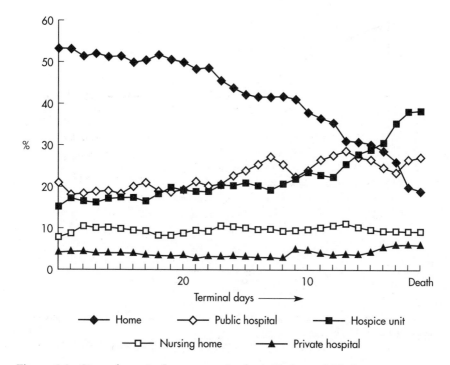

Figure 6.4 Sites of terminal care over the final 30 days of life for 171 Southern Community Hospice Programme cancer patients who died between January and April 1989

designated hospice facilities (Figure 6.5). Between 1981 and 1986, a time of expansion of hospice services, the proportion of deaths occurring in hospitals decreased markedly for cancer patients, and deaths in hospice facilities increased, while for non-cancer cases there was no change in place of death (Hunt *et al.* 1989). Between 1990 and 1993, a period during which there was less increase in the number of hospice beds, the proportion of cancer deaths in public hospitals remained relatively stable. The proportion of the state's terminally ill cancer population involved with hospice services was 56 per cent in 1990 and 63 per cent in 1993.

Equity issues in palliative care

Cancer and other diagnoses

About 90 per cent of hospice patients in South Australia have cancer, and only 10 per cent have an array of non-cancer diagnoses, including motor neurone disease, AIDS, and end-stage organ failure of various kinds (Hunt

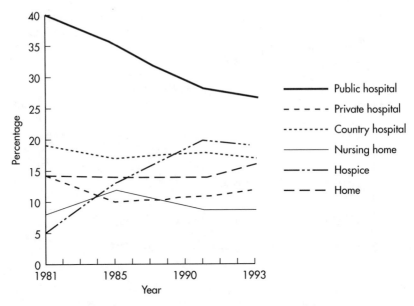

Figure 6.5   Places of death of South Australians dying from cancer in 1981, 1985, 1990 and 1993
Sources: Roder *et al.* 1987; Hunt *et al.* 1993; Hunt and McCaul 1996.

and McCaul 1996). This figure applies to most hospice services, and is related to the nature of malignancy and to cultural perceptions about it. Several writers, including Sontag (1991), have commented on the pervasive fear of cancer in modern society.

The trajectory of decline in cancer is more predictable and progressive than for many other diseases, and its discomforts – pain, nausea, constipation, delirium, etc. – are confined to a relatively short terminal phase, so that intensive efforts to relieve distress and provide intimate family support are not demanded indefinitely. Cancer patients, particularly the young or middle-aged, exercise a special appeal, their anticipated and relatively predictable decline seems unfair, tragic and deserving of the best care. Hospice services are seen to address these problems effectively.

It has become possible to state 'You are lucky if you have cancer', since that diagnosis authorizes entry to a network of informed concern and comprehensive skill which can sustain patient and family throughout the course of the final illness and into the time of bereavement. But a slow and uneven decline from emphysema, cerebral or peripheral vascular disease, chronic renal failure or cardiac failure, advanced arthritis or dementia offers little hope of winning admission to a hospice programme. In a current study of palliative care in nursing homes, staff in the nursing homes have been found to class as 'palliative' many patients who do not have cancer,

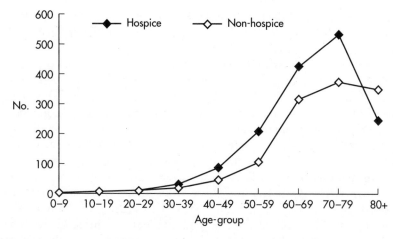

Figure 6.6   Hospice service involvement with cancer patients occurred more often than not in all but the oldest age-group, South Australia, 1990

and they advocate for them levels of nursing time and skilled support similar to what is allowed for cancer patients in a hospice.

Age

People 80 years or older with cancer were half as likely as those younger to be involved with a hospice service (Figure 6.6). Perhaps elderly patients have less need for specialized care, since older people seem generally less troubled by a cancer diagnosis than younger people (Feifel and Branscomb 1973; Funch and Marshall 1983; Hunt et al. 1990a). Alternatively, it may be that elderly cancer patients unfairly miss out on the benefits of hospice involvement. This raises questions about the extent to which age should be used as a criterion for determining the type of care a patient receives (Hunt 1993; Hunt and Maddocks 1994). Hospice philosophy suggests that services should be determined on the basis of need, and remain flexible, rather than be constrained by policies based on the criterion of age.

Opportunity to die at home

Patients of hospice services, particularly the home-based services, generally spend more time at home than non-hospice patients. In a Western Australian study, for example, patients of a home care hospice service had significantly fewer days of institutional care in the last 90 days of life than matched controls (MacAdam et al. 1985). Despite the high coverage of the population of cancer patients by hospice services in South Australia, the overall proportion of deaths at home (about 14 per cent) is quite low. A Victorian study showed that 19 per cent of cancer deaths occurred at home in 1988 (Clifford *et al.* 1991).

A survey of 462 South Australians showed that almost 60 per cent of South Australians would prefer to die in their homes if they were terminally ill (Ashby and Wakefield 1993). Some of the discrepancy between the preferred (60 per cent) and actual (14 per cent) proportion of home deaths may be due to the younger age of the survey sample and the tendency for younger persons to state a preference for home care. Also, a person's preference may change when actually trying to undertake terminal care at home.

Death at home is more likely for younger than older cancer patients, those with partners, males, and those from higher socio-economic areas (Clifford *et al.* 1991; Hunt *et al.* 1993). This reflects the availability of home support for terminal care. Younger patients are more likely to have an able home carer, whereas older patients are more likely to be widowed or have a frail home carer (Seale 1991). Females may be more prepared and able to take on the role of home carer for their partner than are males (Roder *et al.* 1987). Patients from higher socio-economic groups are more likely to have private resources which can be used to maintain them in the home setting. It is possible that the provision of home support services at a reduced cost to clients, or without direct charge, would increase the overall proportion of time spent at home during the terminal phase and enable a more even distribution of home terminal care across the community.

Nursing home terminal care

The proportion of all South Australian deaths in nursing homes increased from 1 per cent in 1960 to 20 per cent in 1990 (Figure 6.3). Elderly people, especially those without partners, are more likely to die in nursing homes (Roder *et al.* 1987; Clifford *et al.* 1991). Nearly three-quarters of nursing home residents are female, and half of these are in the 80–89 age-group.

The number of nursing home beds has failed to keep pace with the growing population of elderly persons. This has resulted in more stringent criteria for nursing home admission, a more dependent resident population, and an increased turnover of admissions and deaths. The pressure to transfer dying patients from hospitals to nursing homes is likely to increase with the implementation of case-mix funding for hospital care, and the trend for more nursing home deaths seems set to continue into the future (Hunt and Maddocks 1994). Nursing homes are assuming a slow-stream hospice role, particularly for people dying from non-cancer causes.

The hospice standard for nursing staff which has become generally accepted in Australia is 45.5 hours per patient per week. Nursing home care in Australia is funded through a Resident Classification Instrument, which assigns between 9 and 27 nursing hours per week to each resident on the basis of a formula which focuses on mobility and behaviour needs. It makes little allowance for the skilled nursing response to physical and emotional need which terminal cancer care demands. Three-quarters (74 per cent) of nursing home directors stated that extra nursing hours were necessary to provide satisfactory terminal care for their residents (Hunt and Bond 1990).

Referrals to hospice agencies for cancer patients resident in nursing homes increased from 20 per cent in 1990 to 45 per cent in 1993, suggesting a greater awareness in nursing homes of the value of skilled palliative care support. The provision of relevant education for general practitioners and nursing home staff, more regular specialist hospice consultations and additional specific funding for those patients whose needs are not satisfactorily met by existing arrangements needs to be advocated (Hunt et al. 1990a).

Country patients

Health service provision is difficult in the vast, sparsely populated areas of outback Australia. Although not all country regions can be served by a designated hospice programme, South Australia has funded 12 country services, which vary from no more than a part-time nurse up to a multidisciplinary team with medical, nursing, social work and volunteer components. Travel times are sometimes long, and major use is made of the telephone with an emphasis on education and support of the caring family. There is a lower proportion of home deaths in country regions, and a lesser involvement of country residents with hospice services (Roder et al. 1987; Hunt and McCaul 1996). This may reflect the more flexible use of small country hospitals, which are less alienating for patients than are large city hospitals. The patient in a country hospital knows it well, and caring staff are often friends or relatives. It can be difficult for nursing staff in such facilities to develop confidence in the skills of pain management and symptom control, because the number of terminal patients they see is small, and the needs of their patients range from neonatal care through road trauma to geriatrics.

A population with special needs is the aboriginal population. The significance of death within aboriginal communities and the practices and rituals which accompany terminal illness are not well understood by white care providers. Taboos reflecting differences in moiety or gender may inhibit the care which can be offered. Higher mortality in younger age groups and a high prevalence of diabetes, renal disease and hypertension limits the numbers of aboriginal persons who die of cancer.

Several initiatives have sought to improve palliative care for rural populations. Video-conferencing with groups of country nurses discussing cases and common problems with city experts has been appreciated. In 1996 a major allocation of Commonwealth funding for new initiatives in palliative care was directed at educational activities for rural medical and nursing practitioners. Close links with urban palliative care services are encouraged so that relevant advice can be readily offered to patients and their carers in country regions.

Types of cancer

Patients with a haematological malignancy are less likely than patients with other malignancies to receive hospice care, and more likely to die in a major hospital (Roder et al. 1987; Clifford et al. 1991; Hunt et al. 1991; Maddocks 1994; Hunt and McCaul 1996). Patients with haematological malignancy develop close relationships with the oncology units of the major hospitals through frequent contact for chemotherapy, often continuing into the last month of life (Malden et al. 1984), and the complications of infection and haemorrhage, that would tend to precipitate readmission to the acute care hospital, are frequently the cause of death.

Cancer patients with a relatively short survival time from diagnosis to death are more likely than other patients to die in a major public hospital, or in a hospice (Hunt and McCaul 1996). Those with a longer survival time are more likely to be referred to a nursing home. Commonly a patient is admitted to a hospice unit whose condition subsequently stabilizes with a revision of the initially short prognosis. This is particularly likely with non-cancer diagnoses, but may also occur with cancer. Transfer of a patient from the well-staffed hospice to the frugally funded nursing home causes considerable distress to families and discomfort for hospice staff, yet the demand on hospice beds requires that a patient with major symptoms and rapid deterioration be given priority.

Affluence and insurance status

The ability of palliative care programmes in Australia to offer inpatient care in publicly funded beds varies widely. In South Australia, of five hospice units, three are located within public hospitals, and offer free care. One is in a private hospital and one in a nursing home complex; both receive substantial block grants from the state to provide for the admission of non-insured patients. The Department of Veteran Affairs provides a daily grant to Daw House Hospice of A$440 to cover care for terminally ill veterans. This amount is higher than the estimated daily cost of an acute medical bed, and was calculated on the basis of the actual care offered in the hospice. As case-mix funding becomes a major determinant of the care which either public or private hospitals will offer, an increasing discrepancy emerges between the expressed aim of palliative care to meet patient need and the requirement that funds available for any patient have a defined cap.

In this climate, there is advantage in being enrolled in a private hospital insurance scheme, but even that is closely monitored and may limit a dying patient to no more than 35 days' inpatient care. Private insurance will sometimes pay for home nursing, usually for a limited number of hours per day, though at least one insurer in South Australia is prepared to offer a lump sum which may be expended over longer or even continuous shifts. Non-insured patients can usually rely upon district nursing support, but this allows only visits of brief duration (up to four or more per day, if necessary), not prolonged shifts. Overnight nurse support for two or three nights can be funded through limited charitable resources offered by the Anti-Cancer Foundation.

Conclusion

Within the relatively stable community of South Australia, hospice and palliative care has been promoted effectively and has developed strongly. Its impact can be appreciated in the number and timing of referrals to hospice services, changes in the sites where death occurs, and the acceptance of palliative care services as a government responsibility. Although a high level of coverage of the population of terminally ill cancer patients by palliative care services has been achieved in South Australia, there remain some issues of inequity. Patients dying from diseases other than solid cancer, those who die in rural areas or in nursing homes, and those who do not have private cover may all have less access to the levels of support seen as appropriate for patients referred for palliative care. Governments which responded to the persuasive advocacy of the hospice movement in its early years will not be expected to extend hospice and palliative care services readily, since the cost of those services is considerable and is increasingly visible. The benefit of palliative care to patients who do not now receive it will need to be argued on the basis of sound research and accurate estimates of cost. Requirements for reporting in South Australia should provide an accurate and continuing monitoring of demand and services for terminal care, and will inform the planning of the appropriate balance of services to meet the needs of persons dying in the next decades.

References

Ashby, M. and Wakefield, M. (1993) Attitudes to some aspects of death and dying, living wills and substituted health care decision-making in South Australia: public opinion survey for a parliamentary select committee. *Palliative Medicine*, 7: 273–82.

Bird, B., Humphries, S. and Howe, A. (1990) Hospice care in Victoria: a profile of programs and patients in 1988–89. A report from the Aged Care Research Group, La Trobe University, to the Health Department of Victoria, 1990.

Clifford, C.A., Jolley, D.J. and Giles, G.G. (1991) Where people die in Victoria. *Medical Journal of Australia*, 155: 446–52.

Feifel, H. and Branscomb, A. (1973) Who's afraid of death? *Journal of Abnormal Psychology*, 81: 282–8.

Funch, D.P. and Marshall, J. (1983) The role of stress, social support and age in survival from breast cancer. *Journal of Psychosomatic Research*, 27: 77–83.

Harris, R. and Findlay-Jones, L. (1987) Terminal care in Australia. *The Hospice Journal*, 3: 77–90.

Hunt, R.W. (1993) A critique of using age to ration health care. *Journal of Medical Ethics*, 19: 19–23.

Hunt, R.W. (1994) Palliative care: the rhetoric-reality gap, in H. Kuhse (ed.) *Willing to Listen – Wanting to Die*, Harmondsworth: Penguin.

Hunt, R.W. (1996) 'The origins and impact of hospice care: investigations in South Australia', *thesis in preparation*.

Hunt, R. and Bond, M. (1990) Terminal care in nursing homes: a survey of South Australian directors of nursing. *Geriaction*, 9(1): 7–8.

Hunt, R. and McCaul, K. (1996) A population-based study of the coverage of cancer patients by hospice services. *Palliative Medicine*, 10: 5–12.

Hunt, R.W. and Maddocks, I. (1994) Review of nursing home terminal care. *Geriaction*, 13(1): 23–5.

Hunt, R., Roder, D. and McHarper, T. (1989) The impact of hospice services on the place of death in South Australia. *Cancer Forum*, 13: 110–13.

Hunt, R.W., Bond, M. and Pater, G. (1990a) Psychological responses to cancer: a case for cancer support groups. *Community Health Studies*, 14(1): 35–8.

Hunt, R., Radford, A., Maddocks, I., Dunsmore, E. and Badcock, K. (1990b) The community care of terminally ill patients. *Australian Family Physician*, 19(12): 1835–41.

Hunt, R.W., Bond, M.J., Groth, R.K. and King, P.M. (1991) Place of death in South Australia: patterns from 1910 to 1987. *Medical Journal of Australia*, 155: 549–53.

Hunt, R.W., Bonett, A. and Roder, D. (1993) Trends in the terminal care of cancer patients – South Australia, 1981–1990. *Australian and New Zealand Journal of Medicine*, 23: 245–51.

MacAdam, D., Boldy, D. and Gray, D. (1985) A comparative cost analysis of terminal cancer care: a study of expenditure on health care during the last 90 days of life under a home based hospice service and in hospital. *Cancer Foundation of Western Australia*.

Maddocks, I. (1990) Changing concepts in palliative care. *Medical Journal of Australia*, 152: 535–9.

Maddocks, I. (1994) Quality of life issues in patients dying from haematological diseases, *Annals Academy of Medicine, Singapore*, 23: 244–7.

Malden, L., Sutherland, C., Tattersall, M. *et al.* (1984) Dying of cancer: factors influencing the place of death of patients. *Medical Journal of Australia*, 141: 147–50.

Roder, D., Bonett, A., Hunt, R. and Beare, M. (1987) Where patients with cancer die in South Australia. *Medical Journal of Australia*, 147: 11–13.

Seale, C. (1991) Death from cancer and death from other causes: the relevance of the hospice approach. *Palliative Medicine*, 5(1): 12–19.

Sontag, S. (1991) *Illness as Metaphor*. Harmondsworth: Penguin.

South Australian Health Commission (1990) *Hospice Policy Statement*, mimeo.

7 Palliative care in India

GILLY BURN

> If you visit a country for a week you become an expert and can write a book. If you stay for a year you might write a paper, and if you stay longer you do not know enough to write anything.
>
> (Olweny 1994: 56)

In order to appreciate the enormous task facing pioneers of palliative care in the poorest countries of the world, it is important that we identify several challenges which face not only those attempting to deliver the service, but also those needing it. In this chapter attention will focus on India, a country which accounts for one-sixth of the world's population. The issues found in India may resemble obstacles and difficulties present in other countries which are 'poor' and 'developing' in terms of financial or technical resources. These same countries often have a rich potential in terms of spiritual and cultural resources, and this too has a bearing on their capacity to provide care for sick and dying people.

The World Health Organization (WHO) estimates that over 80 per cent of cancer patients in developing countries present in the advanced stage of disease and that by 2015 there will be 10 million new cancer patients per year in countries of the developing world. Escalating tobacco consumption, AIDS and an increasingly elderly population will all exacerbate the problem (Stjernsward 1993). The relevance of palliative care in this context is therefore indisputable. Despite the fact that even today there are millions suffering unrelieved pain, the vast majority are denied appropriate treatment. The reasons for this are both simple and yet paradoxically complex (Stjernsward 1993; see also Stjernsward, Chapter 13 in this volume). When examining the reasons why palliative care is not well established in these countries, even though there is significant research evidence

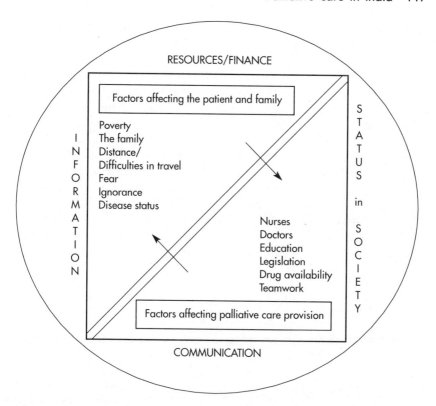

Figure 7.1 The interrelationship of issues affecting patients and families and the provision of palliative care acknowledging wider social factors

to support the need for it, it is necessary to identify issues from both the professional and patient/family perspective (see Figure 7.1). The problems here are very often interrelated. For example, 'lack of resources' may mean that a hospital is under-resourced to provide adequate treatment, or it could relate to the patient who cannot afford to pay for the treatment needed.

Patient/family related issues

Poverty, fear, ignorance of the disease process, lack of information regarding treatment options, communication difficulties and long distances to travel to and from the hospital all mitigate against very sick and terminally ill people having access to palliative care.

Poverty

India has among its 900 million population more poor people than anywhere else in the world. About 80 per cent of India's population live in rural areas with minimal health care facilities (Tulley 1992). Although there is a vast community health network, most of the efforts are directed towards preventative care, hygiene, child and maternal welfare, family planning, inoculation programmes, public health and primary prevention. Cancer detection camps are offered in the community, but these do not include palliative care. Unfortunately such camps are not always able to offer effective therapy, even when a curable cancer is detected.

In India, there is no social security system. No work means no money, and therefore no money to purchase treatment or to provide food for the family. Invariably, the main wage earner will continue working despite warning signs of disease, being unable to afford the time off to visit the doctor or pay the necessary fees (Burn 1990). Eventually, it is the severe pain or other symptoms which prevent such a person from working, and medical attention being sought. Local remedies which are easier to access not only may be inappropriate, but also may drain precious financial resources.

Travel

The problems of poverty are compounded by the fact that most centres offering cancer treatment are in the cities. This may mean travelling hundreds of miles in a hot overcrowded bus, in extreme heat, on a road rutted by heavy monsoon rains. Even major roads are reduced to dirt tracks. The problems of travelling in such conditions with, for example, multiple bone metastases and no pain relief, are beyond the imagination of people in the affluent west. On arrival from a village, patient and family are confronted by strange surroundings and a far higher cost of living. Lack of familiarity with the harsh realities of urban life, and loss of their social network also render them vulnerable to exploitation. Whole families can be seen camping outside the hospitals, complete with primus-stove, as they await admission; even then, patients are not guaranteed a bed and many sleep on the floor in overcrowded wards (Burn 1996).

Fear and lack of knowledge

The world of 'cancer' strikes terror in the hearts and minds of those who suspect they may have it, and their families. Fear of the unknown and a lack of awareness that if detected and treated early, some cancers are curable, means that many, even highly educated people, put off seeking a diagnosis in case their worst fears are confirmed. In India, as elsewhere, there is also a social stigma attached to the diagnosis of cancer and many people with the disease become social outcasts, because other family members are sometimes not able to endure the patient's symptoms and suffering. The problem will be compounded as more people are diagnosed with AIDS which is associated with other perhaps even more virulent forms of stigma and oppression.

Communication problems

India has hundreds of dialects and several official languages. Not all people speak the national language of Hindi. The educated language and the 'jargon' of the medical profession may be totally incomprehensible to the patient who not only may be unable to read or write, but also may not understand what the doctor or nurse is trying to convey. This makes the whole issue of informed consent, for example, particularly fraught and in most instances it is rarely achieved (Burn 1996). One female patient with throat cancer awoke from the operation unable to speak; she was unaware of the implications of a laryngectomy and the first she knew of what had been done to her was when she tried to ask for a glass of water and could not speak. In that particular hospital, a regional cancer centre, there was no speech therapist.

The social status of most patients in relation to doctors makes it difficult to communicate fears, needs and queries, and thereby almost impossible to understand the implications of the treatment. In most instances there are no simple explanatory leaflets – albeit useless for those who are illiterate – and no nurse to act in an advocacy role. Direct and honest communication between patient and doctor is rare. Constraints on the doctor's time make meaningful explanations difficult. In addition, the relatives often see the doctor first and ask the doctor not to tell the patient. So the 'conspiracy of silence' isolates the patient early on, denying the opportunity of attending to 'unfinished business' and creating a sense of imprisonment in a lonely world of silence and secrecy, in which all treatment choices are denied. Even if it proves possible to overcome the obstacles of communication in terms of travel and information, the person may be confronted with the news that there is no treatment available as either the relevant equipment has broken down or the drugs are not available. Recently, in one cancer hospital, equipment had not been functioning for nine months; in another hospital the equipment was so antiquated that its safety and accuracy left much to be desired.

The concept of the strong family support network in India is currently under threat. It still exists but the culture is changing – more women are now working, and more families are becoming 'nuclear'. There is a move away from the village to the cities, where work is perhaps more available. There are now reports of patients with advanced cancer being abandoned by their families. In an unpublished study of head and neck cancer patients from rural areas followed up a year after treatment, 25 per cent of patients had been abandoned by their families. There are several questions here. Is it because financial resources are so drained that the family has gone in search of work in the cities? Or is it because family members cannot cope with their own terrible suffering and feeling of impotence at the sight of someone they love in uncontrollable pain or with the smell of fungating lesions? Supportive palliative care could have enabled those families to cope and share together their burden of suffering.

Palliative care challenges from a professional perspective

There are rarely sufficient resources in any country's health care budget to meet demand. However, in India allocation of funds for cancer care is minimal and those funds are spent disproportionately on primary treatment: 90 per cent of cancer resources benefit only 10 per cent of the population, while the 80–90 per cent patients who require palliation have a mere 10 per cent of the already inadequate cancer budget (Stjernsward 1993). There are eleven regional cancer centres in India offering comprehensive facilities but it is estimated that they see less than 10 per cent of the country's cancer patients. The 'comprehensive' nature of the facilities does not often extend to comprehensive palliative care and many patients still suffer considerably, with their 'total pain' not fully addressed.

Working conditions in the overcrowded government hospitals are generally not conducive to the delivery of competent and compassionate palliative care (Burn 1990). A doctor may be expected to see 120 or more patients in an outpatient clinic and is constantly confronted with the ethical dilemma 'to treat or not to treat'? The language difficulties and the overburdened clinics may mean that a doctor has less than two or three minutes to break bad news, explain treatment options and answer patients' and families' questions. One 25-year-old man was given his diagnosis of cancer of the penis and expected to make a decision of whether to have chemotherapy or surgery during a five-minute consultation. Many patients with treatable cancer cannot afford the cure, while many of those with advanced disease are begging for anything that might relieve their suffering and prevent them from being abandoned. Lack of time or poor communication skills on the part of the doctor and the nurse means that many patients gain no real understanding of either their disease or its treatment.

There are rarely enough nurses to provide holistic care – often only a single nurse per 60 or more patients (Burn 1990). Doctors outnumber nurses 25:1. The status of the nurse varies but is mainly low and there is generally little meaningful communication between either nurse and doctor or nurse and patient. Nurses in hospitals are not generally expected to use their initiative and patient advocacy is rare. In the community, nurses have more autonomy and tend to be more highly regarded.

Education

As in many western countries, in India palliative care has not yet been included in the undergraduate curriculum of either nursing or medicine. Continuing education of staff in palliative care is still uncommon and therefore there is a lack of awareness of what palliative care encompasses. It is often confused with 'pain control', but the concept of 'total pain', which is relevant in any care setting, is rarely appreciated. In spite of the vast body of research which already exists regarding cheap and effective oral analgesia, the professional prejudice of many Indians regarding the use of opiate medication as well as ignorance and fear prevent millions of cancer patients from having their pain controlled adequately. Stjernsward has summed up this state of affairs: 'there is – even in many resource-rich countries – an inadequate application of available knowledge' (Stjernsward 1993: 805).

It is important to understand the different levels of nurse training that exist in India. The diploma nurse (three year training) remains at the bedside, but tends to be regarded by the public and professional peers as a 'second class citizen'. A random survey by the author of 50 nurses showed that less than 5 per cent of them took up nursing as a first choice of career. Reasons for not liking their job included the poor status afforded to their role. At entry, however, many diploma nurses are enthusiastic. They welcome interactive teaching, as opposed to purely didactic sessions in large classes, and their ideals are high. It is not helpful that they are frequently taught by graduate and postgraduate nurses who do not always want to be in nursing, have not had training in teaching methods, nor have access to teaching resources such as up-to-date books or journals. The hierarchical nature of both nursing and medicine means that many keen young people do not have a chance to develop their creativity for the benefit of their patients, and enthusiasm at entry to the profession may soon be dissipated, turning to disillusionment at qualification. Despite this, there are nurses and doctors who do retain their professional enthusiasm and ideals in the face of overwhelming challenges.

Legislation and morphine

Extensive legislation and the numerous bureaucratic hoops through which the medical profession has to jump in order to acquire drugs makes the use of morphine more problematic than less efficacious analgesics (Lal 1994). Many of the laws are outdated and are aimed at preventing drug addiction rather than preventing pain. In India each state has its own laws regarding morphine, including transport, export, import, prescribing, and the holding of licences which need to be obtained before the drug can be used (WHO 1993). In one instance it took four years of bureaucratic battling for a professor of radiotherapy to obtain oral morphine. Even then, he was told that the hospital had a licence to dispense only oral morphine solution, not tablets. In some states licences have to be renewed annually. Not all doctors can prescribe morphine and often only one doctor per hospital has this burden or privilege. This means that even within a hospital which *has* morphine, a patient in pain may not get pain relief if the physician does not have permission to prescribe, or is not able to refer the patient to another doctor who can.

Teamwork

In many hospitals, the concept of teamwork is not evident. Professionals work more as individuals within a group, each with their own tasks and objectives. Doctors may fear losing their patients, as they would also lose the patient's fees, and therefore there is an element of understandable competition with colleagues. Conversely, the atmosphere among nurses is more passive. Both the competition and the passivity appear to block interprofessional communication, and can affect patient care. There is also a lack of awareness regarding what other team members (e.g. occupational or physiotherapists, dieticians, chaplains, etc.) can offer to palliative care. Despite lack of financial resources, patients and their families frequently seek several opinions regarding their treatment. This is often due to lack of information regarding treatment options.

Technology and truth

Saunders has remarked that 'awareness of what quality of life means . . . demands full consideration of both suffering and the appropriateness of various possible treatments and settings in the particular circumstances' (Saunders 1993: vii). One of the problems confronting doctors is the high expectations of both professionals and the public regarding the preservation of life at all costs. Unaware of what palliative care encompasses, some doctors are prescribing a 'living death' for their patients in the mistaken belief that it is the best option (Burn 1996). Western death-denying attitudes have undoubtedly reached countries like India. Of course high technology has its place; just because a country is financially poor does not mean it should be denied advanced technology and professional updating in the latest techniques. For example, in the context of acute life-threatening crises, with appropriate treatment there is a good chance of a positive outcome.

At present, however, health care technology is used indiscriminately and patients with advanced cancer are often dying alone in intensive care units wired up to every possible machine, with no nurse in attendance. Outside the hospital, the patient's family, denied access, wait for the inevitable. Both family and patient therefore suffer the final separation, alone, at a time when they most need to be united. The relatives are left with the recurring nightmare of a loved one's traumatic, solitary death, with none of them able to complete their 'unfinished business'. Unfinished business in the Indian context can mean, for example, a father ensuring that he has found a suitable husband for an unmarried daughter or seeing a family member who lives far away before he dies. Compounding the emotional, social and spiritual suffering, the financial burden to the family can often be hundreds of dollars per day. Inappropriate use of technology, often camouflaged as 'hope', has left families bankrupt. Cows, land, jewellery, tractors, even houses are sold and money borrowed because patients have been denied a true appraisal of the situation. The ethics of informed consent are as relevant in India as anywhere else in the world (Sanwal *et al.* 1996). Feelings such as love, guilt or desperation to stop the suffering on the part of the family, and the fear of abandonment for the patient, make all of them vulnerable to grasping at any treatment, irrespective of whether or not it is medically or ethically sound. Families, carers and professionals alike should acknowledge the wisdom behind the words of Cicely Saunders: 'if he is recognised as the unique person he is, and helped to live as part of his family, and in other relationships, he can still reach out to his hopes and expectations and to what has deepest meaning for him and end his life with a sense of completion' (Saunders 1993: vii).

Professional fascination for high technology means that instead of achieving coverage through the WHO palliative care principles (see Stjernsward, Chapter 13 in this volume), precious resources may be directed to benefit a small proportion of the population of people with life-threatening illness (Burn 1996). In one centre resources were spent on sending doctors to the USA to learn about stereotactic radiotherapy and yet the same centre had no oral morphine tablets and no professional with in-depth knowledge of palliative care to treat the poor and suffering majority. Discussion with professionals caring for people with a life-threatening illness has invariably led to superficial consideration of euthanasia revealing a need for more education about the whole subject. Many doctors have thought that denying patients ventilation and other life support measures are tantamount to euthanasia, even when the disease is advanced with widespread metastases. Others think that prescribing morphine is also synonymous with 'killing the patient'. Often, this misconception is conveyed to the patients and their relatives. Education regarding both ethics and appropriate treatment is urgently needed.

Models of care to meet the challenge

When considering the obstacles that professionals and public alike have to overcome in order to deliver and obtain a humane alternative to suffering, it is encouraging that there are several visionary individuals who have taken up the challenge in India. An example of this is the work of Mother Theresa and the Missionaries of Charity in Calcutta which is a well-intentioned attempt to provide low-tech loving care to destitute dying people. The work has been criticized for not comparing favourably to western-style hospice care (Fox 1994). This fails to acknowledge the good work that is being done in Calcutta and the fact that no attempt is being made to mimic western-style hospice care.

Developing hospices in India

Dr L.J. de Souza, a compassionate and competent surgeon from a major cancer centre, built the first hospice in Bombay, India. In 1986 Shanti Avedna Ashram was opened, the building closely modelled on the design of St Christopher's Hospice, London (de Souza 1981). Since then two further 'Shanti Avedna Ashram's' have been opened in Goa and in Delhi. The hospice in Delhi opened in 1994 and is staffed by dedicated and caring missionary sisters. When the hospice was visited by the author 16 months after it opened, only three out of the 40 beds were occupied despite the fact that there was major public and professional publicity when it opened. Such a low capacity is not due to facilities being unavailable, just that they are underused. This seems extraordinary when one considers that the Ashram is built within a mile of a regional cancer centre and within half a mile of another general hospital with cancer facilities. The patients from both these hospitals would benefit greatly from admission for symptom control and psychosocial support at some point during their illness trajectory. The policy of the hospice at that time was that patients receiving 'active' treatment could not be admitted, even if these needed symptom control as well. One patient with incurable cancer was sent home from the cancer centre to die with no supportive care. She lived near the hospice and fortunately her husband found out about it by chance. The patient was admitted and enjoyed considerable benefit. All this begs certain questions. Is it because doctors are not informing their patients of available facilities? Is it due to lack of awareness or inability to collaborate with colleagues? Is it ignorance of the potential of palliative care? Does it represent 'defeat' on the part of the referring physician or surgeon or is it the stigma and fear sometimes associated with such places by an uninformed public?

Other hospices are developing in India. A community-based team in Bangalore aims to have inpatient facilities in the future. Another hospice, Jeevodaya, in Madras, opened in 1995. Already they have plenty of patients who want and need to be admitted but as yet the hospice is unable to function to its full capacity because of lack of funds. Good preparatory work in terms of working relationships has been undertaken with both professionals and public to generate support. Collaboration with medical colleagues has ensured a steady supply of oral morphine. The hospice also offers a community outreach service. Community palliative care is vital if coverage is to be achieved, especially as 80 per cent of India's population lives in rural areas.

Hospital-based palliative care

Several regional cancer centres are endeavouring to develop palliative care alongside curative therapy. However, it has been the hospital-based pain and palliative care clinic set up by Dr M.R. Rajagopal at Kozhikode that has been singled out by the WHO for its work. It is unique for a variety of reasons. Dr Rajagopal visited the UK for training in palliative care in 1993. On returning to India he converted an old anaesthetic store-room at the teaching hospital into a clinic for pain and palliative care advice. With his excellent team-building skills, Dr Rajagopal created a dedicated team, made up mostly of untrained volunteers including medical students. There is one full-time paid doctor who has taken more than a 50 per cent drop in salary in the private sector to bring him in line with government salaries. Since opening in 1994, the clinic has seen over 1,000 new patients (inpatients and outpatients). The team works on a referral basis, giving advice, not taking over other consultants' patients. Team members visit the wards daily and teach by role-modelling. Potential professional and public communication barriers are prevented by skilful interaction from team members. Colleagues, patients and families alike are empowered to deliver care. The team includes over 20 volunteers – something that is virtually unheard of in India. This innovative and far-sighted unit was declared a model for developing countries by the chief of the Cancer and Palliative Care Unit of the WHO during a visit there in 1995. Individuals thinking of setting up palliative care services in India are encouraged to visit this centre, which has introduced a culturally sensitive model of palliation.

Comparison of several initiatives around India leads one to discern features which enable effective delivery of palliative care. Inspired leadership, teamwork, empowerment of colleagues, patients and families, humility, recognition of the importance of communication skills, constant review of progress, acknowledgement of the dynamic and the diverse nature of palliative care, makes continuing education a vital component. Contrary to commonly held beliefs, buildings *per se*, big budgets, and high technology are low on the list of priorities. Stjernsward rightly observed that 'institutions, organisations and countries have no excellence in themselves . . . and therefore individuals and their initiatives remain essential' (Stjernsward 1993: 813) and this is clearly apparent in this context.

Educational challenges

Education of professionals regarding the philosophy and relevance of palliative care is vital in order to change entrenched and often erroneous misconceptions, and to encourage a change in behaviour.

Education and thus empowerment of the families is also vital. The Cancer and Palliative Care Unit of the WHO is working to develop family guidelines for delivering palliative care at home in under-resourced countries where a vast number of the population may be illiterate (J. Hockley, personal communication, 1996). Those teaching the families need appropriate information and the skills to impart it. Information needs to be provided on how to access services and what to do at 'community' level.

In order to address both professional and public educational needs, an organization, Cancer Relief India, was established by the author in 1990 with education as its main aim alongside the provision of palliative care (Webb 1993). Since then the director has been involved with major educational initiatives. Multiprofessional workshops have been held alongside clinical teaching. In the main both classroom and clinical teaching has been undertaken by a nurse/doctor team thus placing equal importance on the contribution of different professional skills and in order to act as role-models. The importance of clinical teaching cannot be overemphasized. It is not enough merely to deliver a lecture: people new to palliative care need to see it in action. Clinical work is ideally undertaken in the morning so that the afternoon teaching bears relevance to the local situation. What is relevant in the well-resourced west may have little meaning in a country where even the basic necessities of life are not available. Teaching must be culturally sensitive if it is to have any chance of being implemented.

Since 1990 the author has arranged educational opportunities in the UK for over 50 Indian health care professionals. These courses have included principles of palliative care theory, teaching communication skills, clinical attachments, and how to 'manage change on return to the workplace'. After completing one such course several of the course members have returned with renewed enthusiasm and have made a significant difference to their local situations, and have access to ongoing support. One nurse has written a booklet about palliative care for the local people in their own language, as well as giving services to develop a rural centre. A nurse/doctor team has set up a hospice and outreach programme including education of professionals. Doctors and nurses are now including palliative care in the teaching of undergraduate students. To disseminate the knowledge and skills they have learned they are setting up multiprofessional palliative care interest groups, and communication workshops on 'truth telling' and 'breaking bad news'. There is value in seeing palliative care in action in a well-developed setting, provided the experience is 'tailored' to the needs of the visitor.

Recognizing the importance of education in order to disseminate knowledge and improve care, the CIPLA Cancer and AIDS Foundation is building a Palliative Care Centre in Pune together with an education department. The intention is that the education centre will organize a variety of courses, not only clinically sensitive and appropriate to the Indian setting, but also closely integrating the theory and practice of palliative care. It is envisaged that palliative care research relevant for India will also emanate from the centre which is due to open in 1997.

Ethical challenges

Semblhi observed that 'having survived the risky passage into this world, surely a person has a right to skilled and compassionate care . . . regardless of his/her country of residence' (Semblhi 1995: 48). It is vital that palliative care is incorporated into mainstream medicine and integrated into both institutional and community care. The compassion, competence, courage and commitment of individuals who are struggling to ensure that palliative care will achieve coverage for the millions that need it, is to be respected. In order to succeed, the philosophy of teamwork and partnership must underpin all endeavours. Partnership is needed, not only with our patients, families and colleagues but also between those countries where palliative care is established and those which are struggling to develop it. However, emulating a purely western model is not the answer and may lead to disillusionment if the goals striven for are unrealistic and unattainable. Again, Stjernsward reminds us that each country must work out its own philosophy for palliative care according to its culture and resources. Palliative care, even in under-resourced countries must not be thought of as a luxury, but as a necessity. As Semblhi puts it so tellingly: 'palliative care cannot be considered a luxury when it is the only option' (1995: 49). The earlier quote from Olweny brings into stark focus the infinity of learning and the richness of what is gained by sharing the human experience. Accordingly, this chapter raises more questions than definitive answers. Those in the western world have much to learn from their eastern counterparts. The western way of life, with its nuclear families, death-denying attitudes and materialistic values has much to learn from the strength of the extended family and communities in which spiritual aspects of life are an integral part of daily living and are not merely relegated to festivals and funerals. Despite the differences in culture, creeds and castes that exist in the world, certain human needs are basic to all. To be able to live with dignity and to die where one chooses, without pain, is a fundamental human right, wherever a person is born.

References

Burn, G.L. (1990) A personal initiative to improve palliative care in India. *Palliative Medicine*, 4: 257–9.
Burn, G.L. (1994) Mother Theresa's care for the dying defended (letter). *Lancet*, 344: 1098.

Burn, G.L. (1996) From paper to practice: quality of life in a developing country: the challenges that face us, in *Annals Volume: Communication with the Cancer Patient: Information and Truth*, New York.

Fox, R. (1994) Mother Theresa's care for the dying. *Lancet*, 344: 807–8.

Jeffrey, D. (1994) Palliative care in India: an educational challenge. *Proceedings from the Royal College of Physicians (Edinburgh)*, 24: 462–5.

Lal, A. (1994) *Proceedings of 1st International Conference of the Indian Association of Palliative Care*. Varanasi: Indian Association of Palliative Care.

Mumford, J.W. and Mumford, S.P. (1988) The care of cancer patients in a rural south Indian hospital. *Palliative Medicine*, 2: 157–61.

Olweny, C.L.M. (1994) Ethics of palliative care medicine: palliative care for the richer nations only (letter). *Journal of Palliative Care*, 11(1): 56.

Sanwal, A., Kumar, S. *et al.* (1996) Informed consent in Indian patients. *Journal of the Royal Society of Medicine*, 89: 196–8.

Saunders, C. (1984) *The Management of Terminal Malignant Disease*. London: Edward Arnold.

Saunders, C. (1993) Foreword, in D. Doyle, G.W.C. Hanks and N. MacDonald (eds) *Oxford Textbook of Palliative Medicine*. Oxford: Oxford University Press.

Semblhi, K. (1995) Palliative care in developing countries: luxury or necessity? *International Journal of Palliative Nursing*, 1: 48–52.

de Souza, L.J. (1981) The hospice movement worldwide: Asia, in C. Saunders, D. Summers and N. Teller (eds) *Hospice: The Living Idea*. London: Edward Arnold.

Stjernsward, J. (1993) Palliative medicine: a global perspective, in D. Doyle, G.W.C. Hanks and N. MacDonald (eds) *Oxford Textbook of Palliative Medicine*. Oxford: Oxford University Press.

Stjernsward, J. and Teoh, N. (1993) Current status of Global Cancer Control Program of the World Health Organisation. *Journal of Pain and Symptom Management*, 8: 340–7.

Tulley, M. (1992) *No Full-Stops in India*. New Delhi: Penguin.

Webb, P. (1993) Cancer relief in India. *European Journal of Cancer Care*, 2(2): 53–4.

World Health Organization (1993) Guidelines for opioid availability, in *The Report on the Expert Committee on Cancer Pain Relief and Active Supportive Care*. Geneva: WHO.

8 | Palliative home care

GIORGIO DI MOLA

Home, it may be argued, is where many people feel most truly themselves; in a context where home is perceived to be the centre of a person's life and closest relationships (Rybczynski 1986; Ruddick 1994). In the western world the concept of 'home' has developed around certain fundamental principles, including the recognition of home as a 'social place', the recognition and sometimes respect for traditional family hierarchies, as well as a sense of social and community security represented by 'home'. The situation that develops around these concepts is a synthesis of the social rules of aggregation, interacting with the environment in which individuals have been born, grown up, looked after themselves and lived until death. During the course of the twentieth century society has assumed most of these functions, but until the end of the nineteenth century they all took place at home.

Home is the place in which most of us first receive nourishment, including psychological sustenance. It is a place in which we receive our first education and the help necessary in overcoming the first difficulties we face in life. Symbolically it represents a primordial place, which offers a sense of social and physical security.

Historically, the home has not been the 'private' place as we know it today. It used to be a social meeting place, a place of exchange of both material objects and emotions – where illness and death were situations that were faced in a spirit of solidarity. Due to the frequency with which they occurred, illness and death were moments of learning. Both were seen as natural events, to be faced with a precise rituality according to codes that were taught and passed on through the family. People who were weak in body and soul, because of a fatal illness, lived in conditions in which they were sure of the support of the entire community, not just the family.

Only a faint memory of this tradition lives on in western society, apart from a very few areas where there is still a sense of solidarity built around the family nucleus. Individuals are usually obliged, in an attempt to preserve their privacy, to behave according to a series of taboos which surround death and disease.

The increasing length and prevalence of chronic disease and the increasing numbers of elderly people have reawakened interest in the family and the home as a place in which to care for sick people. The most recent surveys in health care indicate that most people would prefer to receive medical care in the home, especially when considering the economic aspects. In the case of dying patients, this desire also reflects their wish for a better quality of remaining life. The home environment may provide sick people with greater control over their lives than they sometimes have in medical institutions (Dunlop *et al.* 1989; Ventafridda *et al.* 1989; Townsend *et al.* 1990; Lubin 1992; Chambers and Oakhill 1995; Samaroo 1995). The home is thus resuming its ancient role of a place to care for sick people. This is an important factor in achieving the goal of palliative care with its emphasis on quality of life and expert care.

Home: comforting rituals of everyday life

There is a tendency to medicalize the home environment, subjecting the traditionally private sphere of the home to the intrusion of medical personnel, timetables and equipment. However, home care is rarely organized into an efficient, coherent and comprehensive package (Hastings Center 1994). If, therefore, the home is assuming the role of the preferred place to care for dying people, one needs to ask what variables might interfere with such a goal being attained. Identifying these variables requires a critical appreciation of those factors which may cause the home to suffer unpleasant intrusions and a medicalization which is not appropriate to the goals of caring for the patient. Certain elements are particularly critical such as

- the way in which medical staff are present and assist the patient;
- the obligation of indications and/or prescriptions;
- the type and quantity of medical equipment.

Patients often prefer to be looked after at home because it represents a place where they may feel safe, and have most control over decisions. The circumstances and the language that exist in the home represent a comforting daily ritual for the patient. The features of the family environment which patients appreciate, and prefer to see kept intact, may be listed as follows:

- sense of belonging (to the place, to the family, to one's role in all this);
- communication (familiar language, honest information);
- sense of security (essential interventions, control in decision making);
- presence (company of family members, of friends);
- distractions.

These features of home life are often disturbed by the presence of health care personnel, who behave in the home as if they were in a hospital, forgetting or ignoring the fact that they are no longer in an environment in which the hierarchy demands that they are superior to the patient, but in the place in which the patient commands. The home obliges health personnel to completely rethink their roles. The doctor and other staff are no longer in the limelight, but in the background of a scene which has as its main character the patient and his or her home environment. Sankar (1991) has noted the power of the doctor in hospital, whereas at home it is the patient who is in charge and who must be asked permission. This transformation, which in behavioural terms may be defined as a change in 'gestalt', is of crucial importance to the delivery of medical care. It sees the patient as being in charge, something which does not change when the patient is dying.

Taking care not to disturb the equilibrium of the domestic environment, the home must, however, be reorganized to cope with the needs and choices of the patient. Such needs will change periodically, and ultimately, in the last days of life, necessitate a reassessment of the care programme on a daily basis. This entails a careful interpretation of the patient's and the family's requests, recognizing that it is important not to disrupt the home environment too much by the necessary medical and nursing care. It might be suggested that a good response to the needs of a dying patient is one in which patients recognize their own role right to the end, within a home environment which is not transformed into a hospital, but rather kept as it has always been.

International developments and high-tech home care

Home care has developed on an international basis and is more commonly known as 'Hospital at Home'. It emerged out of the problem of increasing pressure on hospital beds – a factor which is often overlooked in discussions about the idea of 'home care'. The aim of 'Hospital at Home' is to cut costs, by reducing the number of inpatients and the length of hospitalization (Shepperd and Iliffe 1996). This aim is only partially compatible with that of home care for dying patients, where the real goal is not to save resources but rather to improve the quality of life.

The development of domiciliary health care was welcomed internationally, especially after the World Health Organization report *Hospital for Health*.

The report proposes strategies that emphasize the relationship between public health services and the community. Faced with a change in the demand for health care, the WHO considers domiciliary treatment (home health care) to be the synthesis of the new demand, integrating the medical with the wider aspects of caring.

This new trend in 'home care' in many ways is re-inventing the care being given before the Second World War, when health care was usually given in the home. It was only after the war, with the advent of the technological hospital, that there was the emphasis on hospital care services. Recent reports on the scarcity of resources, which affect the health services to a great extent in nearly every western country, have given new life to the idea of health care in the home. In the future one can almost certainly predict that a fair proportion of health care will take place out of hospital; and that general practitioners and district health services will be most involved (Orton 1994). An example of such a tendency is seen in Europe, especially in the Mediterranean basin, where health care resources are frequently penalized by national budgets. However, despite limited economic resources and a shortage of hospital beds, there is a steady increase in the number of palliative care services helping to support families in the care of dying people at home (Di Mola 1995).

The development of home care in 'high-tech' countries is just as evident, where the market for hospitalization at home, given the high profits, allows and maintains the spread of such services. There is an ongoing debate in these countries not only about the necessity of applying technology to the field of palliative care, but also about the problems related to the application of high-tech home care for many non-fatal diseases. This provokes reflections on the ethics of certain attitudes in the health care field, which are under discussion in the context of bioethics (Noddings 1994).

The high-tech home care industry and the medicalization of death

High-tech home care can raise the issue of the continuing medicalization of death. Whether or not a particular deployment of high-tech home care is problematic will depend upon various contextual features of the situation such as, for example, intensity, duration, difficulty, family support, benefit and burden (Hastings Center 1994). The problem of the use of technology in the home must be faced in the context of domiciliary palliative care for two reasons, one ethical and the other clinical. The first refers to the high-tech choice that industry tends to impose on health care, or in fact medical developments allow, and how this is put to use in the home care context. The second concerns the role of palliative care more directly in the potential 'medicalization' of death.

Inherent problems in the use of advanced technology in home care not only raise ethical issues but also involve contextual variables which are features of this type of health care, such as:

- the intensity and frequency of interventions;
- difficulties in using technology because of organizational constraints;
- the presence of effective family support;
- costs and benefits.

The assessment of these variables will determine to what extent the use of high-tech equipment in home care is ethical. Many home interventions, such as total parenteral nutrition with peristaltic pumps or the continuous administration of drugs for pain or other symptoms by electronic micro-infusion, might be considered disproportionate to the aims of good palliative home care. Such interventions need continually to be monitored by specialists and often require the constant presence of a family member. There are also the concomitant costs, both in terms of the equipment and human effort involved.

In some countries this is a very common problem within the health care system, especially when the choice of the patient is based on incorrect information, is influenced by business interests or by a member of the family who feels that any intervention which can possibly be afforded should be carried out. Some people ask why dying patients should be deprived of technical interventions (such as oxygen therapy, intravenous drips, parenteral nutrition, administration of drugs by continuous infusion, etc.) and even technological treatments (such as mechanical ventilation in cases of respiratory failure or dialysis) which under certain circumstances are normally given to many patients. What limits should be imposed? This question was at the centre of a debate on the medicalization of the dying (McNamara et al. 1994) and is of direct relevance to the organization of palliative home care services.

Practically speaking, what is under discussion is the extent to which the mandate of 'low-tech and high touch' should be followed. It would appear that one side of the debate favours the return of palliative care to the fold of traditional medicine, while the other side feels that this tendency towards the medicalization of death would lead to a loss of identity for palliative care (Field 1994). Many groups concerned with the care of dying people tend to classify themselves as 'technical' or 'non-technical' according to the percentage of doctors on the staff or team. However, it appears that teams have proved more efficient according to the numbers of doctors on their staff, a fact which could be considered a parameter in assessing the efficacy of home care interventions for dying patients (Johnson et al. 1990).

The answers to these problems are complex, especially where it is impossible to deny the advantages that technology confers, not only because of the increased frequency and intensity of the interventions, but also because of the increased quality of the treatment and the improvement in the patient's quality of life. However, by referring expressly to the quality of life, talking to the sick person, and listening to what the patient is saying about personal needs and choices, it becomes clear what is the most effective and appropriate care. One should not exclude the possibility of using technological treatment, generally reserved for acutely ill patients, otherwise correctly informed terminal patients would be deprived of the possibility of choosing more 'active' medical interventions.

Hospital versus home in the care of terminally ill patients

The worst home is not necessarily better than the best hospital or medical institution. The best way to respond to the question of which health services should be made available is to say that we shall aim at providing whatever people need. Society should therefore devote more thought and economic resources to the establishment of new institutions which are intermediate between hospital and home. While it is true that the majority of people express the desire to be cared for and to die at home, an objective assessment of the environment and the family circumstances sometimes reveals that the best home is not always preferable to the worst hospital and vice versa. Many studies report contrasting conclusions. Often the choice of dying at home or in hospital is reached because of the force of circumstances, such as shortage of hospital beds, swift discharge from hospital and even the type of cancer (Clifford *et al.* 1991; Hunt *et al.* 1991; Dudgeon and Kristjanson 1995). Circumstances that often influence the ability to care for a dying patient have been documented (Townsend *et al.* 1990; While 1992; Hansen 1994 *et al.*; Hinton 1994; McWhinney *et al.* 1995). These include:

- favourable family environment (acceptance of death);
- supportive members of family;
- availability of voluntary and capable carers;
- possible reimbursement from the health service;
- patient's preference;
- paediatric diseases.

There are, however, circumstances which prevent or render it impossible to care for a dying patient at home and favour a hospital solution (Tsamandouraki *et al.* 1992; Mann *et al.* 1993; Kawaguchi *et al.* 1994; Johnson 1995; Seamark *et al.* 1995). These include:

- lack of family support;
- excessive burden for the family of a dying patient confined to bed for a long period;

- sudden changes in the patient's condition;
- patient's preference;
- poor control of pain or other symptoms;
- type of primitive cancer;
- AIDS (in certain countries);
- active treatment and specific planned therapy.

The data on hospital deaths would seem to contradict any attempt to uphold the home as a place to die or where one would prefer to die. In the latter decades of the twentieth century there has been a considerable increase in the number of hospital deaths and many patients still express the desire to be cared for in a hospital for the following reasons:

- better health care;
- lower risk in emergency conditions;
- better treatment;
- more company (in the absence of family support);
- greater security.

The data reported, the observations made and, most importantly, the desire of the patient continue to indicate that in order to guarantee dying patients a dignified end to their life at home, it is necessary to adapt the home to the patient. When the home cannot fulfil all the needs of a dying patient, hospitals ought to be able to make up for any shortcomings in the home, and offer a familiar environment as part of the humanization of medical care. The possibility of receiving medical care in a hospice should also be available for dying patients, where scientific and technical quality is combined with respect for the patient's quality of life.

The patient in the hospital is often perceived as a stranger in a strange land. As Ruddick (1994) notes, hospital is often experienced as a place of insecurity, discomfort, intrusion and demands for compliance and conformity. However, some hospitals are trying to become more homelike and some terminally ill patients prefer these redesigned wings to hospice units.

Hospitals tend to normalize disease and, in a sense, death too. The comparison with an illness experienced in the home environment makes individuals in hospital feel deprived of their importance as patients. Unfortunately there is a danger that a patient in hospital becomes a number and no longer the unique protagonist of the situation. Hospital patients are relieved of their daily tasks, beginning with the responsibility for any medical care. In the home environment, however, deteriorating ill health and death may provoke a certain degree of confusion concerning the true state of the patient's health. In hospital it could be said that patients are generally more able objectively to assess the extent of their illness because of easier access to doctors and nurses.

These positive features of hospital care have been reassessed due to, among other things, the critical analysis of doctors' attitudes compared with the reality of home care (Sankar 1991). Some hospitals have therefore equipped themselves to seem more homelike without, however, assuming completely the principles of the hospice. Many patients prefer these new kinds of hospital structures to hospices. Hospitals are changing, but the image of the traditional hospital is still the motivation of many patients' and families' preference, who consider it a place of institutionalized care as opposed to the home. The hospital represents the place where medical staff and technologies function most efficiently, rather than a place designed for the comfort of the patient. Because its goal is to cure the patient, it inspires more confidence in dealing with illness and death.

In conclusion, if it is going to be possible for someone to die at home, hospital staff must organize 'good discharge planning'. We also have to provide the social and symptomatic support and, above all, gently talk about dying with our patients and families when given the right opportunity.

Models and development of the home palliative care services

The wide dissemination of palliative care throughout the world has resulted in various interpretations of care to accommodate different local situations. Resources available to each country have not always allowed for an ideal development of palliative care i.e. a multidisciplinary approach to address the physical, social and spiritual needs as well as integrating both hospital and home care services.

The development of palliative care based on the principles of the hospice movement shows two main practical approaches: care within dedicated structures (hospital-based, hospices) and home care (hospice at home and hospital-based home care) (see Beck-Friis, Chapter 9 in this volume). According to the political and institutional situation – as well as available resources – a terminal patient may be cared for mostly or exclusively within one or the other structure, or within a system integrating both models (Greer et al. 1983; Di Mola 1995).

A review of the literature shows a great variety of palliative home care models. Doyle (1993) suggests calling these specialist home care services 'domiciliary palliative care services or teams', so that they are not confused with the more generic term 'home care service'. Such specialist teams in the UK generally consist of one or more doctors and specialist nurses (Doyle 1993). More often than not, these teams report back to and work with a hospice, or a palliative care unit, although sometimes they operate independently. Other models, such as those in Italy, report to the oncological or pain therapy services, or community health care services. These teams are nearly always made up of a basic unit of one doctor, one or more specialist nurses and numerous volunteers. The more complete teams have a psychologist, social worker and a person responsible for pastoral care. Not all the doctors who work in these teams have a specialist qualification in palliative care, as happens in some countries (UK, Australia, Canada) where palliative care is recognized as a specialty in its own right. However, they are experts in palliative care and pain management, having undertaken postgraduate courses or worked with chronically ill and/or dying patients (elderly people, patients with cancer, AIDS, Alzheimer's disease, or other degenerative chronic diseases). The same is true for the nurses in these teams. Similar structures are operative in various countries, including Canada, USA, Australia, New Zealand, England and Italy.

The situation in Italy is a good example of different models which have been developed according to available resources and local application. A comparison of the way in which various domiciliary palliative care teams work in other countries shows that Italy, although not one of the leading countries in palliative care, has none the less developed a considerable network of palliative home care units (Corli 1995). In the same way as other countries, the Italian home palliative care service developed because of swift hospital discharge, in particular cancer patients, and the lack of beds in hospices. However, as we have noted, often this was because of the choice and desire of patients and their families.

All the home palliative care service units in Italy provide specialist doctor and nurse input, medical equipment (beds, chairs, commodes, etc.) and everything that is necessary for the patient's comfort that the family cannot provide. The strong point of this model is the weekly planning and revision of patient care with the community health centres in which most members of the team work. These centres do not have beds as such, but have recently introduced a hospital hospice system, to which the home care service is connected, thus providing the missing link between 'home care' and the places a patient might be cared for other than at home. This model reproduces the recommendations given on an international basis for the development and diffusion of models for the care of terminal patients (see Stjernsward, Chapter 13 in this volume).

The future for palliative home care services

Data on the experience of receiving care and dying at home vary widely, because of the different ways home care is provided; namely, the different specialists available, and the availability and use of the resources offered by the community. The problem of resources is linked to that of 'standards' of home care. This is a fundamental issue to which an answer must be given in order not only to obtain the best results from home care but also that these results may be compared.

Another problem which needs to be resolved and assessed carefully is the control of symptoms. While it is certain that psychological well-being is in most cases improved in terminal patients at home – given the presence of family and volunteers – the same cannot be said about an improvement in certain symptoms. It has been shown that physical symptoms are often less well controlled in the home compared to the hospital. The main cause of hospitalization of these patients is in fact poor symptom control (Parkes 1985; Lunt and Neale 1987; Field and James 1993). However, even when control of symptoms is achieved there are other problems to solve, such as those concerning the capacity of family members to deal with some of the patient's needs. These aspects are a real challenge for the future of specialist palliative home care.

A Canadian study carried out in the Regional Cancer Centre, Hamilton, Ontario (Broadfield 1988) highlights the seriousness of the increasing number of cancer patients in the future. He also reported the dramatic increase in national health costs for dying patients, reaching 1 per cent of the GNP during the last year of life. Broadfield states that such a trend should be considered carefully by experts, along with a systematic evaluation of the effectiveness of palliative care. He also noted that the use of randomized controlled trials in palliative care goes back only to 1984 (Kane et al. 1984), where no significant difference in both control groups was observed. Broadfield claims that the quality of life issues examined in the study were not sufficient, and that the study could not be applied in other circumstances. He concludes that the benefits offered by the USA National Hospice Study, to researchers and those wishing to study palliative care, are more descriptive than conclusive.

Clearly we cannot disregard how difficult it is to report reliable data and their conclusions. In medicine we should be able to apply the golden standard of the randomized controlled trial to prove whether a new intervention in the medical field is better than the lack of it. However, if there are so many problems to accommodate in evaluating a single, specific service, how much more difficult is it to assess home care which offers a number of different services. This is why there are no reliable randomized controlled trials of hospital at home services, which is a serious problem. Every medical intervention should require a suitable assessment of outcome, in order to evaluate its cost-effectiveness. The difficulty in assessing a particular complicated intervention might be seen as an excuse for not assessing other complex interventions. Could this mean that the randomized controlled trials are not the right way to obtain the results expected in palliative home care? Certainly there are related ethical problems, such as the moral impossibility in palliative care, of randomly assigning a group to what appears de facto to be inferior care. This obstacle could be overcome by comparing two models of care, neither of which is acknowledged as being the best (McQuay and Moore 1994). This applies to single or multiple interventions which could be randomized even in individual patients (n of 1 trials) (Guyatt *et al.* 1986).

Conclusion

The historical role of caring for sick people in their homes has been addressed and its relationship to the work of home care services in the 1990s has been considered. Clearly, there are certain features both in the home environment and the disease process that are essential if a dying patient and family are to feel 'safe' with being cared for at home. A discussion on the issues associated with 'low-tech and high touch', and hospital versus home in the care of the dying patient, clarifies the importance of talking and listening to the dying patient's request for information and choice of care. Finally, the need for vigorous evaluation of palliative home care services has been highlighted.

References

Arno, P.S., Bonuck, K.A and Padgug, R. (1994) The economic impact of high-technology home care. *Hastings Center Report*, 24(5): S15–S19.

Broadfield, L. (1988) Evaluation of palliative care: current status and future directions. *Journal of Palliative Care*, 4(3): 21–8.

Chambers, E.J. and Oakhill, A. (1995) Models of care for children dying of malignant disease. *Palliative Medicine*, 9: 181–5.

Clifford, C.A., Jolley, D.J. and Giles, G.G. (1991) Where people die in Victoria. *Medical Journal of Australia*, 155(7): 446–51.

Corli, O. (ed.) (1995) *Realtà esistenti e operanti in Italia nel campo delle Cure Palliative* (Reality and operating systems in Italy in the field of palliative care). Milan: Società Italiana di Cure Palliative.

Di Mola, G. (1995) Role and evaluation of Palliative Home Care Services. *Progress in Palliative Care*, 3(1): 1–6.

Doyle, D. (1993) Domiciliary palliative care, in D. Doyle, G.W.C. Hanks and N. McDonald (eds) *Oxford Textbook of Palliative Medicine*. Oxford: Oxford University Press.

Dudgeon, D.J. and Kristjanson, L. (1995) Home versus hospital death: assessment of preferences and clinical challenges. *Canadian Medical Association Journal*, 152(3): 337–40.

Dunlop, R.J., Davies, R.J. and Hockley, J. (1989) Preferred versus actual place of death: a hospital care support team experience. *Palliative Medicine*, 3: 197–201.

Field, D. (1994) Palliative medicine and the medicalization of death. *European Journal of Cancer Care*, 3(2): 58–62.

Field, D. and James, N. (1993) Where and how people die, in D. Clark (ed.) *The Future for Palliative Care*. Buckingham: Open University Press.

Greer, D.S., Mor, V. and Sherwood, S. (1983) National Hospice Study analysis plan. *Journal of Chronic Disease*, 36(11): 737–80.

Guyatt, G., Sackett, D. and Taylor, W.D. (1986) Determining optimal therapy: randomised trials in individual patients. *New England Journal of Medicine*, 314: 889–92.

Hansen, J.B., Jensen, M.K. and Nielsen, G. (1994) The role of social factors in the place of death of cancer patients in the county of Nordjylland. *Ugeskr Laeger*, 156(12): 1789–91.

Hastings Center (1994) *The Technological Tether*, Executive Summary of Project Conclusions, 24(5): S2–S3.

Hinton, J. (1994) Which patients with terminal cancer are admitted from home care? *Palliative Medicine*, 8(3): 197–210.

Hunt, R.W., Bond, M.J., Groth, R.K. and King, P.M. (1991) Place of death in South Australia: patterns from 1910 to 1987. *Medical Journal of Australia*, 155(8): 549–53.

Jimeno Aranda, A., Catalan, R. and Garcia Ruiz, M. (1993) Where does the terminal patient die? *Aten Primaria*, 11(3): 120–2.

Johnson, A.S. (1995) Palliative care in the home? *Journal of Palliative Care*, 11(2): 42–4.

Johnson, I.S., Rogers, C. *et al.* (1990) What do hospices do? A survey of hospices in the United Kingdom and Republic of Ireland. *British Medical Journal*, 300: 791–3.

Kane, R.L., Wales, J. and Bernstein, L. (1984) A randomized trial for hospice care. *Lancet*, 1: 890–4.

Kawaguchi, Y., Tamura, H., Hattori, M., Ebihara, T. and Sugita, H. (1994) Problems and solutions of home care for a terminal cancer patient: cooperation as a team approach. *Gan To Kagaku Ryoho*, 21: 533–5.

Lubin, S. (1992) Palliative care: could your patient have been managed at home? *Journal of Palliative Care*, 8(2): 18–22.

Lunt, B. and Neale, C. (1987) A comparison of hospice and hospital: care goals set by staff. *Palliative Medicine*, 1: 146–8.

McNamara, B., Waddel, C. and Colvin, M. (1994) The institutionalisation of the good death. *Social Science and Medicine*, 39(11): 1501–8.

McQuay, H. and Moore, A. (1994) Need for rigorous assessment of palliative care. *British Medical Journal*, 309: 1315–16.

McWhinney, I.R., Bass, M.J. and Orr, V. (1995) Factors associated with location of death (home or hospital) of patients referred to a palliative care team. *Canadian Medical Association Journal*, 152(3): 337–40.

Mann, W.J., Loesch, M., Shurpin, K.M. and Chalas, E. (1993) Determinants of home versus hospital terminal care for patients with gynecologic cancer. *Cancer*, 71(9): 2876–9.

Noddings, N. (1994) Moral obligation or moral support for high-tech home care? *Hastings Center Report*, 24(5): S6–S10.

Orton, P. (1994) Shared care. *Lancet*, 309: 1413–14.

Parkes, C.M. (1985) Terminal care: home, hospital or hospice? *Lancet*, 1: 155–7.

Ruddick, W. (1994) Transforming homes and hospitals. *Hastings Center Report*, 24(5): S11–S14.

Rybczynski, W. (1986) *Home: A Short History of an Idea*. New York: Viking Penguin.

Samaroo, B. (1995) Comfort levels with the dying. *Canadian Nurse*, 91(8): 53–7.

Sankar, A. (1991) *Dying at Home: A Family Guide for Caregiving*. Baltimore, MD, and London: Johns Hopkins University Press.

Seamark, D.A., Thorne, C.P., Lawrence, C. and Gray, D.J. (1995) Appropriate place of death for cancer patients: views of general practitioners and hospital doctors. *British Journal of General Practice*, 45(396): 359–63.

Shepperd, S. and Iliffe, S. (1996) Hospital at home: an uncertain future. *British Medical Journal*, 312: 923–4.

Townsend, J., Frank, A.O. and Fermont, D. (1990) Cancer care and patients' preference for place of death: a prospective study. *British Medical Journal*, 301: 415–17.

Tsamandouraki, K., Tountas, Y. and Trichopulos, D. (1992) Relative survival of terminal cancer patients in home versus hospital care. *Scandinavian Journal of Social Medicine*, 20(1): 51–4.

Ventafridda, V., De Conno, F. and Vigano, A. (1989) Comparison of home care and hospital care of advanced cancer patients. *Tumori*, 75: 619–22.

While, A.E. (1992) Consumer views of health care: a comparison of hospital and home care. *Child Care Health and Development*, 18(2): 107–16.

9 A Swedish model of home care

BARBRO BECK-FRIIS

Sweden has a population of 8.9 million with approximately 18 per cent of its people aged 65 years or older. Since 1980 there has been a 44 per cent increase in people living to over 80 years of age, with an indication that this percentage will increase to 60 per cent by the year 2000. With elderly people living longer this is likely to lead to a substantial rise in the national incidence and prevalence of cancer. The need for good palliative care for all has therefore been the subject of a Swedish parliamentary commission (Swedish Government 1995).

In most Scandinavian countries, the majority of deaths occur in hospital. Sweden is no exception. Because of the lack of comprehensive day and night community services for severely handicapped or dying patients at home, 85 per cent of deaths in Sweden take place in hospitals or comparable institutions (Beck-Friis 1993a). The development of inpatient hospice units is an aspect of palliative care in Sweden; however, in this chapter I shall detail a model of home care, focusing upon one of the regions of Sweden, the county council of Ostergotland, where home care teams are based within the main acute hospital of each district. Such a system has been developed in relation to the constraints created by the absence of a comprehensive day and night community service. The hospital-based home care team (HBHCT) provides 24-hour care for dying patients and their families at home and has the back-up of beds in the hospital whenever a need arises. These hospital-based home care teams are designed as an *alternative* to hospital care and not merely to complement the existing health services. Although the model described here is rooted in the particular context of a region of Sweden, it may well have applicability in other settings.

Table 9.1 Organization of HBHCTs in Ostergotland, Sweden

Hospital + population	No. of beds	HBHC team members
Motala (eastern district) 88,200	309	59 full-time equivalents including 4 doctors + 6 beds at their disposal
Linkoping (central) 159,000	838	95.5 full-time equivalents including 8.25 doctors + 12 beds at their disposal
Vrinnevi (eastern) 145,000	567	42 full-time equivalents including 2 doctors + 7 beds at their disposal
Finspang (eastern) 24,000	58	14.8 full-time equivalents including 1.5 doctors + 2 beds at their disposal

Regional organization

The county of Ostergotland, in southern Sweden, has a population of 416,000 people (one-twentieth of Sweden's total). The county is divided into three districts which form the basis for the organization of HBHCTs (western, central and eastern). Within these districts there are four teaching hospitals from which the hospital-based home care teams work: western district with a population of 88,000 at Motala; central district with a population of 159,000 at Linkoping; and eastern district with a population of 169,000 at Norrkoping and at Finspang. Each hospital has its own HBHCT, except for the hospital at Motala which has now expanded to two teams, thus making five HBHCTs. At present, these teams cover 90 per cent of the population within the county of Ostergotland.

The county council of Ostergotland has decided to concentrate its palliative care resources in three ways:

- financial provision for HBHCTs in the four main hospitals in the county;
- the importance of education and writing of guidelines by specialists involved in palliative care;
- establishment of a chair in palliative medicine at the University Hospital of Linkoping.

All four of the hospitals are attached to the University of Ostergotland for work relating to the education of doctors, nurses and paramedical staff. Apart from this, the hospitals are run independently. The HBHCTs are organized from a hospital base out into the community (see Table 9.1).

Model developments within hospital-based home care

The four HBHCTs have evolved differently according to how, when and where they were first started. The team care started at Motala in 1977 and has been widely acknowledged (Beck-Friis 1993b). The Motala HBHCT, albeit now subdivided into two teams but still primarily resourced and staffed from Motala Hospital, and latterly the Linkoping team in the central district, both grew out of an increasing interest in the care of dying people from within the department of geriatrics. However, over the years some of the teams have taken on their own identity rather than remain within a department of geriatrics. At the University Hospital of Linkoping, the team is now a department in its own right and called the Hospital-based Home Care Clinic. In the eastern district, the HBHCT at Finspang is based in the department of internal medicine, while at the larger Norrkoping Hospital the newly based team works from its own department, like the Linkoping team, but includes a ward of seven beds.

Day-to-day team practice

Each HBHC team/unit operates a 24-hour, 7 days a week home care service for dying people and their families, and is fully funded by the county council of Ostergotland. A core team consists of a consultant, doctors and nurses who will respond to a call from a patient within 20–30 minutes. All the consultants and nearly all the doctors are trained in palliative care. Those few who are not trained specifically in palliative care are provided with appropriate supervision. Most patients are suffering from advanced malignant disease, but the teams will accept referrals where patients are in the terminal stage of severe chronic heart or pulmonary disease. An important condition of referral to a HBHCT is that the patient and the family are willing for care to be carried out in the home. However, a team will offer qualified palliative care and advice to patients in a nursing home or a home for aged people, as and when requested.

Expert palliative care with attention to meet the physical, emotional, social and existential needs of the patient and family are a priority. Wherever appropriate members of other health care disciplines (for example social workers, clergy, anaesthetists, dentists) will be asked for their advice and contribution to the care. Because of the close association of working from a hospital base, resources and expertise are easily accessible. Blood transfusions, paracentheses, the provision of pain relieving pumps, and so on, will be provided in the home if such a procedure is appropriate to aid the quality of life of the patient. However, the philosophy of palliative care is not compromised and like any palliative care service, bereavement follow-up with families after a patient has died is also offered.

In 1995 a report from the county council of Ostergotland (Emtinger 1996) into the practice of the HBHC teams/units within Ostergotland region revealed that 412 deaths occured at home (70 per cent from cancer and 18 per cent from severe cardiac and vascular disease). Statistics show that this was 10 per cent of deaths for that region which, for Sweden, is an extraordinary high number of deaths occurring at home.

A 'spot check' of HBHCT patients in the region of Ostergotland during one week in October 1995 revealed the following statistics:

91% patients were referred from hospital (70% from acute departments);
80% patients being cared for were 66 or more years old;
65% patients lived with a next-of-kin;
53% patients were women;
40% patients had support from home helps and meals on wheels;
38% patients still attended their referring department (i.e. surgery, onco-logy, etc.).

(Emtinger 1996)

Although up until recently HBHCTs have cared only for patients with advanced disease, the Motala HBHCT and the unit at the University Hospital of Linkoping have been attending patients at home who are recovering from recent prostatic, thyroid or breast surgery (Brote *et al.* 1994). This has been as a response to requests from surgeons within these hospitals and seen to be a vote of confidence in the service provided. These patients are not terminally ill and some do not have a malignancy, but HBHCT members visit for a short time at home (averaging six days) after the initial post-operative night in hospital. Two aspects can be highlighted from such a service: first, that team members get to care for some patients who are not imminently dying; and second, that it shows the flexibility and possibilities of advanced HBHC organizations.

Future visions

What has been achieved in the county of Ostergotland is being looked upon as a model for palliative care/medicine throughout Sweden. There are four vital aspects to this:

● The general improvement of palliative care throughout the country, with the emphasis on specialist palliative care at home alongside primary care and social services.
● The integration of palliative care services which advise on patients with advanced disease in the hospitals and outpatients rather than just at home.
● The inclusion of specialist palliative care for patients dying from non-malignant diseases at home, incorporated into the HBHCT.

- The establishment of a professorial chair in palliative medicine at the University of Linkoping. The post will be able to promote education and research in palliative medicine according to recommendations contained in the *Palliative Medicine Curriculum*.

Early in 1996 the county council of Ostergotland stressed the importance of developing specialist palliative care within the acute hospital setting. This awareness has probably been highlighted by the developments from the home care programme first started at Motala in 1977. According to the final report of the Swedish Parliamentary Priorities Commission, palliative care has high priority (Swedish Government 1995). The commission has stated that the treatment of acute life-threatening conditions and palliative care be equally important in the allocation of resources:

> How we live is important, but so, too, is the way in which we die. Most of us in Sweden will die slowly. This being so, the end of life is an intensive period for us. A dignified end to life ought, in the Commission's opinion, to be among the cardinal rights of the individual in health care. When cure is impossible and a fatal outcome is expected shortly, the aim should be to give the patient quality of life in the form of a calm and dignified death. This can be achieved through active holistic care, with relief of pain and other troublesome symptoms, and by giving psychological, social and spiritual support to the patient and his or her next-of-kin, to offer effective help against somatic discomforts or anxiety when necessary, not least when the patient is being cared for at home. It is unacceptable that relief should not be offered for severe pain or that terminally ill patients should be discharged from hospital against their own wishes, especially if there are not guarantees of next-of-kin or the local authority being able to provide adequate palliative care.
>
> (Swedish Government 1995: 5)

What has developed in the county of Ostergotland has been followed by other districts. There are now 28 HBHCTs throughout Sweden. Palliative care of highest quality can be given only with competent and expert knowledge. Improving the care of dying people, in their own homes, as in Ostergotland, is a big step forward in a society where a death-denying attitude still prevails.

References

Beck-Friis, B. (1993a) 'Hospital-based home care of terminally ill cancer patients: the Motala model'. *Acta Universitatis Upsaliensis*, Dissertation 393.
Beck-Friis, B. (1993b) The organisation of hospital-based home care for terminally-ill cancer patients: the Motala model. *Palliative Medicine*, 7(2): 93–100.

Brote, L., Beck-Friis, B., Rosenquist, A. and Gustafsson, G. (1994) Prostatakirurgi. *Lakaritidningen*, 91: 1606–11.

Emtinger, B.G. (1996) *Varda och Vardas hemma* (To care and be cared for at home). A report from the county council of Ostergotland (Landstinget i Ostergotland).

Swedish Government (1995) *Priorities in Health Care*. Final report by the Swedish Parliamentary Priorities Commission, Stockholm.

10 Rational planning and policy implementation in palliative care

XAVIER GÓMEZ-BATISTE, M. DULCE FONTANALS, JORDI ROCA, FRANCESC MARTINEZ, ELISABETH VALLES AND PERE ROIGE-CANALS

In this chapter we describe the key elements of a rational planning approach to palliative care policy development and implementation. Within this broad process we shall highlight several key aims, including assessment of needs; introduction of specific services; measures to improve generic services; education and training; models of finance; the evaluation of results; public coverage; equity; quality; and satisfaction with care. In examining these themes we shall draw upon our own experience within a five year programme of palliative care development, organized in Catalonia as a World Health Organization (WHO) demonstration project. We shall show that efficacy, efficiency and the improvement of the global effectiveness of the health care system can be achieved after the introduction of palliative care. In addition we find that the implementation of palliative care services also adds positive cultural and organizational values to the public health care system.

Palliative care as a public health topic

To begin, we identify several themes that are relevant to the understanding of palliative care as a public health issue.

The rising tide

It is evident that across the world, and particularly in the more affluent countries, we are facing a rising tide of increase in the incidence, prevalence, mortality and resource use associated with many chronic, progressive and incurable conditions. These not only include the 'classic' palliative care diseases, such as cancer and AIDS, but also incorporate a wide range of other conditions such as chronic lung and liver disease and the chronic diseases and conditions of old age. These present some striking issues within the current context: 25 per cent of deaths due to cancer; 15–20 per cent of the population aged over 75 years; extensive use of acute and casualty beds by terminally sick and chronically ill patients; increasing demands for home care; rising health care costs; and millions of persons infected with HIV. Such a picture also presents us with a common set of clinical features associated with diseases which are long term, progressive, incurable and which may have many physical symptoms. Alongside such problems we must also consider the emotional impact of these conditions, the increasing dependency and disability which results from them, as well as their impact on patient, family and the clinical team. Other non-clinical features can also be identified in common, associated with the pattern of resource use, and the need for care in a variety of settings (home, hospital, long term and hospice). To these we must add the frequent misuse of resources associated with these areas, together with the difficulties in defining goals of care (curative versus palliative). There are also problems in the delivery of care for people with these conditions in settings which are predominantly curative (especially acute hospital beds). Beyond these lie ethical issues and difficulties associated with the appropriate balance between over-treatment and abandonment, and the difficult ethical dilemmas that are raised for clinicians.

Within this spread of issues there are also important differences. For example in the clinical area there will be variations in the prevalence of cognitive disturbance, incontinence, constipation and diarrhoea, as well as in causes of pain. We would also expect to see variations in emotional response (for example between young people and older adults), as well as differences in social adaptation to disease. Within this broad spectrum of health problems there are considerable variations in experience. For example the isolation of elderly people or the family problems associated with problem drug use and dependence. These lead in turn to differences in the 'atmosphere' of care settings. Nevertheless we have to emphasize that the model of care is based substantially on the same principles and aims and its planning, organization and provision have many things in common. These would include, for example, palliative goals, quality of life, symptom control, emotional support, comprehensive systems, the multidisciplinary team, and the importance of interactions with the wider society. It is our contention therefore that for such health care problems a rational public health policy approach to palliative care is needed which can guarantee coverage, equity and quality. This approach would seek to introduce palliative care for a wide range of conditions as a routinely available

in the provision of palliative care if such services are to receive support from health care budgets.

From the public health perspective, the original conception of hospice provision raises a number of problems (Gómez-Batiste 1987). Several themes can be identified here, including the issue of 'need' versus 'demand' planning and the impact of this on coverage, equity and cost-effectiveness. There are also problems associated with the stable long-term financing of palliative care in mainstream settings compared with the financial situation experienced in hospices which make use of substantial voluntary contributions. From the public health perspective similarly there are wider questions relating to academic training for palliative care, the implementation of research findings into practice and the wider 'credibility' of the discipline within mainstream medical culture. Against this of course must be weighed the very high levels of public support and acceptance associated with the independent hospices. Since the 1980s therefore important developments have been taking place, for example in the UK where there has been less emphasis upon the creation of new hospices and much more attention given to the development of community and hospital-based palliative care services.

In many other countries, the introduction of palliative care has begun in hospital and community settings. This has often been associated in the first phase with the deployment of very basic support teams as an initial measure. Such teams will operate in the acute bed hospital or within long-term care settings where their work is in each case made possible by the reallocation of existing resources. In-patient specialist palliative care beds are seen as a longer-term goal. Such a team approach seems to be reasonable. It requires relatively low investment of new resources and yet can have a great impact on coverage, for example through interaction of professional colleagues, through training, through policy development. All of these can produce valuable effects which we might term 'indirect coverage'. In this way support teams not only act as good caregivers to patients and families but also undertake vital work as assessors of need, as case managers and as change agents within the organizational context. Here they can promote the team approach, the comprehensive district approach, family intervention, continuing care, the idea of the patient's goals as the team's goals, explorations of ethical issues in practice, and good communication between users and providers. We believe that this approach has widespread potential and can lead to changes in the care of other client groups, such as elderly people or those with advanced, progressive illnesses associated with high dependency, where in all cases similar models of care may be appropriate. This model of palliative care development serves to promote radical change within the host health care system and allows for the creation of new conceptual thinking and practical change management at field level (Table 10.1).

Table 10.1 Principles and elements of palliative care planning and implementation

1 Public health problem	⟶	Planning methodology • palliative care as a mainstream service • evaluation essential
2 Needs and aims	⟶	'Cure to care' • organization • innovation
3 Coverage and equity	⟶	Global approach • measures in all settings • inserted within health system • network > individual services
4 Few services	⟶	Rational strategy • combined measures • clear comparisons
5 Combined measures	⟶	Place • time • type • short/mid/long term

1 By considering palliative care as a public health topic, we establish the importance of rational planning, implementation and evaluation.
2 The philosophical and practical differences between palliative care and other health services must be acknowledged; these are rooted in the notion of 'cure to care'. It is important that this approach is introduced into other services.
3 The aims of coverage and equity require the use of a global approach to implementation, with palliative care provision inserted at different levels of the health system, with clear service targets.
4 When few services exist, there is a need for a gradual and rational strategy for extending them. Government and policy makers may be wary of the cost of new provision, in which a high priority should be placed on the introduction of cost-effective measures in selected settings, coupled with education and training.
5 From the outset, it is important to combine new measures by type and across place and time: service development, education and training and needs assessment must proceed together.

The elements of a palliative care programme

The likelihood of success both for palliative care planning and the delivery of individual services is complex and multifactoral. In this section we shall describe the elements that might be incorporated into an effective plan for palliative care, which may be implemented at a number of levels: country, region, health district, or individual service. For the successful development of any new palliative care initiative a degree of political commitment is essential. The initiative must be prioritized, financial support must be achieved and it is also crucial that there is an element of political and policy 'protection' during the initial phase. Palliative care will not achieve the goals of coverage and equity without a substantial degree of political and policy endorsement. Professionals, organizations and governments therefore need to work together in order to build rational plans for the development of palliative care in any country or region. The main factors involved in achieving political commitment are as follows:

- Identification of the importance of clinical improvement relating to widespread and common problems within the health care system; pain is the paramount example.
- Highlighting the efficiency and cost-effectiveness of palliative care within a strategic approach; our preliminary results show that the palliative care programme is in fact self-financed through dramatic improvement in the efficiency of care for non-curable patients. We find that these results can be achieved at all levels, for example a reduction in the use of emergency wards, length of stay and the increased prevalence of home deaths, together with a reduction in inpatient care and pharmacy costs.
- New values are added to the health care system, accompanied by wide recognition and improved work satisfaction on the part of the professionals; examples here would include the impact of new roles associated with the multidisciplinary teams, the perceived value of a comprehensive approach, or the reduction of burnout.
- High levels of satisfaction on the part of patients and families. This can have a major impact at managerial level. In a context where health care managers are faced with problems of provider competition, low satisfaction with services and conflicts over resource allocation, then the introduction of low cost services with high user satisfaction provides an important element of recognition and appreciation.
- High level social and cultural regard; this is associated with clear improvement in the quality of care, with wider discussion of ethical issues, with the humanitarian values associated with palliative care as well as with deeper and more personal issues, for example relating to individuals' fear of suffering, pain, isolation, and death in society.

We would acknowledge that there have been difficulties in obtaining political commitment to palliative care, sometimes resulting from the mistakes of its adherents. There has been lack of consensus between professionals, conflict between individual health care developments (for example oncology versus primary care versus pain clinics). There have also been differences between individual and general views, problems associated with individual goals and egotism, as well as the lack of a public health approach and adequate training. All of these issues must be addressed if coherent plans and broad agreement are to be achieved.

Clear professional leadership

Especially in the early days of a new palliative care development within a region, clear professional leadership is crucial. In most cases the synergistic combination of well-trained, strongly committed and respected professionals is a key factor and determinant of success. The involvement here of individuals with clinical, educational, planning and managerial abilities is vital. In particular we would emphasize the need for clinicians to be effective trainers, to develop managerial skills, to emphasize quality assurance and the value of strategic planning. In some contexts local opinion or corporate resistance and misunderstanding may block palliative care initiatives over long periods of time. Our own experience includes some common examples: 'we are already providing this form of care'; 'this is only a British need'; 'we only need to train general practitioners'; 'we do not have enough money for this development'; or even 'we don't have these types of patients in our area' (Health Minister of Spanish Region, personal communication, 1991). Such remarks are frequently heard and relate to a range of individual and corporate resistance to the benefits which can be achieved. To respond to this situation we need a combination of good teams with clear ideas and the ability to build on earlier successes in order to achieve worthwhile results.

Sometimes, corporate resistance is very strong and it is vital that we understand the reasons that underpin it and work towards achieving a consensus of views. One example concerns the importance of a focal point for care. This can help to distinguish between palliative care services and, for example, pain clinics or oncology services, in a context where palliative care standards have been clearly defined. This is particularly important where there is a political dependency of one service on another, rooted in local power positions. Once a number of good initiatives is underway, however, and these have been consolidated, local experience is frequently the most effective rejoinder to criticism. It then becomes possible to focus more on issues of extension and coverage. Very good examples exist of palliative care leaders who have come from backgrounds in oncology, pain, primary care, geriatrics, internal medicine. This wide variation is testimony to the value of good quality common training in the palliative care approach, coupled to strong commitment. The issue of initial leadership in a new palliative care development also raises the question of protection from overload, battle fatigue and burnout. These can be real problems in

Table 10.2   Types of descriptive baseline studies

- Prevalence
- Mortality
- Symptoms
- Symptom control
- Morphine use
- Resource use

Table 10.3   Dying from cancer in Catalonia: a study

Aims	To assess in the last month of life: prevalence and control of symptoms; resource use; morphine use
Method	Interviews with family members of a consecutive series of 380 cancer patients

Results   *Symptoms:*   weakness, anorexia, weight loss (> 80%)
                                            pain (70%)
          Place of death: hospital (65%)
          Hospital emergency use: 44%
          Morphine use: 68%

situations where individuals and teams have excessive responsibilities for clinical delivery, together with high demands to deliver training, along with the day to day rigours of teamwork and clinical delivery. Where only one team exists in a region, then its effective deployment in relation to a number of demands becomes an important issue.

Baseline studies to assess needs

There are undoubtedly problems in combining immediate action to implement new services with the business of undertaking effective needs assessment studies which may provide vital information on the kinds of services that should be promoted. Typically, most of the energy goes into building up teams and obtaining local support. It is also true, however, that objective assessment of need and analysis of the baseline context are crucial, especially if there is to be effective monitoring of the results of a new initiative. Our view is that these activities can be undertaken concurrently and that needs assessment should never be an excuse for inaction on policy development. Needs assessment, however, may have an important impact upon the views of policy makers (see Tables 10.2 and 10.3).

Defined aims: coverage, equity, quality, comparability and user satisfaction

The global aim of the introduction of palliative care services is the improvement of quality of care for patients with advanced non-curable disease. More concrete public health aims include coverage, equity, quality, comparability, and the introduction of changes into the organization of health care services.

Public coverage

Public coverage refers to the highest proportion of patients achieving adequate care with reasonable service provision. We could describe direct coverage as referring to the patients cared for by specific teams, and indirect coverage as relating to benefits achieved for patients through improving the standards of all services, including provision for those with cancer, AIDS, chronic diseases and the diseases of old age. It is clear that the goal of a public plan has to be extended to all patients, but adequate and cost-effective direct coverage is controversial. We do know systems with high direct coverage (MacIllmurray *et al.* 1986; Gómez-Sancho *et al.* 1995; Gómez-Batiste *et al.* 1996) usually in well-defined rural or urban areas with highly committed teams. It is difficult, however, to establish the correct balance between direct and indirect provision. A good recommendation could be to achieve around 50 per cent direct coverage and then to assess indirect effects, for example by monitoring morphine use. In some areas with good primary care and oncology services, a low direct coverage, coupled with flexible models of intervention and a strong emphasis on training and general measures, could be sufficient to improve overall standards of care.

A further dilemma relates to the extension of palliative care beyond cancer and to the development of a more integrated approach across a spectrum of diseases. Due to the need for specific and visible interventions, or because of the nature of local specialization in cancer institutes and large teaching hospitals, it is clear that an initial approach which focuses upon cancer has a good deal to commend it. In a district-based, more global strategy, however, the mid- or long-term goal must clearly be to include all patients who would benefit by the palliative care approach. It is vital that the principles and practices of palliative care are extended to other patient groups. The dilemmas here relate to *When? How?* and *Where?*

Our experience in Catalonia (Gómez-Batiste *et al.* 1996) shows clearly that on a district basis, with the standard prevalences of such diseases as cancer, AIDS, and the diseases of old age, it is possible to develop a cost-effective long-term and comprehensive plan for palliative care. For example in one large teaching hospital, with a high prevalence of all these conditions, specific teams attached to or linked with their specialties are beginning to be developed. As a general recommendation we would suggest that any palliative care plan must include specific measures for cancer, AIDS, geriatrics and other conditions and that local or individual services must decide how this can be achieved. Large hospitals with high specific prevalences and needs will require additional resources in order to achieve this. A fundamental strategy for achieving coverage, especially in short periods of time, is to prioritize development in areas of high prevalence, such as cancer centres or hospitals for cancer.

Equity

Equity is a basic ethical principle of any public health based programme. The principle refers to the idea that no differences in the quality or accessibility of care will result from social status, location, age, sex, or race. To this we might also add type of disease and stage in the disease progression. The other key principle of equitable coverage is that it should be financed publicly and available to all persons, free of charge. Private sector health care, however, must also take on board the need for good palliative care for its own group of patients. Our central argument here is that the accessibility of palliative care is related to its insertion within the mainstream of public health care provision, coupled with adequate and known referral mechanisms designed to avoid inequities. This incorporation of palliative care into the 'normal' service of the health system will require flexibility and a willingness to prioritize in relation to specific needs and dilemmas.

Quality

The new palliative care programme must also ensure the quality of its services through the elaboration of standards and processes of accreditation (National Council for Hospice and Specialist Palliative Care 1992; Ingleton and Faulkner 1994; Gómez-Batiste et al. 1995). In the initial phases of the development of a palliative care service, clear definition of client group, structure, process and outcomes of services is crucial if misunderstandings are to be avoided. Assuring quality for patients is also a mechanism for assuring equity.

Comparability

Palliative care programmes and projects must also be based within clear, objective, measurable and scientific principles which can be compared, adapted and applied elsewhere. In the case of WHO demonstration projects, the principle of comparability is very important for others contemplating similar work. On a more local basis, the concept of reference teams which serve as models and tutors for newcomers to the field can assist health administrators in implementing new initiatives flexibly and safely. This approach has been adopted in the eight health care areas of Catalonia in which reference units are charged with training and support responsibilities for new teams, using techniques of modelling and mentoring.

User satisfaction

Finally, it is worth repeating that visible and measurable satisfaction of patients, families and professionals with a palliative care service is itself an important political aim and will serve as a key indicator of success when building support for the programme.

Deployment of specific palliative care services

Those contemplating the development of new palliative care services typically have a range of questions: Which type? Where? How many specific services are needed in a country, region, district or specific health care setting (hospital or community)? In our experience the initial targets and judgement of what is achievable often differ from the final proposals.

The most basic type of resource for palliative care development is the support team acting individually or together with other teams in a specific place or as part of a wider system. The direct care activities will include care in hospital (peripatetic team or specific unit), day unit, outpatient clinic, home care and activities relating to families (for example bereavement care). To these support activities we must also add the work of training and of research as well as the more widespread promotion of palliative care philosophy and practice.

A reasonable planning position is to begin with a basic team (one doctor, two nurses, one social worker) and to develop activities gradually. We have experience of such an approach and it is one which commends itself as probably the most efficient option. Such a team can act as a good provider of care, but also as a describer, planner and change agent in specific settings. Initial low investment in this kind of team may also help to reduce potential corporate resistance. Our experience shows that within two to three years such teams are able to consolidate themselves, building both internal and external support and consensus, and during this time will also have achieved acceptable clinical results. From such a position the development of specific palliative care units could be a realistic next step, if appropriate.

The process of building teams and the phases of team consolidation are depicted in Table 10.4.

Table 10.4 Building and consolidating teams

• Project definition	
• Selection	**Key phases**
• Internal training	
• Internal consensus	1 Project definition
• External consensus	2 Initial development
• External training	3 Consolidation
• Research	4 Advanced development
• Evaluation	

Both of these are vital phases in any development and both require institutional support and commitment. The chosen sites for initial implementation are also significant and may be controversial, depending upon the local situation. Again we need to combine concerns with rational coverage with considerations of commonsense and local feasibility, not least because the ideal places from which coverage may be achieved are usually more complex and initially resistant, for example cancer institutes and large hospitals. Conversely, situations with a supportive local environment and attitudes, where initial developments may flourish, can sometimes be relatively isolated from mainstream health care.

The palliative care teams, in order to be effective, must be inserted in all elements of the health care network. In Catalonia, these include hospitals, socio-health centres (for long-term care) and the community. In the context of health care for elderly people (Horroks 1986), the district is the basic unit of intervention for specific teams, with a comprehensive and flexible approach focused on direct coverage and training. Within this context the specific provider or physical base for the teams is less relevant than the strategic goals of the global intervention. Teams based in hospitals need to link with the community and others based in hospices or socio-health centres must establish liaison with hospitals and the community, and conversely. The efficiency of such teams in the provision of continuing palliative care depends upon their ability to intervene in all settings. In our organizational standards therefore, effective liaison with other services is one of the activities which must be demonstrated in order to achieve accreditation. When different health care providers are involved, the role of health authorities in fostering consensus and liaison is crucial if resource use is to be optimized.

Determining the specific level of resources required in any local context is a complex issue, in part dependent upon the prevailing pattern of health care organization. In the Spanish context there are examples of high coverage, comprehensive systems, such as Las Palmas and Vic. These are usually in rural or urban areas and can obtain coverage of over 80 per cent using two basic teams and 10–20 beds for 150,000 inhabitants. Alternatively in

Table 10.5   Catalonia: specific palliative care resources (1990–5)

	1989	1992	1995	1997*
Hospital support team	—	7	16	20
Palliative care beds	22	120	350	450
Hospital palliative care unit	—	—	2	6
Socio-health centre palliative care unit	2	7	16	25
Home care support team	1	25	42	55
Districts with a palliative care team	2/55 (4%)	—	44/55 (80%)	55 (100%)
New patients per year	350	—	5000	8000
Coverage	5%	—	40%	60%
Global morphine consumption (kg/million/yr)	3.5	>11.4 (1994)		18

(*estimated)

areas of low coverage the principal emphasis would be upon education and training. In our view the number of basic teams could be a more precise indicator of coverage than the number of beds. In 1996 actual coverage in Catalonia consisted of one basic team per 100,000 inhabitants (i.e. 65 teams for 6 million population); however, distribution was patchy. Districts with any specific palliative care resource numbered 44 out of a total of 55 (i.e. 80 per cent). The WHO demonstration project in Catalonia has resulted in 16 hospital support teams, 18 units (2 based in acute bed hospitals, 16 in socio-health centres, 350 beds), and 42 specific sectorized home care teams, with a coverage of 40 per cent for cancer and AIDS (see Table 10.5).

The support teams in the community have a mixed caseload of advanced geriatrics (50 per cent), terminal cancer (40 per cent), AIDS (5 per cent) and other patients (5 per cent) (Gómez-Batiste et al. 1994a, 1994b).

The number of beds is also a controversial issue. Cultural factors, family support, availability of other resources for home care, and length of stay are determining factors here. Figures for cancer are around 50–70 beds per million population but the inclusion of geriatric patients, those with chronic illnesses, and people with AIDS has the potential dramatically to increase the number towards 150–200 beds per million. Actual figures in both Catalonia and the UK are currently around 50 beds per million population.

Table 10.6   General palliative care measures: hospitals and community

---

1 Time and place of patient care
2 Training: basic, intermediate
3 Policies: symptom control, communication
4 Promotion of multidisciplinary approach
5 Availability of opioids
6 District liaison/referral policies
7 Hospitals: presence of families
8 Community: support for families

Any plan for palliative care development must include its promotion within current health care delivery and resource use (see Table 10.6). Targets for this must be selected rationally and prioritized. In hospitals, surgical wards and oncology wards for cancer and in general medicine wards for geriatric and AIDS patients, there exist clear targets to implement such an approach. This can have a striking effect on coverage and also provide care at earlier stages of the disease process. For example, a typical oncologist in Catalonia will look after 200 new cancer patients per year, and a typical surgeon between 50 and 100; more than 50 per cent of these patients will be characterized by an advanced stage of disease. We have found also that nurses are important advocates for the implementation of good palliative care in the general ward setting. In the community, high coverage of a general palliative care approach must be achieved through a district strategy, not least because individual general practitioners look after relatively few advanced cancer patients (the mean in Barcelona is four such patients per year). The introduction of a more generalist approach therefore includes action on training, the definition and implementation of standards and the establishment of clear referral policies for specific teams. In local, regional and national plans the monitoring of services which have adopted palliative care approaches is important.

Education and training

In the initial phases of palliative care development, the training of a core nucleus of teams both in the development of practice and in the techniques of education, seem more rational aims than those of direct coverage. Initially teams will require strategic planning of their training activities, based on a coverage approach and reflecting local needs rather than simply responding to demands. An emphasis on efficiency is important throughout this process.

At the mid- to long-term stage strategies for training must begin to include the definition of targets, levels, methods and the accreditation of services to provide training (see Table 10.7).

Table 10.7   Elements of an educational plan for palliative care

1 Level
2 Targets
3 Activities
4 Methodology
5 Accreditation
6 Evaluation

Table 10.8   A tailored methodology for training

Goal	Structure	Approach
Initial dissemination	Basic course	Lecture
Practical implementation	Project	Placement Modelling Tutorials Demonstration teams
Specific topic	Workshop	Consensus-building Joint policies Joint research

Targets should be chosen according to their impact on patient coverage. As we have seen, oncological and surgical services in hospitals are excellent targets in this respect. Other professionals may constitute fertile ground for development and may be characterized by a positive disposition towards palliative care but may have less impact on direct coverage. Two examples of this relate to training for general practitioners and undergraduate training. In the case of general practitioners, training is crucial to promote the improvement of care, but its impact upon coverage is at the mid- to long-term level since individual doctors see small numbers of patients. Similarly undergraduate training will achieve significant coverage in five to ten years but it will also need maintenance activity and the support of specialist teams during those years if full benefit is to be achieved. Three levels of training activity can therefore be identified. First, basic training with 100 per cent coverage at the undergraduate level. Second, intermediate training targeted upon oncologists, geriatricians and (optionally) general practitioners. Third, advanced, expert or specialist training for professionals involved full-time in palliative care (MacDonald 1994). Training activity therefore needs to be tailored to specific aims and targets at the local or general level (see Table 10.8).

Definitions of training activities and accreditation of services (especially for intermediate and advanced training) are good methods for quality assurance for palliative care educational providers.

The definition of organizational standards

In order to avoid confusion at the early stages, the definition of specific services and their standards must be made clear in any palliative care plan (Gómez-Batiste *et al.* 1995). Confusion between palliative care, pain services, oncology, and long-term care is a frequent dilemma for professionals and policy makers in many countries, particularly at the early stages of development. Our preference is to define standards as the consensus between professionals, providers, health administrators and clients on the definition of specific services. A health care service can be defined and identified by a combination of several factors, including the types of clients, the aims, the 'functional data' (number of patients, intervention pattern, median survival, length of stay), the structure, the activities, the results, and the level of knowledge needed for its delivery.

Types of clients

Palliative care services look after those with advanced or terminal cancer, with AIDS, with the diseases of old age and with progressive chronic disease. Such services are defined by a combination of advanced, non-curable disease, multiple symptoms, together with the potential for complex emotional impacts of illness. In addition such conditions are characterized by a low probability of response to specific therapies and limited prognosis.

Aims and principles

The key aims of such a palliative care service are those of comfort and quality of life for patients and families. The principle is one of total care, in which the patient *and* family are seen as the focus of care and where there is an emphasis on symptom control, emotional support and communication, as well as the adaptation of the organization to the needs of patients and families through a multidisciplinary team approach and the provision of continuing care.

'Functional' data

We would argue that a minimal number of patients (around 150 per year) is needed in order to achieve efficacy and efficiency. Median survival is a good indicator of the type of service and serves to differentiate palliative care from oncology, long-term care and pain services. The average median survival of patients receiving palliative care services is less than three months. Taking median survival and the pattern of intervention, we can differenti-ate two forms of palliative care service (Gómez-Batiste 1987). These can be described as on the one hand hospice or terminal care, with median survivals of less than one month, and continuing care services, with median survivals of two to three months. Median survival is also related to the proximity of referral services and the pattern of intervention.

Length of inpatient stay is another useful indicator for distinguishing palliative and long-term care. In our data, length of inpatient stay in pal-liative care services is always under two months (4–60 days) and will also depend upon the type and complexity of patients admitted, together with family needs and the availability of home care. Palliative care inpatient units providing terminal care in the last days will have a median length of stay of only a few days. Those providing care for 'chronic' patients will have lengths of stay of 40–60 days, while those devoted to 'acute complex' patients (i.e. those admitted for symptom control or psychosocial prob-lems) will have a length of stay of around 15–20 days. In practice most units have a mix of all three types of patients (Catalan Health Service 1995). Linked to type of patient admitted and the availability of home care, mortality rates provide another important indicator. Inpatient units will have mortality rates varying between 50 and 90 per cent. These will be lower if a substantial level of service is provided to those in the 'com-plex acute' category and where good home care is available. Conversely they will be higher among units which primarily admit patients for care in the last days and/or those with chronic long-term needs and poor avail-ability of home care.

Structure and type of services

Support teams, if they have no specific beds, may operate in either hospital or community settings. Wherever they are located, adequate selection, training based on previous experience and support are crucial factors in achieving success.

Again, a 'basic team' could be considered to consist of a doctor, one or two nurses and a social worker. We feel strongly that such a team consti-tutes the minimum level to avoid the burnout or ineffectiveness of indi-vidual workers. Of course, more complex teams will be needed in palliative care units which have inpatient beds. In Catalonia the size of such units varies from 6 to 28 beds per ward and the emphasis is upon the comfort of patients, the presence of families, showing sensitivity to cultural pat-terns, and staff support. Such units seek to create a home atmosphere with a high level of adaptation to individual needs.

Table 10.9   Activities of palliative care teams

---

1 Care of patients
2 Care of families (including bereavement care)
3 Multidisciplinary team
4 Evaluation of results
5 Support of teams/sectorized liaison
6 Internal team training
7 External training
8 Research
9 Volunteers
10 Spiritual/pastoral care

The activities of palliative care teams are set out in Table 10.9, in which each element is designed to be open to monitoring and documentation. In this context 'process' standards are useful to define the range of activities in a single service, while 'results' standards serve as a method for comparing the activities and outputs of similar teams and services in different locations.

In Catalonia since 1991, we have sought to develop palliative care services, adapted where appropriate to differing local situations. Our experience shows the variability of palliative care organization even in a small region of 6 million inhabitants. Several models of organization are in evidence:

- *High coverage comprehensive model* (Vic, Terrassa, Valls, Mataró, Sabadell, Vilanova). These services are mainly based in well-defined urban or rural areas, with a unit based in the socio-health centre, together with two support teams in the community and in the acute bed district general hospital. Coverage is high at around 70 per cent of patients with cancer, AIDS and illnesses of old age.
- *University hospital large cancer centre* (Catalan Institute of Oncology, Hospital Duran-Reynals). This unit is located in an urban area of southern Barcelona and is based at the Cancer Institute with a support team working in the oncology wards and in the hospital Ciutat Sanitaria de Bellvitge. There are also seven community support teams based in the surrounding district and closely linked to the unit. 'Chronic' inpatients are cared for in three units based in socio-health centres. All of this care is exclusively for cancer patients, due to the high level of need. Coverage within the hospital is around 50 per cent, although the population coverage is difficult to establish.
- *Support team based in a comprehensive oncology service* (Girona, Reus). Here a support team is inserted in the oncology service and linked to several surrounding support teams in hospital and in the community.
- *Special organizations*. These are designed to meet specific and concrete needs. For example, the paediatric hospital support team (St John of

God Hospital, Barcelona) acts as a support team internally and provides training and consultation on specific cases. At the same hospital there is also a unit for AIDS patients who have been in prison; this has 12 beds and strong links with the prison medical services. In another hospital (Ciutat Sanitaria de Bellvitge) a support team focuses on the needs of patients with chronic advanced respiratory disease, working in the large teaching hospital and in the community using the palliative care model.

Opioid availability

The availability of opioids is a crucial measure of success in implementing a palliative care strategy in any country or region. In our view the best opioid regulation is no regulation. Nevertheless, many governments have strong resistance to the promotion of opioid availability, and this often lies in ignorance, prejudice and negative myths associated with dependency, tolerance, the precipitation of death, and illegal misuse. Change of legislation relating to opioids can be a slow process, it is therefore important to establish agreement on urgent measures which can be achieved in the short term. Direct distribution of morphine from district-based teams can be useful initially. In our experience, Spanish legislation was improved dramatically in 1994 but even in a study of dying from cancer in Catalonia, conducted in 1993 (Viladiu *et al.* 1995), 68 per cent of patients had morphine in the last month of life and 78 per cent of 300 families reported no difficulty in the availability of morphine. This reflected the achievement of agreement about morphine use which was a feature of the work of the specific palliative care teams.

Another important aspect is to promote the prescription and availability of opioids through education and training. In the absence of other factors, education and training can explain substantial regional differences in morphine consumption, even where (as in Spain) the same federal laws apply.

Cost benefits of palliative care implementation

Where there is a strong managerial commitment to the introduction of palliative care, as we have indicated, it is possible for the 'reconversion' of resources to take place and for palliative care services to begin with no additional resource requirements. The financing of palliative care services is a clear duty of the public health system, which must take responsibility if equity, quality, coverage, efficacy and cost-benefit improvement are to be achieved. We estimate that the palliative care programme in Catalonia has been substantially 'self-financed' through radical improvement in the use of health resources. Based on the most measurable and clear indicators

Table 10.10   Costs and savings of the Catalan programme in 1995

	Million pesetas
Estimated costs	
Support team + units' beds[a]	2200
Estimated savings	
Different daily costs of palliative vs acute care beds (×350)[b]	1500
Reduction of length of stay[c]	1375
Total	1875

Notes: [a] Includes 42 home care support teams, 16 hospital support teams, 350 palliative
care beds
[b] Mean cost of acute beds: 25,000 pesetas/day
Mean cost of palliative care beds: 10,000 pesetas/day
[c] Estimated reduction of length of stay inpatients,
5 days/patient × 2500 patients (50%) × daily cost
Source: Catalan Health Service 1996

(bed costs and mean reduction of length of stay) our figures for 1995 (see Table 10.10) show that around 80 per cent (1800 million pesetas) of the total cost of the programme (2200 million pesetas) could reasonably be self-financed following changes in the pattern of resource use and lowered costs. This is clearly a preliminary estimate, but suggests a powerful argument. Additional savings, such as reduction in the use of hospital emergency wards, lower cost of medication and investigations, are not included. The Catalan health care system, with the separation of purchasing and providing, daily fees for beds and team services, allows us to form a clear picture of the costs of new initiatives.

The impact of new developments in palliative care on the efficiency of the general health care system is a fascinating area for research and represents a key question for us in the coming years, not least when competition for resources will become an increasingly important factor. We are seeking to develop the argument that the best possible justification for palliative care may well be the low cost of its implementation. Such an argument would therefore be based upon appeals to a rational and efficient system of health care delivery in which palliative care could be seen to be cost-effective *vis-à-vis* other services.

Evaluation of palliative care programmes

It is important to select appropriate and simple indicators for the measurement of progress in the development of palliative care services. As we have seen, baseline studies will be crucial in measuring the impacts of implementation. Several possible indicators exist, including:

- number of specific resources;
- percentage of specific resources achieving the required standards;
- population coverage (e.g. for cancer, AIDS, geriatrics, others);
- efficacy in provision (e.g. percentage of pain control achieved);
- morphine consumption;
- training coverage;
- impact on other patterns of resource use.

Conclusions and recommendations

The introduction of palliative care services requires a rational strategy involving assessment of need, definition of aims (short, medium and long term), resource use within the existing health care system, measures of improvement, definitions of levels (basic, intermediate and specialist), clear definition of services and organizational standards, and evaluation measures. The basic principles which we have outlined in this chapter are those of coverage, equity, quality, scientific validity and satisfaction of patients, families and professionals. Palliative care must be considered as a service routinely available within mainstream health care.

The measurable impacts of palliative care implementation are the improvement in the efficacy, the efficiency and the cost-effectiveness of the provision of care for those with advanced disease and terminal conditions. We have argued that this can be achieved through improved and more rational use of existing resources. Using this approach, specific palliative care developments can be brought about at low additional cost. Additionally, palliative care gives further value to the health care system through the promotion of a total care approach, of patient autonomy and dignity, through the reintroduction of families into the care process, through the philosophy of the multidisciplinary team, and through the satisfaction of patients and families. Particularly when linked to a comprehensive district system of health care, the introduction of palliative care provision can add a sense of social and cultural dignity and make a positive contribution to debates on euthanasia. In our view, the existence of palliative care services is not only a good indicator of the efficiency of the public health care system, but also an important measure of the dignity of society itself.

References

Catalan Health Service (1996) *Life to the Years Program*: internal reports from units and teams. Barcelona: Catalan Health Service.

European Association for Palliative Care (1993) *Report and Recommendations of a Workshop on Palliative Medicine Education and Training for Doctors in Europe.* Brussels: European Association of Palliative Care.

Gómez-Batiste, X. (1987) *Terminal Care: Basis for Therapeutics and the Organisation of Care in the UK.* Vic: CIRIT, The British Council.

Gómez-Batiste, X., Fontanals, M.D., Vía, J.M., Roca, J.M., Trelis, J., Porta, J., Stjernsward, J. and Trías, X. (1994a) Catalonia's five year plan: basic principles. *European Journal of Palliative Care*, 1(1): 45–9.

Gómez-Batiste, X., Fontanals, M.D., Vía, J.M., Roca, J.M., Trelis, J., Porta, J., Stjernsward, J. and Trías, X. (1994b) Catalonia's five year plan: preliminary results. *European Journal of Palliative Care*, 1(2): 98–102.

Gómez-Batiste, X., Fontanals, M.D., Vía, J.M., Roca, J.M., Trelis, J., Porta, J., Stjernsward, J. and Trías, X. (1995) *Estandards de cures palliatives.* Servei Català de la Salut, Societat Catalanobalear de Cures Palliatives, EUMO editorial, Vic, Barcelona.

Gómez-Batiste, X., Planas, J., Roca, J.M. and Viladiu, P. (1996) *Ciudados Paliativos en Oncología.* Barcelona: Editorial JIMS.

Gómez-Sancho, M., Ogeda Martin, M., Garcia Rodriguez, E.D., Navarro Marrero, M.A. and Marrero Martin, M. del S. (1995) *Escasez de recursos: mejor argumento para la implementación de la medicina y cuidados paliativos.* Abstracts of the Fourth Congress of the European Association for Palliative Care, 6–9 December, Barcelona, Spain, 74–5.

Horroks, P. (1986) The components of a comprehensive district service for elderly people. *Age and Ageing*, 15: 321–42.

Ingleton, C. and Faulkner, A. (1994) *Quality Assurance in Palliative Care*, occasional paper no. 14. Sheffield: Trent Palliative Care Centre.

MacDonald, N. (1994) Educational programmes in pain and palliative care. *Journal of Pain and Symptom Management*, 8(6): 348–52.

MacIllmurray, M.B., Gorst, D.W. and Holdcroft, P.E. (1986) A comprehensive system for patients with cancer in a district general hospital. *British Medical Journal*, 292: 669–71.

National Council for Hospice and Specialist Palliative Care (1992) *Quality and Standards*, occasional paper no. 2. London: NCHSPC.

Viladiu, P., Gómez-Batiste, X., Roca, J.M., Lafuerza, A., Alcalde, R., Lozano, A., Borras, J., Beltran, M. and Castellsague, K. (1995) *Dying by Cancer in Catalonia: A Population Study.* Barcelona: Catalan Institute of Oncology.

11 Palliative care in eastern Europe

JACEK ŁUCZAK

The impact of political and economic reforms upon the development of hospice/palliative care

In the 1980s and the beginning of the 1990s, Poland and other central and eastern European post-communist countries, including the Soviet Union, underwent profound political and economic change following the rejection of totalitarianism and the widespread acceptance of reforms leading to democracy and the free market economy. The revolution started in Poland, was taken up by the then Czechoslovakia and by Hungary, finally reaching the cradle of world communism, Russia and the former Soviet Union countries.

The final revolution had long been preceded by national independence movements protesting at the economic situation. The most significant events of that period were the riots, strikes and demonstrations in Berlin, Poznań, Budapest, Prague and, notably, the events on the Polish Baltic coast in which the prolonged strike of shipyard workers in Gdańsk, led by Lech Wałesa, resulted in Solidarity, the first independent trade union, with nearly 10 million members. Further important events or factors in the struggle were the collapse of the Berlin Wall, Gorbachev's conciliatory policies and the epoch-making Round Table talks leading to the first Solidarity-based government, with a mandate for political, economic and social reform.

Health care under totalitarianism had excluded care for terminally ill people. Oncological institutes were few and poorly developed; there was a lack of any palliative care education; health care, generally, was bureaucratic and inefficient. Hence, dying patients and their families had been totally neglected.

However, the bloodless revolution was to have a profound impact upon attitudes in society. It brought to oppressed nations a freedom of political expression and helped to realize individual potentials, so long suppressed. It should be remembered that the Roman Catholic Church had always been a bulwark against Soviet communism. Now, following the overthrow of communism, several church-inspired and secular organizations were set up in a spirit of enthusiasm and hope. Prominent among these new organizations were groups of people calling the attention of society to the needs, hitherto ignored, of suffering and dying people (Drazkiewicz 1989; Cassileth 1995a).

The political and economic reforms were crucial in creating a favourable climate for the growth of palliative and hospice care in post-communist countries. Positive factors included deeply seated ethnic and cultural conditions based upon tradition and family ties. There was also a new spirit and new attitudes which charismatic leaders greatly encouraged. Negative factors, however, comprised poor health care and, particularly, the ignorance and prejudice prevailing in the system at all professional and administrative levels. Another obstacle to progress was widespread poverty.

An important backdrop to these changes was the existence of clear policies for palliative care on the part of the World Health Organization (WHO). In order for these to be realized it has been necessary to recognize and implement WHO's three main objectives: education in palliative care and cancer pain relief; availability of basic analgesics, oral morphine in particular; and legal regulations for licensing palliative care organizations and cancer pain centres (WHO 1990; Foley and Portenoy 1993). These WHO recommendations call for action by governments and health ministries. It therefore remains vital that all three recommendations are implemented comprehensively, and that palliative care and cancer pain relief programmes are given the highest priority (WHO 1990; Foley and Portenoy 1993).

At a more local level, it is also important to note that the introduction of palliative care into Poland and other countries could not have been done without the vigorous help of an informal voluntary hospice movement. The achievements of the pioneering hospice teams in embracing holistic care, in educating professionals and volunteers, as well as the wider society as a whole, cannot be overstated. These pioneers have popularized palliative care, have established its place in national health care programmes, and in so doing have implemented the three important WHO recommendations.

In this chapter, I shall try to summarize a wide-ranging process of development taking place across the whole of eastern Europe. This is a rapidly changing scene and factual information on services in particular countries is likely to become quickly out of date. It is nevertheless important to attempt some sort of overview of the development of palliative care in this part of Europe. In doing so, I have drawn on a considerable quantity of 'grey' literature in the form of newsletters and other documents currently in circulation, as well as personal communications from a wide range of colleagues in several countries. Inevitably, my detailed knowledge is greatest in relation to the situation in Poland, my own country, and this is reflected in the contents of the chapter. I hope nevertheless that my attempted overview proves of benefit to those seeking to develop their understanding of the growth of palliative care in eastern Europe and, indeed, that it may serve as a stimulus to further action and involvement on the part of colleagues elsewhere in the world.

The status of palliative/hospice care in eastern Europe

Bulgaria

Palliative care in Bulgaria was started after two oncologists from the National Cancer Institute in Sofia took part in a course (on psychosocial oncology and palliative care) organized by the European School of Oncology (ESO). They then attended a course organized by the International School for Cancer Care (ISCC) in 1992. The knowledge and skills thus gained led to publications and courses in palliative care in Sofia in 1993. A palliative care service within the Sofia National Cancer Institute is now being established. Booklets on *Cancer Pain Relief* (WHO 1996), *Oral Morphine in Advanced Cancer* (R.G. Twycross) and *Practical Guide to Palliative Medicine* (C. Deckers) have been translated and given to all medical professionals. Articles on palliative care and cancer pain relief were also published in the *Bulgarian Medical Journal* and in the medical journal *The World*.

In 1993, the controlled-release opioids DHC and MST-continus were imported and administered to cancer patients. For 18 months of pre-registration clinical trials 98 patients received DHC and MST-continus. In 1994 these preparations were registered and their consumption gradually increased. Although highly effective and convenient, these medications are very expensive and their use is limited to a small number of selected patients. Liquid injectable morphine and pethidine are actually the most used opioids. In general, there is a trend towards increasing use of opioids. Morphine consumption was 3.65 kg in 1992 and had risen to 25 kg in 1994.

Palliative care is a relatively new approach to overall treatment of cancer patients in Bulgaria. The country is divided into 12 areas and there are 12 oncologic dispensaries, responsible for treatment of cancer and the care of terminally ill people. Bulgaria has 8.5 million inhabitants and 15,000 deaths occur each year from cancer. For example, Sofia district has 1.2 million inhabitants and in 1995 26,700 cancer patients were registered; 660 of them, terminally ill, needed palliative care at home. Sofia district dispensary has a staff of two doctors and three nurses experienced in home care for terminally ill people. Unfortunately no beds are provided from national health authorities for symptom control in medical institutions.

Courses in palliative care are now being organized regularly in Bulgaria. In 1993, the controlled-release opioids DHC and MST-continus were imported from Austria and given to cancer patients, so that in May 1994, the first 100 patients received adequate pain relief for the first time (Gancheva 1994). The introduction of MST continus led to a gradual but significant increase of morphine consumption in Bulgaria from 3.65 kg in 1991 to 25 kg in 1994. Bulgaria has 8.5 million inhabitants and 15,000 deaths each year from cancer. Given the successful achievements so far of Dr Gancheva and others, we can expect further developments in palliative care in Bulgaria.

Czech Republic

According to information given in *Hospice Worldwide*, there are, in the Czech Republic, seven organized or planned hospice/palliative care units (Hospice Information Service 1995). Most teams provide home care. Two home care teams are working in Brno; one of these, based at the University Hospital, is cooperating with the pain control department there. A 21-bed inpatient palliative care unit has been established at Babice. Inpatient units or home care services are to be set up at Hradec Kralove, Kamenici and Trebic. The Strasburk Hospice in Prague has 20 in-patient beds; home and day care started in 1996. All drugs recommended by the WHO for symptom control/cancer pain relief, including oral morphine, are available in the Czech Republic.

Hungary

The Hungarian Hospice Foundation, registered in 1991, played the leading role in the formation and development of the Hungarian hospice movement. The founders of palliative care here include politicians, oncologists, psychologists and other academics. In 1995 the Hungarian Hospice Association was established; it aims to link hospices to business federations and to educational, publishing and publicity enterprises (Hegedüs 1994; Hungarian Hospice Foundation, personal communication, 1996).

Hungary has a population of 10.34 million. In 1993, 32,201 people died of cancer; Hungary has one of the highest death rates from cancer in Europe.

At present, there are twenty-seven hospice organizations and initiatives in Hungary, including the Hospice for Children in Budapest. Five of them, including those in Budapest, Gyula, Szombathley and Miskolc, have in-patient palliative care units. Most hospices provide home care by professionals and volunteers. The exemplary service in Budapest is run by two physicians, eight nurses, two psychologists, two physiotherapists, one chaplain, thirty-two volunteers and two secretaries.

The Soros Foundation has been instrumental in giving financial assistance to the Hungarian Hospice Foundation, which, with three other hospice organizations, has also been financed, since 1994, by the Department of Social Insurance. The other hospices obtained financial support mainly from the Ministry of Public Welfare and, to some extent, from Social Insurance, which department recently announced a competition for the development of hospice activity (Hungarian Hospice Foundation, personal communication, 1996).

From 1991 onwards, the teaching of hospice philosophy was initiated by the National Alliance of Cancer Patients and the Hungarian Psychological Society. In 1993, there was a successful congress on palliative care; and training programmes for nurses and doctors were also organized in October of that year. In 1994, the Hungarian Hospice Foundation implemented a multidisciplinary, nationwide educational programme in palliative/hospice care. This programme consists of:

- foundation course;
- vocational training for doctors, nurses, physiotherapists, volunteers;
- advanced courses for hospice trainers; foreign lecturers; training abroad.

Since 1995, the Hungarian Hospice Association has been responsible for the continuation of this programme, now linked with the Budapest Semmelveis Medical University and the Health Continuation Course Institute. The latter organization has accepted the hospice nurse training programme as one of its officially recognized courses. Information about hospice courses is distributed to hospitals and universities by the Ministry of Public Welfare. Any doctor, medical student, nurse, social worker, psychologist or member of a relevant profession may be admitted to these official courses and receive certificates. In Hungary, it is not however possible to take an independent medical examination in palliative care.

Since 1994, cooperation between the Hungarian Hospice Foundation and the University Department of Palliative Care in Poznań, Poland, has brought about the beginnings of a postgraduate research and education programme in Hungary.

Opioid analgesics, including MST continus and adjuvant drugs, are available free of charge to cancer patients in Hungary. Analgesics are administered according to WHO guidelines contained in the 1986 booklet, *Cancer Pain Relief*, which was translated into Hungarian in 1992, with supplementary information from *Pain Killers and Adjuvants*, by Borsi Mate (Hungary). Established in 1989, the Cancer Pain Relief Unit of the National Cancer Institute offers a clinical service for 2000–3000 cancer patients in pain every year (Embey-Isztin 1993). This unit also offers postgraduate courses paying special attention to cancer pain treatment and practical training to cancer pain treatment and practical training. In 1994, the consumption of morphine in Hungary was 50 kg orally and 7.9 kg by injection.

Hospice activity in Hungary does not conform to existing health legislation and this gives rise to certain problems. For example, any doctor can prescribe morphine to a patient for a period of ten days but, if the patient remains at home, only the same doctor may prescribe a new dose. The effect of this protocol is that some hospice doctors are not allowed to control the palliative therapy of hospice patients in the home situation. A new health regulation is in course of preparation, which should amend these protocols according to recommendations made by the Hungarian Hospice Foundation (personal communication, 1996).

Factors supporting the growth of a dynamically developing hospice movement since 1992 include the activities of the Hungarian Hospice Foundation and the Hungarian Hospice Association, many enthusiastic professionals and volunteers, good public education and the financial support of the Ministry of Welfare and Social Insurance. The next important task of the Hungarian Hospice Foundation is to work out a national programme of palliative care development which is acceptable to the government. This programme should include standards of care, quality assessment, financial strategies, principles of education and organization. It must also incorporate recommendations for mandatory training in palliative care for medical students. The cooperation of international organizations such as WHO, the European Association for Palliative Care (EAPC), ISCC, hospice charities, hospice-twinning projects and pharmaceutical companies is an important aspect of this process.

Latvia

Christel Pakarinen (1995) from Kiruna, Finland, has described palliative care developments in Latvia. Her article, 'Starting palliative care', focuses on two important issues: the refusal of most doctors in Latvia to discuss death with patients, and the willingness of a group of doctors and nurses from a new private clinic to be trained in palliative care. This training is to be provided by Pirkanmaan Hospice in Tampere, Finland. The clinic group is fund-raising with a view to starting a hospice programme and widespread discussions are underway to help bring about the organization of a course in palliative care for doctors and nurses. It is envisaged that such a course would cover a range of topics, including the work of hospices and pain clinics, medication for symptom control, ethical issues, home care and caring for families and staff.

Another important initiative, the Hospice of Latvia, was created by the Department of Oncology at Gailezera Slimnica Hospital, in Riga (Hergt 1995). Plans are now afoot with MOST (Mission Opportunities Short

Term) in Michigan, USA, to arrange training in US hospices for Latvian doctors and nurses.

Lithuania

The Lithuanian palliative care movement was founded after a successful two-day seminar organized in Kaunas in October 1993 in association with palliative care specialists from Norway. In 1994, the first (21-bedded) hospice in Lithuania was established in Kaunas, followed by the opening of the Pain Clinic at Vilnius University Santariskes Hospital and a palliative medicine service at the Lithuanian Cancer Institute. In 1995, a hospice was set up in another Vilnius hospital; and the Lithuanian Society for Palliative Medicine was started, which now has 50 active members (Poniskaitiene 1995).

There are six members of staff at the Vilnius pain clinic: two anaesthetists, one psychologist, one part-time neurologist and two nurses. During the course of the first year, the staff cared for 274 patients. Continuous subcutaneous infusion of morphine was given to 50 per cent of patients. Oral morphine is not available in Lithuania (Poniskaitiene 1995).

The team at the palliative medicine centre consists of oncologists and several volunteer nurses, caring for both inpatients and outpatients with advanced cancer. Efforts are made to care for patients in their own homes and home calls are made when needed. Physicians from this centre provide information about palliative care to the medical profession, by visiting various hospitals throughout the country, by giving lectures and involving local health services.

The population of Lithuania is 3.72 million. In 1995, 7500 patients died of cancer; 66 per cent of cancer patients died in the year following diagnosis. Important future plans are to

- change policies regarding the availability and prescription of weak opioids and oral morphine;
- achieve funding for the provision of hospice care (the health service is under-funded because of the crisis in the Lithuanian national economy);
- improve information about, and education in, palliative care with the support of international organizations such as EAPC, ISCC and the Soros Foundation; visits by international lecturers would be appreciated;
- procure standard textbooks and other literature on palliative care and pain management (requested particularly by the Vilnius Palliative Care Centre).

Poland

Despite the political and economic reforms, the old communist system of health care is substantially still in place in Poland (Łuczak 1993a; Łuczak *et al.* 1995). However, the system of funding has recently passed from central government to the regional and community health authorities; family medicine – a new specialization for doctors – has been introduced; and it is planned to increase the number of beds for chronic patients. There are twelve regional cancer centres – large new centres were recently opened at Bydgoszcz and Warszawa – but access for patients who require palliative radiotherapy or palliative chemotherapy in the other 37 Polish regions is often difficult to achieve. Oncology is a speciality and programmes of oncology are implemented in the student syllabus of twelve university schools of medical science. However, palliative medicine is in the syllabus of only seven of them.

The population of Poland is 38 million. In 1993, 76,000 patients died from cancer: 44,000 in hospital and 32,000 at home. There are 171 hospice and palliative care units in the country as a whole; of these, 66 are independent voluntary hospice teams and 105 are NHS palliative care services. There are 162 home care services and over 100 pain and palliative care outpatient clinics, all working closely with home care services. There are 30 inpatient units, either freestanding or within hospitals; these comprise 250 inpatient beds, 20 support teams, 12 day care centres and 15 bereavement services. Overall, specialist palliative care is provided for 25 per cent of patients with advanced incurable cancer, but in certain places the percentage availability is higher: Poznań (80 per cent), Sieradz (70 per cent). In Gdańsk, Kraków, Wrocław, Włocławek, Bydgoszcz, Częstochowa, Toruń and Szczecin the percentage is 50 per cent.

There are many registered and non-registered charities in Poland, either secular or founded by the Roman Catholic Church. All provide home care; a few offer inpatient care, day care and bereavement services. Most of these hospices provide education. Some have a contractual link with their local health authorities, from which they receive funding, generally for salaries. Other funding is raised in the community. National Health Service units provide hospice or palliative care in the same way as the independent hospices.

In recent years a significant contribution to palliative and hospice care developments has been made by the Catholic charitable organization, Caritas. Caritas has funded a hospice home care service in Lódz and is supporting a freestanding hospice in Tarnów. The organization has also funded mobile hospice home care teams, especially in Opole. More than a hundred nurses and doctors working in these services took part in the foundation course in palliative care organized in 1996 in Opole by the Poznań Department of Palliative Care.

The exemplary model developed in the Department of Palliative Care, Poznań University of Medical Sciences, consists of a pain clinic, palliative home care service, inpatient unit and bereavement service. This model is being reproduced in other hospitals – in six instances in oncological centres – or in community-based teams within the structure of outpatient services (Łuczak 1990; Łuczak et al. 1990; Łuczak 1993; Łuczak et al. 1995). The community satellite model developed by Professor Edmund Orszański in Sieradz is an exemplary rural model of palliative care and has been implemented in other, similar, regions (Łuczak et al. 1995).

Some hospitals have wards specifically designed for palliative care which supplement the work of the pain and palliation clinics and home care services. Units sited in acute hospitals also provide supportive care for hospice patients. A few units provide day care and bereavement services. All of them employ both paid and volunteer professionals giving home care. In addition to these, there is a Sue Ryder Home at a newly opened oncological centre at Bydgoszcz, a children's hospice in Warszawa and a hospice for AIDS patients at Rembertów.

In three of the seven university schools of medical science where palliative medicine is taught, there are palliative medicine teaching units within medical faculties; in such cases, the teaching team works in the local hospice or palliative care service.

Nevertheless, in Poland, some myths still prevail. Many still feel that the truth should often be evaded in the doctor–patient relationship (Corr 1991; Łuczak et al. 1995) – a belief actually shared by a professor of oncology. There is also the myth of morphine abuse as well as ill-founded beliefs in the superiority of pethidine as an analgesic for cancer pain relief (Luczak et al. 1995). There are also obstacles: in a city where palliative care is well developed and the staff highly skilled, the Rector of the Medical Faculty decided not to include palliative medicine in the syllabus for medical students. However, there have been advances in medical and lay education which, it is hoped, will change the attitudes of doctors, professors of medicine, health care officials and politicians. Books and articles have been published about death and terminal care and the hospice philosophy, showing the benefit to patients' families. Programmes have also been broadcast on radio and television.

When looking at the overall development of hospice and palliative care in Poland it is possible to identify three key phases.

Early phase: the voluntary hospice movement (1981–8)

The formation of the Society of Friends of the Sick Hospice, in Kraków, in 1981, was the first hospice in central and eastern Europe – at that time under the communist regime – but had been preceded by many preparatory attempts in the early 1970s. According to the charismatic leader, Haline Bortnowska, journalist, philosopher and inspiration of the Polish hospice movement: 'The beginnings of the Kraków hospice were not totally imported from abroad and from the West' (Drazkiewics 1989; Sikorska

1991). The surge of interest in hospice ideas was strongly associated with the Kraków Diocesan Synod (1971–8). During that period, a group of parishioners of the Lord's Ark Church in Nowa Huta-Bienczyce (Nowa Huta is a large industrial district of Kraków, built in the 1960s, during the communist regime) formed a study group. The group composed ordinary citizens, employers of a nearby foundry and their families, and one doctor, who discussed the problem of 'how to find a clear expression of our desire for effective compassion'. This discussion group looked at ways of expressing love for the suffering, the sick and, especially, the dying (Kujawska-Tenner 1990). Influenced by Halina Bortnowska, they formed a group of volunteers providing care for sick and dying patients at a local hospital at Nowa Huta. Those volunteers established the first informal hospice team in Poland (Kujawska-Tenner 1990). Their work was based on principles of holistic care, including the kind of respect for the dignity of the dying person developed by Nurse Hanna Chrzanowska, the founder of Kraków's home care nursing centre in the late 1960s. The impact of their work was felt by Heinrich Pera, a Catholic priest from the former German Democratic Republic. Father Pera joined the Nowa Huta group and lovingly tended the sick as a chaplain and lay volunteer. The group practised approaches to the care of dying people that were in clear opposition to the non-caring communist doctrine (Drazkiewicz 1989; Kujawska-Tenner 1990; Sikorska 1991).

The Nowa Huta hospice team established basic principles and objectives and a future model for Polish hospices that would suit local communities. Members drew on their experiences as caregivers and used a model of home care deriving from traditional rural culture, that is, to care to the end of life. Poor and overcrowded housing conditions, however, particularly in industrial areas, made home care very difficult. The Nowa Huta team contacted Dame Cicely Saunders, the British founder of the modern hospice movement. The visit of Dame Cicely to Poland in 1978, and her meetings with people interested in hospice care in Warszawa, Gdańsk and Kraków, stimulated the plan to build a freestanding hospice in Kraków (Kujawska-Tenner 1990).

Initially, the founding group intended to make the hospice a part of the parish church, and were supported in this aim by the Solidarity trade union at the Lenin Foundry. However, the hospice project, which was one of Solidarity's demands, met with opposition from the city and church authorities, so the group went along a different legal route and established an independent charitable society (Kujawska-Tenner 1990).

The promulgation of martial law in December 1981, and the entrenchment of the communist regime, delayed the start of the St Lazarus freestanding hospice in Kraków until 1991. Instead, the team concentrated its efforts on the development of a volunteer training programme, started in 1983, and a home care service of voluntary doctors and nurses and lay caregivers. In 1984, the first patient was offered home care and this was also the first time that oral morphine was successfully used (Kujawska-Tenner 1990). Another voluntary home care service, the Hospicjum Pallottinum, was established in Gdańsk in 1984 by a Pallotine priest, Father Eugeniusz Dutkiewicz, who used his long experience of serving patients who were abandoned and dying at home or in hospital. In this he was supported by Professor Joanna Muszkowska-Pension, who, as a director of a medical department, was familiar with the problems presented by the discharge from hospital of patients with progressive illnesses who had no support thereafter. Professor Muszkowska-Pension gained experience of palliative care in the UK and brought back some educational materials. An important contribution was also made by Dr Ewa Stolarczyk, a radiotherapist, who combined her hospital work with directing the Gdansk home care team. Dr Stolarczyk reinforced her skills in palliative care through a placement at a UK Hospice (St Christopher's, London). Another catalytic factor was Dame Cicely Saunders's visit in 1978, which motivated people to make use of the hospice philosophy she so vividly expounded (Drazkiewicz 1989; Sikorska 1991).

The Gdańsk home care team, comprising doctors, nurses, students, priest, psychologists and lay persons, all working voluntarily, spent many hours a day caring for elderly, disabled, sick and dying patients. This team helped to start other hospices, including St Jan Kanty Hospice, in Poznań (Drazkiewicz 1989; Łuczak 1993a). This hospice from the very first based its service upon the Church, interpreting its role as fulfilling the Church's mission. Its underlying principle, to preserve the unity and faith of the church, is observed by all who work for the hospice. Father Ryszard Mikolajczak, the hospice director, was co-organizer of the first European conference for hospice chaplains, held in Poznań in 1992.

Second phase (1988–93)

Even well-organized hospice teams, using only non-paid caregivers, are unable to provide home care for more than 50–100 patients a year, a small proportion of those in need of palliative care. Between 1981 and 1990, 40 voluntary teams cared for 2500 patients.

With this in mind, the hospice pioneers of the late 1980s set to working out a community programme which would be much more widely available to patients. This was linked to a programme of fund-raising and education involving both the NHS and the voluntary hospice movement (Zylicz 1991; Łuczak 1993a; Łuczak et al. 1995).

The first outcome of this planning was the pain clinic and palliative home care team started by the author in 1987 at the University Oncological Hospital, Poznan (Łuczak et al. 1990; Łuczak et al. 1995). This was followed by the palliative medicine clinic created in 1989 in Gdańsk; a palliative care service organized by the District Railway Hospital in Niwka, near Poznań; and the rural model of palliative care organized in the Sieradz district, to which reference has been made (Łuczak *et al.* 1995). The Poznań model has now been replicated in several settings: Kraków, Włocławek, Częstochowa, Toruń, Szczecin, Kielce, Walbrzych, Bydgoszcz, Zamosc, Radom, Łodź, Slupsk, Suwalki, and in many other towns and cities (Łuczak *et al.* 1995).

In 1987, the pain relief clinic and home care team (now a department) was started at the Department of Oncology at the Karol Marcinkowski University of Medical Sciences in Poznań. In its first six months, this team, under the leadership of the author, cared for 22 patients in their own homes. This great impact on the development of palliative care also owes much to Malgorzata Okupny, a junior doctor working as an assistant in the palliative care service. She graduated in 1989 from an ISCC course in Oxford and transferred the new modern system of palliative care – including the WHO guidelines and patients' charts – to Poznań. In 1988, the team of two doctors, two nurses, a social worker, a priest and lay caregivers, all working voluntarily, and using their private cars for patient transport, cared for 88 patients. The number of patients increased to 1040 in 1994 (Łuczak *et al.* 1990; Łuczak 1993a; Łuczak *et al.* 1995).

The Poznań unit was the first palliative care service in Poland to be organized within the NHS structure and supported by a specially created charitable society, the Aleksander Lewinski and Antonina Mazur Association for the alleviation of suffering in cancer patients. This exemplary service, developed according to principles originally set out by Ventafridda (Łuczak *et al.* 1990; Łuczak 1993a), was complemented by a seven-bed palliative ward in 1990, a bereavement service in 1991 and an intervention team in 1993. All these services are combined into a university department for palliative care, and provide continuous care for patients with advanced incurable cancer. In 1995, the multidisciplinary home care team consisting of doctors, well-educated nurses, psychologists, social workers, physiotherapists, a chaplain and lay caregivers took care of approximately 1100 patients, 90 per cent of these died at home and the remainder in a palliative care ward. The team is also providing palliative care to terminally ill children and adolescents. In Poznań, a city of 588,000 inhabitants, 1540 people died of cancer in 1994. There has been a hundredfold increase in the consumption of oral morphine – about 10 kg per 1 million persons – compared with that in the pre-hospice period (Łuczak *et al.* 1995).

Following the courses and training in UK hospices of Poznań doctors and nurses, an academic link was forged, in 1991, between Sir Michael Sobell House in Oxford and the Department of Palliative Care in Poznań. This academic link facilitated the organization of foundation and advanced courses for doctors and nurses, with prominent speakers from the UK; it also encouraged the extension and improvement of undergraduate and postgraduate education in Poland and eastern Europe, together with the development of research (Łuczak *et al.* 1992; Łuczak *et al.* 1995).

The first informal care team in the Sieradz region was established in 1989. Only a few patients received hospice care in the early stages. In 1990, the Association of Hospice Care of the Sieradz Region was registered. Its main aim was to establish home care teams in all towns in this region of 412,000 inhabitants. In 1992, newly created teams in Wieluń, Zdunska Wola, Łask, Poddebice and Złoczew cared for 160 patients, rising to 260 patients in 1993 and 413 patients in 1994. By the end of 1995, a further increase in patient numbers was noted, covering up to 70 per cent of all those who were terminally ill. Established in 1994, the hospice care ward in Sieradz Hospital carries out inpatient treatment for those patients for whom home care is almost impossible. The inpatient care is supplemented by day care and a bereavement service. After the hospital ward had been operational for a year, it was found that with good home care, eight palliative hospital beds were sufficient for the whole region. There are 73 members of staff working in the hospice ward and in the home care teams, 27 employed full-time and 46 working voluntarily. Average patient time in home care is 49 days and in the hospice ward 14 days (Łuczak *et al.* 1995).

The rural satellite teams regularly meet with the 'parent' unit, which provides outstanding education. All the district nurses and district doctors in Sieradz city and province are trained in palliative care; and the co-operation between rural palliative home care services and local primary care teams is very good.

In the Sieradz region, the dissemination of hospice principles has been led by Professor Edmund Orszański, who founded the model of hospice care in the region, a model which has now been replicated elsewhere. It is based on the assumption care of the patient should be made as local as possible, thus ensuring quicker and better help. This is important, since one of the main obstacles in Poland to effective home care is lack of transport.

In 1991, the initiatives of a temporary council consisting of active hospice physicians appointed by the Polish Ministry of Health and Welfare, led to the implementation of palliative/hospice care in the programme of the Ministry's Department of Health Care, and to government funding for hospice/palliative care services. The funding rose from US$0.06 million in 1991 to US$10 million in 1996. This degree of financial support allowed for the preparation of contracts between independent hospices and regional health authorities. However, funding from the NHS is still insufficient, salaries are very low and caregivers have to use their own cars, often without reimbursement. Many units, therefore, have to raise additional funds in their own communities (Łuczak *et al.* 1995).

Third phase (1993–5)

Besides state financial support, there are now other sources of funding. There is support from charitable institutions and local initiatives have also been successful, notably in Kraków, Warszawa (Oncological Hospice), Bydgoszcz and Poznań (Palliative Care Society). There is support in the UK for education, from the Polish Hospices Fund, soon to be assisted by the Batory Foundation. There is now a great deal of education in palliative care for professionals, volunteers and the public. All this activity has stimulated a huge development in palliative/hospice care in the period from 1993 to 1995. There has been a threefold increase in the number of units and a twofold increase in the consumption of oral morphine (Łuczak *et al.* 1995).

Financial and organizational assistance

The current work of several Polish and foreign organizations merits special attention.

- The Polish National Council for Palliative and Hospice Care – of which the author is chairman – was established on 25 October 1993 as a body affiliated to the Ministry of Health and Welfare. The 12-person council comprises pioneers in, and organizers of, hospice and palliative care. The Council's tasks include making recommendations, consulting, advising, qualifying and coordinating organizational activities as well as supervising the medical and economic status of hospice and palliative care in Poland. The Council's activities are based on cooperation with the Ministry of Health, with chief provincial physicians, with heads of local hospice/palliative care units, and with regional advisers chosen by local hospice care councils to exercise delegated ministerial authority (Łuczak *et al.* 1995).
- The Forum of the Independent Hospice Movement (ORFM), which represents the voluntary hospice movement, was founded in 1991. It is a meeting place for all independent hospices. It is autonomous and helps its member units to carry out their aims (Łuczak 1993b; Łuczak *et al.* 1995).
- The Aleksander Lewinski and Antonina Mazur Polish Society of Palliative Care was established in 1990 in Poznań (Łuczak 1993a). Branches of the society have been set up in 11 regions of the country and the membership now exceeds 400. Its activities include:
  - propagating hospice philosophy and fund-raising;
  - organizing various forms of education in palliative/hospice care: meetings, courses, conferences;
  - research in palliative medicine;
  - cooperating with the European Association for Palliative Care (EAPC).

Several foreign units or organizations are assisting in the development of palliative and hospice care in Poland.

- The Polish Hospices Fund, administered by Gillian Petrie Hunter and chaired by Muir Hunter QC, a charitable organization in the UK provides outstanding administrative and financial support for Polish palliative and hospice teams, mainly for the education of doctors and nurses in British hospices (Petrie Hunter 1992; Łuczak 1993b; Łuczak et al. 1995; Petrie Hunter 1995).
- Since 1991 Sir Michael Sobell House in Oxford, UK, has been collaborating with the Department of Palliative Care in Poznań. This academic link, partly supported by the British Council, has resulted in the organization of many advanced courses for doctors and nurses in Poland (Łuczak 1993a; Łuczak et al. 1995). The International School for Cancer Care (ISCC, finances scholarships for leading Polish hospice doctors and special training courses in the UK (Twycross 1992; Łuczak et al. 1995).
- St Christopher's Hospice, London, cooperates with St Lazarus Hospice in Kraków and provides education, information and materials to Kraków and other units (Kujawska-Tenner 1990; Forrester 1991).
- The National Council for Hospice and Specialist Palliative Care Services, UK, provides information and educational materials.

Education

In Poland, a cancer pain relief programme is included in the education/training programme of palliative medicine (Łuczak et al. 1995). Undergraduate teaching comprises: palliative medicine/care courses implemented in varying degrees in the curricula of medical students (8–33 hours for the course; 2–6 hours designated for cancer pain) in seven of the eleven university schools of medical sciences. In some university schools, palliative care topics are incorporated in the curricula for nursing, pharmacy, dentistry and theology students, and in a few secondary schools and schools for social workers.

Postgraduate teaching courses and training are available for:

- family physicians and district nurses;
- oncologists;
- nurses, doctors, and staff of hospice/palliative care services.

Volunteer education in varying forms is given in all hospice and palliative care services and a model programme has been developed in Kraków and Poznań. In addition, individual hospices organize their own educational programmes. For example, in Gdańsk Hospice there are courses on psychosocial issues for nurses working in palliative care; foundation courses for doctors and nurses; and the introduction of palliative medicine/care into the curriculum of medical students. Whereas Kraków Hospice provides foundation courses for doctors, nurses and volunteers; courses on lymphoedema; courses with input from nurses from St Christopher's Hospice, London; and a 45-hour course in the Nursing Faculty of the University School for Medical Sciences.

The Department of Palliative Care at Poznań University School of Medical Sciences also runs an undergraduate and postgraduate programme consisting of

- palliative medicine/care courses, based on curricula developed in Canada, complementing existing curricula for medical students (30 hours); nursing students (50 hours); pharmacy students (10 hours); dentistry students (6 hours); and theology students (6 hours);
- 80-hour courses for students at secondary nursing schools;
- 8-hour courses for social workers;
- foundation courses/practical training (15 per year) for doctors, nurses and volunteers, attended by over 7000 participants;
- 60-hour course of tuition and practical training for family doctors;
- advanced courses for doctors and nurses in English (two per year) and conferences attended by international speakers;
- diploma courses with extending programme for doctors and nurses working in palliative care/hospice teams (programme is developing);
- educational activities for eastern Europe;
- a 50-hour course for volunteers;
- a broad programme of public education, in conjunction with the Polish Society for Palliative Care (Łuczak et al. 1992; Łuczak 1993b; Łuczak et al. 1995).

Research activity includes topics on pain and symptom management, the introduction of new drugs, the assessment of patients' needs and the quality of life of terminally ill patients, family education and spiritual issue.

In Warszawa, the first Polish hospice for children was founded in 1994. Teachers from this unit, led by Dr Tomasz Dangel, give two to four courses a year on pain management and hospice care for children.

Public education is effected in various ways by

- most hospice/palliative care units;
- Society for Palliative Care and the Department of Palliative Care in Poznań, by means of booklets, information and educational materials;
- National Council for Palliative and Hospice Care Services;
- Ministry of Health and Welfare;
- journalists (newspapers, TV and radio) cooperating with various services or organizations.

A prerequisite of pain management and palliative care at home is a good family–patient understanding and involvement; advisory manuals for families are very valuable in this process. Many units therefore provide families with practical advice, training and support, booklets and printed material.

National policies for palliative care/cancer pain relief

The National Council for Palliative and Hospice Care Services and ORFM (Forum of the Independent Hospice Movement) and the Polish Society of Palliative Care have all been crucial to the development of national guidelines for palliative care by the Ministry of Health, and of national policies for cancer pain relief.

In accordance with Polish health services law, which entitles citizens to *die in dignity and peace*, the government is obliged to provide support for palliative and hospice care services.

In 1994, the Ministry of Health approved the guidelines for a cancer pain relief programme according to WHO (1986, 1990a) principles; 160,000 copies of a booklet on cancer pain relief – written by Professor J. Kujawska-Tenner, Professor J. Łuczak, Dr M. Okupny, Dr A. Kotlińska and Dr T. Dangel and recommended by the Ministry of Health – were sent, free of charge, to all Polish doctors, district nurses and pharmacists. In addition:

- *Principles of Pain Relief* (WHO 1990b), translated by Dr Zbigniew Zylicz, and *Cancer Pain Relief and Palliative Care* (WHO 1990a), translated by Professor Janina Kujawska-Tenner, were posted to all hospice medical directors.
- *Therapeutics in Terminal Cancer* by Dr Robert G. Twycross (Twycross and Lack 1990) was translated into Polish by Dr Ewa Stolarczyk and Professor Julian Stolarczyk.
- *Lectures in Palliative Care*, also by Robert Twycross, was translated into Polish by Dr M Krajnik; and both are recommended for undergraduate and postgraduate education.
- In 1994 and 1995, all leading palliative care services were provided by the Polish Hospices Fund with a copy of the *Oxford Textbook of Palliative Medicine* (Doyle *et al*. 1993), and subscriptions to *Palliative Medicine* and *Progress in Palliative Care*.
- The Ministry of Health nominated Professor Jacek Łuczak as the national specialist in palliative medicine and declared palliative medicine a new medical specialty in Poland (Łuczak *et al*. 1995).
- Morphine consumption rose nationally from 87 kg in 1992 to 137 kg in 1994.
- The fifth edition of the Polish Pharmacopeia, published in 1993, changed the policy relating to morphine prescription and allowed physicians to prescribe, on a single prescription, up to 1 g of oral or 0.6 g of injectable morphine.

The availability of all analgesics and adjuvant drugs recommended by WHO is very good (WHO 1990a), including tramadol, oral immediate-release morphine and MST-continus. MST-continus will, in the near future, be available free of charge to cancer patients. New policies are being prepared which will allow physicians to prescribe unlimited doses of opioids.

Future programme

Looking back on the 15-year history of hospice and palliative care development, started originally by a few enthusiasts in Kraków, the city in which St Lazarus Hospice, a 36-bed modern freestanding hospice will be opened in 1996 (Kujawska-Tenner 1990), many hospice pioneers are happy about the huge achievements so far, but have some concerns about the future. There is a need for more units to be established in order to give patients greater access to palliative care; the quality of patient care must also be continually improved.

The programme of palliative and hospice care development to the year 2000, worked out by the National Council for Palliative and Hospice Care Services, has been accepted by the Ministry of Health and Welfare (Łuczak *et al.* 1995). The programme includes:

- Standards of palliative and hospice care.
- An increase in the number of inpatient units by 500–750 beds by the year 2000; an increasing number of day care centres, support teams, bereavement services; and more small home care community teams based on the Sieradz satellite model.
- The establishment of palliative medicine sections in every university school of medical sciences; the implementation of palliative medicine as a separate discipline with examinations in the student syllabus in every medical school; and an educational programme for family doctors, oncologists and nurses.
- The establishment of the Hospice Pallium in Poznań, a university unit providing research and nationwide education for Poland and for eastern Europe, to include a programme of specialization in palliative medicine for doctors and palliative care for nurses. This educational and research programme will be developed in conjunction with other leading centres in Poland, and with palliative services in Kraków, Gdańsk, Bydoszcz, Katowice, Lublin, Łodz, Sieradz, Szczecin, Wrocław, Warszawa, Włocławek and Zamosc; there will be close cooperation with Sir Michael Sobell House, Oxford (a WHO-collaborating centre in palliative care), with St Christopher's Hospice, London, with the Palliative Medicine Section at the University of Sheffield, with Princess Alice Hospice, Esher, with the Sloan-Kettering Memorial Cancer Center, New York, with the

Cleveland Clinic Palliative Care Foundation and Marie Curie Cancer Care, UK.
- The development of a system of evaluating the quality of care.

To achieve these goals, close co-operation should be guaranteed between the Council for Hospice and Palliative Care Services, the regional and local branches of that Council, the Palliative Care Association, the Forum of the Polish Hospice Movement, the Ministry of Health and Social Welfare, local health authorities and rectors of university schools of medical sciences. The outstanding support of international organizations or charities such as WHO, EAPC, ISCC, Polish Hospices Fund, the Batory Foundation and pharmaceutical companies will no doubt be of continuing importance in this process.

Romania

An article 'A hospice for Brasov' (Perolls 1992) contained a report from the first Romanian Conference on palliative care. Perolls also described the Casa Sperantei project, which was to start in a small ward at the Brasov Oncology Hospital and act as a training centre in palliative care for doctors and nurses. According to information provided by an oncologist from Mures, Dr R. Lupsa, who attended the Vienna Satellite Symposium on Cancer Pain Relief in eastern Europe in 1995 and the Poznań advanced doctors' course in October 1995, there are still many obstacles in Romania to the delivery of appropriate care for terminally ill patients. A serious problem is the lack of immediate-release oral morphine, even though MST-continus will be available. Dr Lupsa has been introducing seminars in cancer pain relief and palliative treatment into the oncology syllabus in undergraduate medical education.

Russia

Hospice and palliative care in Russia started in the early 1990s and is developing despite the difficult economic situation, insufficient funding for health care, poor organization of the public health service, a lack of specialist oncological centres in many regions, a poor standard of hospital facilities and a shortage of drugs and medical equipment: all deficits resulting from the long years of the communist system, which was no respector of human rights. The old communist system of health care, which still exists in Russia and the countries of the former Soviet Union, is very difficult to change, given the economic underdevelopment and the unstable political situation (Gumley 1993; Cassileth 1995a, 1995b; Cerquone 1995).

An important role in the creation and development of the hospice movement in Russia was played by Russian émigré, the late Victor Zorza, a journalist and writer. The first Russian hospice, Lahkta in St Petersburg, was opened in 1992 through Zorza's efforts. He also initiated important Russian and British hospice links and helped to implement other Russian hospice programmes. There are now 13 hospices in Russia and the British-Russian Hospice Society coordinates interest in several projects (Gumley 1993; Karajaeva 1994; Cerquone 1995).

There are six home care services and six inpatient units in the republic – a total of 120 beds. Four of them belong to oncological centres and three more programmes are planned for 1996. In St Petersburg, there are two inpatient hospices (a total of 55 beds) and three home care services. The pain clinic and palliative care department of the Regional Oncology Hospital in Tyjuman (western Siberia) consists of a 10-bed unit, outpatient service and consultancy service. Dr Vladimir Bryuzgin, head of the outpatient clinic in the Centre of Cancer Pain Control in the Russian Academy of Sciences, is involved in planning a pain relief team in Moscow. The Herald of Hope home care team and a self-help group is also operating in Moscow.

In a letter written to the editor of *Progress in Palliative Care* (Frampton 1995), one of the doctors teaching on the first course in palliative care in the former Soviet Union briefly evaluated the impact on hospice development in Russia of ISCC courses and the training offered by Macmillan nurse tutors and British hospice doctors. A most important factor in such developments is the educational programme in palliative care provided by St Christopher's Hospice, London, by Sir Michael Sobell House, Oxford, and by Chelmsford Hospice. Of great educational value also was a five-day ESO conference, at Moldova in 1993, on palliative care and cancer pain relief. Locally organized courses, attended by Russian hospice workers and British visitors, have also helped to improve patient–doctor communication.

In the USA, too, there is an increasing concern for the plight of adults and children suffering from cancer in Russia and Belarus. Two issues of *Hospice* (journal of the US National Hospice Organization: NHO) have published reports of a visit made by members of the NHO to Russian and Polish hospices in May 1995. After that visit, Mr John Mahony, the leader of the delegation, stated that US hospices cannot work in isolation, so it is possible the visit may engender American support for Russian hospices under the auspices of the Citizen Ambassador Program of People to People (USA).

Alongside the personal role of Mr Victor Zorza and the education being provided, mostly by British hospices, local initiatives have been taken by enthusiastic professionals and volunteers, supported by local administrators and health authorities. For example, in St Petersburg, the establishment in 1991 of the first hospice, Lomintsewsky Hospice, was made possible with the backing of the Mayor's wife and funding from the district authority. In the Tula region, a hospice was funded from the central budget of the regional health authority (Karajaeva 1994; Cerquone 1995).

Several factors limit the growth of a palliative/hospice care development in Russia. These include:

- lack of national policies for a palliative care/cancer pain relief programme;
- lack of oral morphine and restrictions in prescribing a sufficiency of strong opioids;
- lack of education about the suffering of dying cancer patients among professionals and the general public;
- lack of understanding of hospice philosophy;
- difficult economic situation and insufficient resources for health care;
- poor and bureaucratic organization of the public health service.

There is an urgent need for the British-Russian Society and other newly established national hospice organizations, in collaboration with the Ministry of Health, to formulate a national programme of palliative care development and cancer pain relief, particularly in respect of the availability of oral morphine and other drugs recommended by WHO, and in respect of undergraduate and postgraduate education in palliative care for doctors and nurses. The sustained support of UK hospices and such organizations as WHO and the European Association of Palliative Care will be needed.

Slovakia

The president of the Slovak Society for the Study and Treatment of Pain, Dr Marta Kulichova, who is also the director of the Multidisciplinary Centre of Pain of Martin Faculty Hospital, provided the author with the following important information.

Slovakia has a population of 6 million. The annual death rate from cancer is about 12,000. Since 1994, there has been a department of palliative care in Bratislava. This year, the Hospice Foundation was created in Martin. The availability of all analgesics recommended by the WHO is very good, and includes oral immediate-release morphine; the cost of MST-continus is refunded by medical insurance. Physicians are allowed to prescribe unlimited doses of opioids.

In November 1995, Dr Marta Kulichova chaired the third annual palliative care meeting, Slovak Dialogue on Pain, under the patronage of EAPC.

Conclusions

Despite considerable initiatives and achievements in palliative/hospice care and cancer pain relief in many eastern European countries, still there are some that do not meet WHO standards.

The main reasons for this can be summarized:

- Difficult economic situation, poor distribution of funding; and lack of governmental money for palliative/cancer pain programmes.
- Old-fashioned, inefficient communist health care systems still persisting in many places, particularly at primary care level. District nurses are overworked and underpaid, and many doctors are uneducated in palliative care.
- Lack of national policies for palliative care or cancer pain relief.
- Myths and obstacles: do not tell the truth to patients with incurable disease; fear of morphine addiction; death as a taboo.
- Underdeveloped education in palliative care and cancer pain management.
- Underdeveloped services for palliative care and cancer pain management.
- Problems with basic drug availability: a lack of oral solution and ordinary tablets of morphine in some countries.

These problems are echoed in the Vienna Message, which was worked out by delegates and participants in the Eastern European Forum for Cancer Pain Treatment, 4–8 September 1995, organized as a satellite meeting of the 24th Central European Congress on Anaesthesiology in Vienna. After a long session, participants from Belarus, Bulgaria, the Czech Republic, Hungary, Poland, Romania, Russia and Slovakia made the following statement:

The Vienna Message

Cancer pain treatment and palliative therapy are insufficiently developed in our countries and do not meet WHO standards.
The main reason for this situation is the lack of national policies for cancer pain treatment and palliative care.
WHO standards are not generally followed in our countries, or are met in certain countries only.
Therefore, we hereby appeal for:

1 Organized systems of undergraduate and postgraduate education of students, doctors, nurses and other medical personnel in the fields of pain treatment and palliative therapy.
Educational initiatives should be focused on:
- introducing and observing the principles of the WHO analgesic ladder
- the elimination of irrational opinions or myths related to applications of morphine
- establishing a specialist task force to deal with cancer pain treatment.
2 Establishing institutional structures which could provide for adequate treatment of patients suffering from cancer-related pain.

The system should be based on the national health service with the close cooperation of the voluntary hospice movement, on the lines of the Polish model.

3 Establishing the legal and financial principles to facilitate the availability of indispensable pain-relieving drugs.

The basic drugs for cancer pain treatment should be made available, free of charge. This applies to selected simple analgesics, weak opioids and morphine. Those drugs should be available in the form of oral solution/tablets, preferably in sustained-release form.

The implementation of the programme outlined in the Vienna Message was started in 1995. Physicians and social workers from Hungary, Romania and Slovakia took part in courses on palliative/hospice care in English organized by the Palliative Care Department in Poznań. A group of Hungarian hospice workers undertook clinical training in Polish palliative care units. Polish speakers took part in advanced courses in Budapest and Debrecen and in a symposium on cancer pain relief in Slovakia. In 1996, the Palliative Care Department in Poznań organized further educational sessions for physicians and nurses from Slovakia, Romania, Hungary, Lithuania and the Ukraine.

The improvement in cancer pain management and the increased consumption of oral morphine, recently observed in many eastern European and formerly Soviet countries, has been achieved by an intensive programme of education and by the introduction of controlled-release morphine (MST-continus). This drug is now available in every eastern European country and, in most of them, is free of charge to the patient.

The future development of hospice and palliative care in eastern European countries will be achieved only by following WHO principles. Much more support for local initiatives is needed from leading foreign hospices and palliative care units and from important international organizations such as EAPC, ISCC, ESO and WHO.

Acknowledgements

The editors are extremely grateful to Gillian Petrie Hunter, of the Polish Hospices Fund, for her assistance in the English language editing of this chapter. The editors wish to thank Dr Nikolay Toporov for his contribution to the section on Bulgaria.

Note

Readers interested in learning more about or becoming involved in the developments described in this chapter are invited to contact the author at the address given below:

Professor Jacek Łuczak
Head of Palliative Care Department,
Karol Marcinkowski University of Medical Sciences
Lakowa St 1/2
61–878 Poznań, POLAND
Tel/Fax   0–048–61–530 106

References

Cassileth, B. (1995a) Hospice and palliative care in Russia. *Progress in Palliative Care*, 3(6): 213–14.

Cassileth, B. (1995b) Euthanasia, bioethics and palliative care in Russia. *Progress in Palliative Care*, 3(4): 123–6.

Cerquone, J. (1995) Ending a long, hard winter. *Hospice*, winter 16–19.

Corr, C. (1991) Some impressions of a hospice-related visit to Poland. *Journal of Palliative Care*, 7: 53.

Doyle, D., Hanks, G.W.C. and McDonald, N. (eds) (1993) *Oxford Textbook of Palliative Medicine*. Oxford: Oxford University Press.

Drążkiewicz, J. (1989) O ruchu hospicjów w Polsce (The hospice movement in Poland), in University of Warszawa, *W stronę człowieką umierąjacego* (Towards the dying person). University of Warszawa.

Embey-Isztin, D. (1993) Hungary: status of cancer pain and palliative care. *Journal of Pain and Symptom Management*, 8(6): 420.

Foley, K. and Portenoy, R. (1993) World Health Organisation – International Association for the Study of Pain: Joint Initiatives in Cancer Pain Relief. *Journal of Pain and Symptom Management*, 8(6): 335–9.

Forrester, E. (1991) Poland 1991. *Hospice Bulletin*, London: St Christopher's Hospice, 3, 8.

Frampton, D. (1995) Letter. *Progress in Palliative Care*, 3(6): 213.

Gancheva, A. (1994) Bulgaria: National Reports. *Newsletter EAPC*, 12, summer.

Gumley, V. (1993) News from Russia. *Hospice Bulletin*, London: St Christopher's Hospice, 19: 8.

Hegedüs, K. (1994) Hungary: National Reports. *Newsletter EAPC*, 14, winter.

Hergt, K. (1995) Hospice in Latvia. *Hospice Update* 5(4): 3.

Hospice Information Service (1995) *Hospice Worldwide*. London: St Christopher's Hospice.

Karajaeva. E. (1994) Out of Russia. *Hospice Bulletin*, London: St Christopher's Hospice, 22: 8–9.

Łuczak, J. (1990) Opieka paliatywna u chorych z zaawansowana choroba nowotworową (Palliative care for patients with advanced cancer). *Nowiny Lekarskie*, 2: 37–49.

Łuczak. J. (1993a) Palliative/hospice care in Poland. *Palliative Medicine*, 7: 68–75.

Łuczak, J. (1993b) News and notes. *Progress in Palliative Care*, 2(60): 256.

Łuczak, J., Okupny, M. and Wesołowska, I. (1990) Organizacja I wyniki pracy Zespołu Opiekii Paliatywnej Katedry Onkologii Akademii Medycznej w Poznaniu (The organization and work of the Palliative Care Service of the

Department of Oncology, Poznań University of Medical Sciences). *Nowiny Lekarski*, 1(7): 7–25.

Łuczak, J., Okupny, M. and Wieczorek-Cuske, L. (1992) The programme of palliative medicine in the curriculum of sixth-year medical students in Poland. *Journal of Palliative Care*, 8: 39–43.

Łuczak, J., Sopata, M., Andrzejewska, J., Kotlińksa, A., Leppert, W., Porzucek, I., Bączyk , E.J. and Gołab, M. (1995) Progress in palliative/hospice care in Poland. *Materia Medica Polona*, 27(1): 85–90.

Pakarinen, C. (1995) Starting palliative care (in Latvia). EAPC Newsletter in *European Journal of Palliative Care*, 2(2): N1–2.

Perolls, G. (1992) A hospice for Brasov: a report from the Romanian Hospice Conference. *Hospice Bulletin*, London: St Christopher's Hospice, 18: 1–2.

Petrie Hunter, G. (1992) Polish Hospices Fund: a charity for Poland. *Hospice Bulletin*, London: St Christopher's Hospice, 17: 12.

Petrie Hunter, G. (1993) Penfriends for Poland. *Hospice Bulletin*, London: St Christopher's Hospice, 21: 12.

Petrie Hunter, G. (1995) Polish Hospices Fund: an educational role. *Hospice Bulletin*, London: St Christopher's Hospice, 21: 7.

Poniskaitiene, I. (1995) Lithuania: National Reports. *EAPC Newsletter*, 16, autumn.

Sikorska, W. (1991) The hospice movement in Poland. *Death Studies*, 15: 309.

Twycross, R.G. (1992) International School for Cancer Care. *Hospice Bulletin*, London: St Christopher's Hospice, 15: 3.

Twycross, R.G. and Lack, S. (1990) *Therapeutics in Terminal Cancer*, 2nd edn. Edinburgh: Churchill Livingstone.

World Health Organization (1986) *Cancer Pain Relief*. Geneva: WHO.

World Health Organization (1990a) *Cancer Pain Relief and Palliative Care*, Technical Report Series 804. Geneva: WHO.

World Health Organization (1990b) *Principles of Pain Relief*, Geneva: WHO.

Żylicz, Z. (1991) Palliative care in eastern Europe: a personal view. *Palliative Medicine*, 5: 171.

12 Is hospice a western concept? A personal view of palliative care in Asia

IAN MADDOCKS

The provision of special places and special rituals of care for persons who are dying is common to many cultures and many times; what is new in the contemporary 'hospice movement' is the close involvement of modern medicine. Until the latter part of the twentieth century, care for the dying was either carried out by non-medical persons, or else subsumed within the institutions created to deliver curative medical care, where death was regarded as a failure, and care for dying persons was inappropriately focused on futile interventions or neglected in favour of those considered more likely to survive.

In Europe, up until the time when scientific medicine began to assert its right to provide care for all illness, religious orders were prominent in offering care for dying persons. The main rationale for this care was obedience to Christ's teaching and example, and the emphasis was more on prayer and preparation for the after-life than on comfort in the remaining days of this one. Mother Mary Potter, for example, whose Little Company of Mary has been so prominent in establishing hospices in the modern era, started her work with just that emphasis, including responsibility for physical care as an appropriate extra, but one which did not call for any specially skilled nursing or medical intervention (Wordley 1976).

The hospice initiatives, which extended at an accelerating rate throughout the British Isles, North America and Australasia from the early 1970s, brought together on the one hand Christian tradition and teaching, and on the other hand a growing recognition of the futility and indignity of continuing expensive and intrusive medical treatments for patients in hospital when they were clearly dying. Many of the first hospice buildings were founded by charitable organizations and trusts, drawing upon funds raised within local communities, and they were often closely linked with the ethos and teaching of the Christian Church. Cicely Saunders, for example, has often made it clear that, for her, the outstanding work of St Christopher's Hospice was a response to the example and command of Christ as she understood it.

> Converted from atheism as a gawky young woman, she went through a period of evangelistic fervour, during which she became a Billy Graham counsellor before she finally settled into the Anglican Church. Her faith created much apprehension among doctors when St. Christopher's first opened.
>
> (*Time Magazine* 12 September 1988)

The recent replacement of the term 'hospice' (with its religious associations) by 'palliative care' reflected an increasing secular interest in special care for dying persons, fostered by professionals who looked for a more effective and appropriate response for patients for whom further heroic efforts at cure were clearly futile. At the same time, there has been a falling-away in regular observance of Christian rituals and practices in most western societies, and a growing agnosticism about any promise of an after-life.

Western medicine, since the 1950s, has become more comfortable with discussing the realities of approaching death, 'truth-telling' has become accepted as a major ethical responsibility, counselling has replaced denial as an appropriate response to severe adversity, and individual autonomy has been accorded a prominence which demands a high level of information and a full measure of consent. Medicine has come to accept the skilled interventions of palliative care professionals with gratitude, since they offer an alternative to the otherwise negative message which they felt bound to deliver in the face of imminent death: 'There is nothing more we can do for you'.

Palliative care in Asia

But do these factors operate in Asia? Asia is at once both familiar and strange to western people. The widespread use of European languages reflects both the domination exercised during the brief colonial era and the persuasive influence of modern science and technology; medicine, in particular, in all its many centres of excellence in Asia is recognizably the kind of medicine that is known and practised in the west, and is fluently explained in English. Western clothing, artefacts and styles run through and beside all that is different, exotic, uniquely Asian.

Palliative care, as it develops in Asia, may not follow the western example so closely. Asia does not have the same pervasive tradition of Christian good works, nor would it seem to have accepted, within medicine, the western ethical imperatives of truth-telling and individual autonomy. Its traditions are different. In parts of Asia, houses for dying were recognized (as, for example, in Singapore), but concern appears to have centred on the avoidance of dying in the home with the attendant bad luck that such an event might bring upon a household. In those houses, no specific medical care was offered; the elderly, frail individual waited fatalistically for the end, perhaps in a simple shelter in a street where coffin makers and persons skilled in funereal rites congregated. In Taiwan, Gudmundsdóttir *et al.* (1996), discussing the rituals that follow the death of a child, note that many are explained as ensuring that the ghost is at peace and does not return to plague the family. They noted great variation in practices following death, but a common component was the understanding that the spirit of the dead one could remain active and be in some form of communication, might influence dreams or interfere in family affairs.

It would be foolish to generalize about Asia, and presumptuous to pretend to have grasped anything beyond the superficial or anecdotal in the few weeks travel which I was able to do in several Asian countries in early 1996. On simple epidemiological considerations alone, Asia will need some form of palliative care services. Among its growing proportion of elderly persons the numbers with uncomfortable cancer must be expected to increase markedly, and they will not be able to rely upon the family structures and supports with the confidence assumed in the past. But the patterns along which those services develop will probably be unique to each country and differ from those of the hospice movement of the west. Determining those differences will be the many aspects of Asian life, culture and history which arouse fascination in the westerner.

The cultural and religious context

Most Asian communities are little touched by Christian ideals or practice. Altruism, a virtue in Christian traditions, is less apparent in Asia. A distinguished academic explained to me: 'In the west, you care for your relatives out of love; in Asia we do it as a duty'. That duty will not necessarily extend to needy individuals who are not within the family.

In cultures and religions outside of European Christianity, and commonly in Asia, giving is reciprocal; it involves some return in kind or implies some future obligation. In Hong Kong it was explained that a businessman who has done well may give generously to a hospice, and part of his thinking will be to maintain the luck which has attended his success. Giving also may demonstrate power and influence. In Hatyai, Thailand, it was the King who gave a major donation to build a dormitory at a local temple where cancer patients receiving hospital therapy could shelter; other donors followed, showing their respect for the royal lead.

Westerners observe a stoicism and fatalism operating in the quiet and uncomplaining response to suffering which seems common in Asian patients, but there is also an abiding Asian interest in avoiding bad luck. To talk of bad things is to make their occurrence more likely; death and dying are clearly topics closely linked with bad luck. An Australian hospice volunteer married to a Chinese man recounts that her father-in-law, after visiting the deathbed of a dear friend, spoke to no one on his return home, and avoided her move towards him to comfort his sadness, going immediately to wash, so that no bad luck would fall from him to the rest of the family.

It is notable that many of the early initiatives in palliative care in Asia have occurred within groups owning a Christian allegiance. They have a ready communication with Christian initiatives in Europe, and affirm the work of care for the dying as obedience to the command to 'love one another'. Very impressive efforts are already in place within places such as Hong Kong and Singapore where Christian institutions are relatively strong.

The religions and religious institutions of Asia have their own traditions of offering refuge and care for the disadvantaged, but they vary enormously. Buddhism, in Japan, looks after funeral rituals; Shinto shrines and practices are more important in the celebrations of birth and marriage. In Kyoto, a Buddhist priest who wished to offer some pastoral support for hospital staff complained to me the nurses sent him away, because his presence implied impending death. The Tibetan Book of the Dead (see Mullin 1986) offers a rich tapestry of sayings and suggestions for achieving the best transition into the next life, which ideally will allow the fullest mental awareness and control right up to the moment of death.

Just outside the city of Hatyai in southern Thailand, in a small Buddhist temple, a charismatic abbot, Venerable Thaveep Punyatachowas, assisted by a small group of monks, is caring for 200 persons with AIDS. They live in simple huts, the 'patients' helping each other to construct new dwellings, cook communal food and attend to the needs of the very sick. The abbot offers traditional medicines (including the use of a magic stone used in conjunction with imbibed coconut water) and he scrounges modern drugs to treat infections as best he can. His charges visit the temple for an hour's meditation and chanting twice a day. The spirit of the place is compelling, and the cost of care per person per day is approximately US$3. It is a powerful model of a very different kind of care.

Professional considerations

In most medical practice in Asia it is not regarded as necessary or helpful to share a bad prognosis with the patient. Tong (1994), commenting on the care of Chinese palliative patients in North America, described a conspiracy of silence which prohibits discussion in front of the patient. He quoted a Taiwan study which found that 73 per cent of patients received treatment only from family members. The family became in effect the treating practitioner, moderating all decisions made concerning care. To discuss dying, in that context, was to wish dying on the patient.

The vocations of medicine and nursing may, in Asia, be less informed by the desire to serve suffering humanity – an idealism which we like to assume in our students – and more attuned to achieving status and income (also important to our students, surely!), working by the rule, avoiding any stepping out of line

Dr Kashiwagi (1991), a pioneer of hospice in Japan, where cancer has been the leading cause of death for some years, summarized factors that were limiting the development of hospices and palliative home care programmes in his country. They included a preference for curative treatment, a confidence in hospital care that encouraged a feeling of security, the lack of space or adequate numbers of family to maintain care in the home, the failure of medical insurance to cover home care, and the relative inexperience of professionals in the provision of home care.

Some of these factors are already changing, and the inauguration of the first national palliative care conference in Japan in July 1996 is an indication of a growing professional and official commitment to palliative care.

The intravenous infusion seems to have become, in some parts of Asia, a defining procedure by which to mark that a person is really ill. In Beijing Hospital I observed patients sitting patiently and apparently comfortably on a bench in the corridor of the Casualty Department, each with an intravenous infusion running. I was told that they were yet to be reviewed by the doctor. In the hospice attached to the Catholic University in Seoul, South Korea, I was surprised to find dying patients receiving intravenous high-calorie fluids, vitamins, protein supplements and fat emulsions on the day of death.

In many parts of Asia government medical salaries are meagre, and doctors have to supplement their wages with private practice, which comes to absorb an increasing proportion of their time. The multidisciplinary teamwork of palliative care which relies on salaried or volunteer staff does not fit easily with individual medical private practice. Teamwork itself is different in Asia, where hierarchies are more obvious, and the easy equality and informality which characterizes palliative care teams and encourages nurse autonomy in Australia, for example, is absent. The status of nursing and its standards of training vary widely. In Thailand there are well-established schools of nursing within universities; in neighbouring Malaysia, university courses for nurses are just beginning.

Political and organizational matters

In spite of sterling efforts by WHO to encourage wider availability and use of simple oral opioids for cancer pain (WHO 1990; Joranson 1993) with the establishment of WHO Cancer Pain Collaborating Centres in several Asian countries, there remains a common official suspicion of prescribed opioids, which are believed to lead to abuse and the promotion of addiction. The long story of opioid addiction in Asia (often vigorously encouraged by the west) has left, in many countries, a public suspicion of the drugs which supports official reluctance to license them.

The degree and type of restriction on the use of opioids varies. In Japan it has been usual to require a new prescription for opioids each day; in Korea and China only a controlled release preparation is licensed for oral use; in Myanmar even the main pain clinic in Yangon can prescribe only a paracetamol-codeine combination tablet. In a university hospital in Thailand I was told that 5 mg was the usual subcutaneous dose of morphine; if not successful, 2 mg might be administered intravenously.

In the smaller affluent states which have well-developed health services and been most strongly influenced by English example there are hospices and hospice programmes readily recognizable to the western observer. Hong Kong and Singapore, for example, have followed the British model and built, with strong community and religious support, lovely hospice buildings and excellent outreach services, which have later received quite generous government support. Yet Asian peculiarities exist even in those post-imperial pockets. In Hong Kong, when I asked to be shown the characters which translated the word 'hospice' on a multilingual brochure, I was informed that it was simply omitted from the Chinese version, since its usual translation, 'good ending' was an unlucky or disheartening phrase. Other Chinese programmes translate 'hospice' with different characters, affirming serenity and comfort, but unsurprisingly no characters carry the connotations that 'hospice' offers to the person steeped in English language and culture.

In Beijing I was taken to see a 'hospice', and found that it housed long-stay patients suffering from dementia or chronic neurological disorders. It was what Australians would call a nursing home. Patients with the discomforts of terminal cancer were being treated in a large hospital and all, it seemed, were receiving supportive intravenous therapy. China faces a major dilemma in the coming generation. Its elderly population and the number of cancer deaths both increase. Accompanying a burgeoning rump of elderly and very elderly people is the legacy of one-child families. In the days of Chairman Mao, youngsters were encouraged to visit elderly people at home after school, in order to undertake small jobs for them, befriend and assist them. The one-child generation has been freed from this obligation; its members are regarded as precious, special (spoiled?). An obvious question is who will care for the elderly parents of the one-child families as those parents move into their 70s and 80s. It is a question that is beginning to trouble both those older generations and the government planners. One possible measure may be that the newly retired, the younger aged, will have to be the volunteer carers. But they will need training, organization and support from professional teams if they are to cope with the multiple discomforts of terminal illness.

Will home care for terminal illness be a feasible option, replacing the current dependence on hospitalization in the more affluent Asian communities? It will not be easy to reproduce the mobile and skilled nurses on whom western societies rely to support families undertaking home care. Many Asian cities are large conurbations with meagre basic services of water, power and waste disposal; transport systems are heavily overloaded; established models for community health care are rudimentary. Although individual dedicated hospice teams have shown that it is possible to deliver good care to persons in shanties and tiny apartments, they are unusual, and touch only a small proportion of the needy population. Cost, urban geography and a lack of nurse practitioners will limit the applicability of this model.

Education for palliative care

Interest in palliative care across Asia continues to grow. The need for specific services which attend to the suffering of those who face death; the responsibility of government to provide such services; the opportunity for communities to create initiatives through giving and volunteering; and the blessing of Asian religions on all this activity are all increasingly being recognized.

Just as the models for delivery of palliative care for Asia need not mimic those of the west, the educational initiatives that are burgeoning in the west should not be taken as necessary models for Asia. Education, no longer a service, is become a business, and universities from the UK, USA and Australia are competing for opportunities to recruit Asian students either for their home courses or within cooperating programmes.

My first intention in making a tour in Asia was to explore interest among potential students there in the graduate courses which are now available in Australia, whether at the International Institute for Hospice Studies or (from 1997) in at least three other universities. Some students, clearly, will look for an early opportunity to complete a university award in palliative care and will also appreciate the prestige which attaches still in Asia to overseas qualifications. There has been a keen interest in the move to teach the Wales Diploma course in Hong Kong, and Adelaide has also received some Asian students for its Graduate Certificate and Master's Courses. Expensive foreign courses will benefit Asia most if they assist the development of local faculty, since, in the longer term, Asia must mount its own courses – for its doctors, nurses, priests, volunteers – courses that reflect the palliative care services developed in Asia. My travels have left me far less confident about what Occidentals have to teach in Asia, and much more aware of what we have to learn. Hospice spread like a charismatic evangel in the west; its introduction was facilitated by many common elements in demography, economics, culture, history, science and medicine. Asia is different; cooperation and mutual exchange, rather than preaching, would seem to be the appropriate pathway by which we may encourage services and education in the new discipline.

References

Gudmundsdóttir, M., Martinson, P.V. and Martinson, I.M. (1996) Funeral rituals following the death of a child in Taiwan. *Journal of Palliative Care*, 12(1): 31–7.

Joranson, D.E. (1993) Availability of opioids for cancer pain: recent trends, assessment of system barriers, new World Health Organisation guidelines, and the risk of diversion. *Journal of Pain and Symptom Management*, 8: 353–60.

Kashiwagi, T. (1991) Palliative care in Japan. *Palliative Medicine*, 5: 165–70.

Mullin, G. (1986) *Death and Dying: The Tibetan Tradition*. Boston, MA, and London: Arkana.

Tong, K.L. (1994) The Chinese palliative patient in North America: a cultural perspective. *Journal of Palliative Care*, 10: 26–8.

Wordley, D. (1976) *No One Dies Alone*. Melbourne, Australia: Little Company of Mary.

World Health Organization (1990) *Cancer Pain Relief and Palliative Care*, Technical Report Series 804. Geneva: WHO.

13 The WHO Cancer Pain and Palliative Care Programme

■ JAN STJERNSWARD

For much of the twentieth century, as research and clinical endeavour focused upon the development of curative interventions for cancer, little attention was given to the issue of cancer pain. Since the early 1980s, however, cancer pain has been recognized increasingly as a major public health problem and, linked to the wider question of palliative care, has become a significant international health issue. The World Health Organization (WHO) has served as an important catalyst in this process, promoting both policies and treatment strategies designed to alleviate the suffering of people with cancer. A wide-ranging WHO Cancer Pain and Palliative Care Programme now exists with support from governments, non-governmental organizations, professional bodies and a strong network of individuals. Although the WHO itself has contracted in recent years, the work that it served to promote is being carried forward, to the benefit of people with cancer around the world.

The WHO Programme was launched out of a conviction that cancer pain relief is among the most pragmatic, humane and realistic goals for health intervention in the developing countries. For in most of these, standard therapies remain limited in availability and the great majority of patients are incurable at the time of diagnosis, if indeed, a diagnosis ever takes place. In such a context, cancer pain, the most common symptom, is seen as a spearhead for the development of a comprehensive approach to palliative care using a public health model designed to reach the greatest possible number of those in need. If such a strategy can be made to work for those with cancer, then ultimately those dying from other diseases may also benefit from the same methods, principles and policies.

In this way WHO has served as a powerful base for a five-pronged strategy, consisting of:

1 The establishment of consensus on a method for cancer pain relief which is considered both scientifically valid and acceptable at community level.
2 The establishment of rational policies for implementing existing knowledge within national cancer programmes.
3 The development of advocacy campaigns.
4 The education of professionals and making drugs, especially oral morphine, available.
5 The creation of a global network of support.

It is these five elements, individually and in combination, that make up the major achievements of the WHO programme.

Consensus on a method for cancer pain relief

A hallmark of the WHO global programme is its emphasis upon a public health approach. This is based upon the principle of putting science into practice in order to reach the maximum number of those in need. This is coupled in turn to a mission to educate health professionals about the need for pain control and palliative care. In addition there is a concern to sensitize patients and families to the notion that pain *can* be managed. This can be done most effectively and with the greatest coverage through the establishment of clear policies and by making available the relevant drugs, particularly morphine. Most significantly of all, WHO's programme has been based upon a concern to impress upon public health authorities the necessity of making palliative care a priority, either in itself, or as part of a national cancer control programme.

A number of key steps can be established within the chronology of the WHO programme (see Table 13.1).

In less than 15 years, therefore, the programme succeeded in generalizing consensus statements, published guidelines and generated global support among experts for its strategy of a simple, inexpensive approach to pain and symptom control, based on uncomplicated technologies.

The implementation of existing knowledge

Even limited resources for palliative care stand a chance of making an impact if the relevant priorities are set and the appropriate strategies are adopted. Three specific measures stand out if drugs are to be the mainstay of cancer pain relief and the WHO pain ladder (WHO 1986) is to be implemented. First, there must be endorsement in government policy. Second, education of health professionals, patients, families and informal carers

Table 13.1   Chronological development of the WHO programme

1980	Cancer pain and palliative care made a priority in WHO's reoriented cancer control programme.
1982	Initial draft of the WHO *Guidelines for Cancer Pain Relief*.
1984	Monograph *Cancer Pain Relief* (WHO 1986), destined to become the standard reference, worldwide (translated into 28 languages; over 500,000 copies printed). When used correctly, the WHO method is capable of controlling pain in 80–90% of patients.
1988	All drugs recommended for cancer pain relief are included in the WHO essential drug list (WHO 1988). Draft policy on opioid availability is formulated.
1989	WHO and United Nations International Narcotics Control Board (UNINC 1989) produce joint report on the opioid needs of cancer patients. WHO expert committee extends the concept of cancer pain relief and produces the landmark *Cancer Pain Relief and Palliative Care* (WHO 1990).
1991	Numerous countries sensitized to the concept of national cancer control programmes and several national or state programmes started, all including palliative care.
1993	A joint WHO-International Association for the Study of Pain (IASP) group begins to draft guidelines on cancer pain relief in children.
1995	Publication of the handbook *National Cancer Control Programmes: Policies and Managerial Guidelines* (WHO 1995). Aimed principally at policy makers, it outlines the scientific basis of cancer control; considers the relative importance of prevention, cure and care; and discusses the creation and management of national programmes.
1996	Second edition published of the WHO method of cancer pain relief (WHO 1996). Monographs on *Symptom Relief in Terminal Illness* (WHO in press b), *Cancer Pain Relief and Palliative Care in Children* (WHO in press a) and a handbook on radiotherapy (WHO forthcoming).

must take place. Three, drugs must be available without undue restriction and at reasonable cost. These measures must be put into effect simultaneously. Together, they can have a massive impact on pain control, while keeping costs low.

The position of WHO is that the relative proportion of resources available for cancer pain relief and palliative care should be increased, if necessary at the expense of resources made available for anti-cancer treatment. Figure 13.1 sets out the desired relationship between governmental policy, education and drug availability in developing countries. It is crucial that palliative care is included as part of total care at the time the cancer is

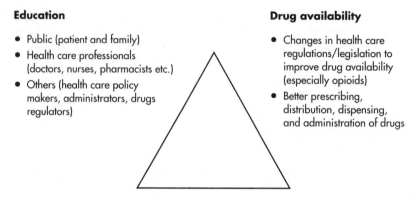

Education

- Public (patient and family)
- Health care professionals (doctors, nurses, pharmacists etc.)
- Others (health care policy makers, administrators, drugs regulators)

Drug availability

- Changes in health care regulations/legislation to improve drug availability (especially opioids)
- Better prescribing, distribution, dispensing, and administration of drugs

Governmental policy

- National or state policy emphasizing the need to alleviate chronic cancer pain through education, drug availability, and governmental support/endorsement
- The policy can stand alone, be part of a national/state cancer control programme, be part of an overall policy on the care of the terminally ill, or of a policy on chronic, intractable pain

Figure 13.1   Fundamental process measures for cancer pain relief: low cost, big effect

diagnosed, and not seen as a measure of last resort. The physician who gives hope for cure should also give hope for freedom from pain and unnecessary suffering.

Because two-thirds of the world's cancer patients are incurable (Stjernsward 1993), the WHO programme suggests practical solutions and approaches, as set out in Table 13.2, and as described also in Gómez-Batiste *et al.* (Chapter 10 in this volume). Although ultimately palliative care should be part of the general health care system, in order to get started it is important to find and support a local 'champion' who can build up a critical mass of excellence, showing that the approach can work. Such centres of excellence can later provide necessary training (see Burn, Chapter 7 in this volume). In turn, these policies can be translated into measurable outcomes which have direct relevance at the community level within each country (Table 13.3).

Growing numbers of governments are recognizing the importance of pain relief and palliative care. Many ministers of health have adopted a national policy on cancer control as part of their countries' health priorities (Stjernsward 1993). Opioid availability, which continues to widen, is an essential component of this.

Table 13.2 Practical policies

- Recruit political commitment and leadership to promote palliative care; find and support a local 'champion'
- Integrate palliative care as part of routine health care
- Ensure adequate access to opioids
- Apply palliative care early in the illness course
- Believe the patient
- Involve the family
- Include pain and symptom control in the standard curriculum of physicians and nurses

---

Table 13.3 Measurable outcomes

- Dialogue exists between health professionals and government representatives to achieve better pain relief and palliative care
- The size of the problem is demonstrated and it is shown that inexpensive methods exist to control cancer pain
- Written national policy exists emphasizing the need to alleviate chronic cancer pain
- Palliative care is linked to previously existing resources
- Oncology and primary care are involved in palliative care
- Curricula are established in palliative care
- Increase in morphine consumption demonstrated
- Increase in patient coverage demonstrated
- Reduction in pain prevalence demonstrated
- Cross-cultural differences integrated positively

Advocacy campaigns

Advocacy programmes are crucial to the process of sensitizing health professionals, cancer patients themselves and the general public to the message that cancer pain can be managed. They are also vital in promoting awareness of the WHO three-step analgesic ladder for pain control. A crucial starting point in the WHO advocacy programme was the simple flyer *Why Not Freedom from Cancer Pain?*, produced in English and French in 1986 and subsequently translated into Spanish, Portuguese, Japanese and many other languages, following the efforts of various non-governmental organizations. A video, bearing the same title, was also produced and has proved to be WHO's best-selling video production. In 1989 a press kit was developed, highlighting the theme 'to cure sometimes, to relieve often, to comfort always', seeking to establish messages about pain relief and palliative care in the public domain.

Since 1988 *Cancer Pain Release* has been published quarterly by the WHO Collaborating Center for Symptom Evaluation in Cancer Care (Madison, Wisconsin, USA). The centre seeks to promote the goals of the WHO programme by reporting on advances in policy, professional education and analgesic availability; printing abstracts of recent research; and by contacts with health professionals in over 100 countries.

The public health approach requires a continuing commitment to advocacy. Numerous international conferences have been addressed, thus promoting awareness of cancer pain and palliative care. In addition, these subjects are being addressed in specialist and other professional journals, and in the mass media.

Professional education

In 1989 the Expert Committee endorsed guidelines on the teaching and training of health professionals in cancer pain relief (Foley 1994). Yet surveys conducted in Japan, Germany, the USA and France continue to document inadequate knowledge and attitudes about cancer pain control among health professionals (Takeda 1993; Van Roenn 1993; Larue 1995; Zenz et al. 1995). A partial explanation for this may be the compartmentalizing of pain and palliative care specialties. It is time for pain control and palliative care to be incorporated into existing systems of care and for those physicians most likely to see chronically ill patients in the first line of duty (general practitioners, oncologists) to adopt these principles within their mainstream practice.

Other WHO initiatives to tackle this problem include the use of prominent individuals with outstanding expertise to serve as 'focal points' for development. To these are added a programme of regional workshops, such as those which have taken place in Latin America in the period 1992–6 (in Argentina, Colombia, Brazil and the Dominican Republic). These have served to reduce isolation and to bring together relevant health professionals for practical discussion (Bruera et al. 1995). In Europe the growth in attendance at bi-annual meetings of the European Association for Palliative Care reflects the dynamism of local, regional and national groups. In the USA the Wisconsin Cancer Pain Initiative has been active in all 50 states.

Outstanding issues

Despite these achievements, a great deal remains to be done. In the developing countries there are specific priorities and needs which must be addressed. Here it will be necessary, in order to achieve meaningful coverage, to involve family members, building on the role of extended family and kinship networks. In the developed countries, it is widely recognized that families have a serious duty to provide care, but families often have to set limits to the care they can give. In both contexts it is important to identify policies which will allow a proper balance between family and government assistance, so that families may continue to respond to the needs of elderly members, knowing that outside care is available when, and if, required. The provision of community and home-based care for elderly people will be essential for effective palliative care, and to achieve coverage. Home care should avoid becoming some version of acute care delivery at home, as this will only be a domestic version of institutionalized care. It should encompass personal care, personal services, social companionship, and applied medical care.

In the economically poorer countries deeply rooted problems still remain to be addressed. For example, in sub-Saharan Africa (with the exception of South Africa) there are fewer than 100 cancer specialists of any description (radiotherapists, chemotherapists, cytologists, cancer nurses, etc.) for a population of more than 300 million. Policies and training in palliative care are non-existent in most African countries. With few exceptions, for example, Zimbabwe and South Africa, no essential drugs, such as oral morphine, are available. This is in spite of the fact that Africa has a cancer incidence of over 100 per 100,000, with 80–90 per cent of its cancer patients incurable.

The most common symptom in palliative care – pain – cannot be controlled adequately without access to opioids. Around the world, there are still 51 countries for which there is no registered morphine consumption. Twenty-seven of these countries are in Africa, nine in the Americas, four in South-East Asia, eight in the eastern Mediterranean region, and three in the Western Pacific. In many countries, such as Pakistan, not even weak opioids, such as codeine, are available (Stjernsward and Joranson 1995).

For example, in Bangladesh, with 120 million people, there is only one cancer unit (established in 1965). Most cancer patients are incurable, if ever diagnosed and no morphine tablets are available. There is no serious will for a palliative care programme.

India, with one-sixth of the world's population, has eleven comprehensive cancer centres. They account for the major part of the cancer care/control resources available, and most of the resources are allotted to therapy (see Burn, Chapter 7 in this volume). However, these centres deal with fewer than 10 per cent of the estimated 700,000 new cancer patients every year. Recently in collaboration with the WHO, and after the establishment in 1984 of a national cancer control programme in which pain relief was made a priority, several Indian states have set rational priorities and strategies through the establishment of state cancer control programmes, in which cancer pain relief and palliative care are always included. Only

16,000 patients are covered yearly by hospitals having expertise in cancer pain in India, while there are an estimated 350,000 cancer patients who suffer daily from moderate to severe cancer pain. By applying the WHO cancer pain relief method, however, it should be possible to achieve coverage relatively simply in 80 per cent of all the 350,000 sufferers.

The great majority of Indian cancer patients is encountered at the district level. India has nearly 400 districts, each with 1 million to 4 million individuals. To increase the impact of cancer control activities at this level, 20 districts have been selected for joint Indian Ministry of Health/WHO demonstration projects. If these activities are found to be effective, the programme can be extended on a national scale. A successful extension throughout India, with one-sixth of the world's population, within a ten year period would have a worldwide impact in palliative care. The activities, common to those of most national cancer control programmes, include anti-tobacco measures; health education; promotion of early detection; early referral to curative treatment; and establishment of cancer units. Radiotherapy also has an important role in cure and palliation. The district demonstration projects will place a strong emphasis on palliative care.

In the course of developing this global network of support, the WHO Cancer and Palliative Care Programme has established links with numerous national and international organizations, NGOs, industry and individuals with leadership, as exemplified in the work by Burn (Chapter 7 in this volume), which have helped to promote regional projects. These initiatives demonstrate the overall maturation of the WHO network. There are now sufficient programmes and networks in all areas of the world to allow concerned health professionals access to advice, support, education and guidance. By focusing on the most common symptom in cancer (pain) a model has been developed to reach the greatest number of those in need. The same method must be used to cover other symptoms to achieve total care. This approach is valid not only for cancer, but for other diseases, and ultimately for the 51 million people who die every year, worldwide. Since 38 million of these 51 million who die are in developing countries with only a fraction of the global resources for health care, the challenge is enormous. Family involvement is crucial. The need for palliative care will increase due to a combination of factors, including an ageing global population, increases in deaths related to tobacco use and the impact of the HIV/AIDS pandemic. In a world of limited or decreasing resources for health care, governments in both developed and developing countries must allocate resources for cancer pain and palliative care in a rational way. In this context the influence of social, economic and cultural factors will prove vital in determining the further development of care for all those in need around the world.

References

Bruera, E., Schoeller, M.T. and Stjernsward, J. (1995) Opioid availability in Latin America: the Declaration of Florinapolis. *Supportive Cancer Care*, 3: 164–7.

Foley, K. (1994) The World Health Organisation program in cancer pain relief and palliative care, in G.F. Gebhart and T.S. Jensen (eds) *Proceedings of the Seventh World Congress on Pain*. Seattle, WA: IASP Press.

Larue, F. (1995) Oncologists' and primary care physicians' attitudes towards pain control and morphine prescribing in France. *Cancer*, 75: 2375–82.

Stjernsward, J. (1993) Palliative medicine: a global perspective, in D. Doyle, G.W.C. Hanks and N. MacDonald (eds) *Oxford Textbook of Palliative Medicine*. Oxford: Oxford University Press.

Stjernsward, J. and Joranson, D. (1995) Opioid availability and cancer pain: an unnecessary relationship. *Supportive Cancer Care*, 3: 164–7.

Takeda, F. (1993) Assessment of physicians' attitudes to cancer pain management in Japan, in G.F. Gebhart and T.S. Jenson (eds) *Proceedings of the Seventh World Congress on Pain*. Seattle, WA: IASP Press.

United Nations International Narcotics Control Board (1989) *Demand for and Supply of Opiates for Medical and Scientific Needs*. New York: United Nations.

Van Roenn, J.J. (1993) Physician's attitude and practice in cancer pain management: a survey from the Eastern Co-operative Oncology Group. *Annals of Internal Medicine*, 119: 121–6.

World Health Organization (1986) *Cancer Pain Relief*. Geneva: WHO.

World Health Organization (1988) *The Use of Essential Drugs*, Technical Report Series 770. Geneva: WHO.

World Health Organization (1990) *Cancer Pain Relief and Palliative Care*, Technical Report Series 804. Geneva: WHO.

World Health Organization (1995) *National Cancer Control Programmes: Policies and Managerial Guidelines*. Geneva: WHO.

World Health Organization (1996) *Cancer Pain Relief: With a Guide to Opioid Availability*, 2nd edn. Geneva: WHO.

World Health Organization (in press a) *Cancer Pain Relief and Palliative Care in Children*. Geneva: WHO.

World Health Organization (in press b) *Symptom Relief in Terminal Illness*. Geneva: WHO.

World Health Organization (forthcoming) *Radiotherapy Handbook*. Geneva: WHO.

Zenz, M., Zenz, T., Tryba, M. and Stumpf, M. (1995) Severe undertreatment of cancer pain: a three-year survey of the German situation. *Journal of Pain and Symptom Management*, 10: 187–91.

PART III

Clinical issues

Introduction to Part III

In Parts I and II of this volume, we have seen the mapping out of palliative care's growth and development, both organizationally and geographically. It will be helpful to keep these perspectives in mind as we approach the third and final part, which covers clinical issues. At first sight, it might seem strange that in a book dealing with patients at the end of life, the medical aspects should come last.

The authors here are writing predominantly from a western (North American and British) standpoint, but the trends and concerns they raise are applicable wherever palliative care is developing. It is fascinating to observe how issues of broad policy and resource use, covered at the beginning of this book, are influencing the clinical arguments put forward in this part. In other areas of the world the recent rapid evolution of the hospice movement, described comprehensively in the second part, are confronting both clinicians and policy makers in developing countries with difficult choices in terms of philosophy and clinical strategy, on top of the local economic and cultural influences which prevail. It is not odd, therefore, to present the clinical section of this compilation at the end: although palliative care is essentially a health care issue, it cannot be seen as primarily disease driven, but rather as a peculiar interaction of medical science, public opinion and governmental reaction.

The five chapters that comprise Part III have three common strands that run through them. First, they discuss the types of patients that palliative care has embraced, and how that client group is changing. Second, there is the question of how these patients' problems are dissected, analysed and managed (the use of biomedical language here being deliberately ironic). Third, and this is the most challenging theme, the authors pose questions in different ways, about what the limits of palliative care might be.

Davis and Sheldon (Chapter 14) explore the meaning and scope of 'therapeutic innovation'. As they point out, innovation is not the same as invention and indeed what is new to palliative care may be well-established practice elsewhere; conversely 'routine' practices in palliative care settings, such as the medical management of bowel obstruction, may be seen as revolutionary in surgical wards. Interestingly, however, they begin their inventory of innovations with non-medical therapies: specifically, the range of cognitive and behavioural interventions which are being transported from psychology into palliative care. Other exotic sounding therapies such as imagework and reminiscence are also described.

They move on to management of symptoms, opening with non-pharmacological approaches. In raising the role of nurses in helping patients control their own breathlessness and with the use of massage and psychosocial approaches to coping with lymphoedema, they anticipate the multidisciplinary teamwork and nurse-led agendas of subsequent chapters by Ingham and Coyle (Chapter 16) and Corner and Dunlop (Chapter 18) respectively. Art therapy and complementary therapies are also reviewed: an important message here is that while more research is needed to prove their effectiveness and safety, the appropriate models of evaluation are still not developed. One problem of assessing the response to exciting new therapies is that all too often the patient is being influenced by other conventional or fashionable treatments, which makes attribution of benefit somewhat problematic.

New drug therapies, new routes of drug administration and high-tech medical interventions such as endobronchial stenting, brachytherapy and laser show that palliative medicine has not forgotten its initial pioneering role with respect to pain and symptom control. These latter innovations have come from anaesthetics, oncology and respiratory medicine, but their inclusion here in the care of advanced cancer patients would represent a substantial widening of their application.

This book has tended to focus on the palliative care of adult patients and their adult families and friends, but Davis and Sheldon highlight also new ideas for tackling the needs of children who are bereaved through terminal illness. Finally, they return to the theme of evaluation, and how this field in itself has had to become more innovative, in response to the diverse faces of palliative care. They challenge the assumption that the randomized controlled trial is the sole gold standard and advocate adding qualitative methods to it.

Chapter 15 by George and Sykes focuses on the subject of diagnostic groups. Starting off with the provocative assertion that 'the hospice movement is too good to be true and too small to be useful', they review its historical development as being initially an innovative concept but, in its coming of age, becoming obstructed from within to further changes. During its growth period, the authors claim, cancer was adopted as its prime focus out of a need to inspire a following, since its malignant nature forms a paradigm for pain, suffering, indignity and death. The following phase of consolidation and routinization of hospice care is discussed further by Corner and Dunlop in Chapter 18.

George and Sykes next put forward the principles of justice and need as complementary rationales for demanding the opening up of palliative care to those with non-malignant conditions. Their arguments are based specifically on equity of access to care, patient autonomy and evidence from GP surveys – their conclusion being that patients who are dying but do not have cancer can be seen as a disadvantaged majority. The logical response to this iniquitous situation, they advocate, is the encouragement of 'generic palliative care'. In these services, medical and other expertise can be offered to all patients who warrant symptom control and the wider benefits. They would operate outside of the established 'specialist' services such as hospices.

The authors propose a three-step hierarchy of service provision, depending on the patient's needs: medically based consultations for symptom control; full multidisciplinary palliative care; and terminal care. To exemplify this proposed approach, which is already being adopted in many UK hospitals and even in some 'progressive' hospice-type settings, several clinical and diagnostic groups are briefly discussed, including elderly people (especially those with dementias), renal, cardiac and respiratory failure; chronic neurological diseases and rheumatoid arthritis.

The vision of George and Sykes amounts to a re-birth of palliative care as a much broader and implicitly less elitist movement, and relies heavily on medical leadership to provide palliation of symptoms at all of their three levels of generic palliative care. The delicate balance of medical and other professional inputs into palliative care is the subject of Chapter 16 by Ingham and Coyle. Writing as a doctor–nurse team, they start from a very conventional medical base: the American Board of Internal Medicine. In response to its drive to obtain a 'broad view' of the physician's role in 'end-of-life' situations, the authors prepared an educational resource document which has been adapted here for this volume.

Their starting point is that physicians are indeed needed at the end of life, but while this should be as part of a team, health care systems do not encourage teamwork at present. They cover the needs of patients with chronic disease as well as cancer, adding weight to George and Sykes's British polemic. Teamwork, they advocate, would enhance continuity of care in long-term illnesses, which currently lead to patients feeling abandoned by physicians when they do withdraw. This could not happen, however, without significant educational changes.

The bulk of this chapter is concerned with the constitution of teams, and their modus operandi. However broad their composition, their members should have a common purpose, which may lead in some situations to an overlap of skills. The types of teams covered include hospices (which in the USA mostly deliver home care) and hospital teams. Some of these services are nurse-led, and the thorny issue is discussed of team leadership in terms of a 'coordinating figure', or key-workers as we would describe them in the UK. The importance of providing 24-hour cover at the end of life is stressed.

Significantly, Ingham and Coyle echo the comments of George and Sykes, and also of Davis and Sheldon, about the need to evaluate and assess their area of work. They view the patient and family as exhibiting common needs, and point usefully to published instruments that could be used to conduct such assessments. It is difficult to know whether one should be heartened to see the leaders in palliative care uniformly advocating formalized assessment, or to be discouraged that they all acknowledge the present lack of evidence for current practices.

The final two contributions draw the reader increasingly away from the clinical scene, towards a more theoretical setting.

It is perhaps indicative of the rapidly changing global attitudes to death and dying that many new texts on palliative care have to include the topic of euthanasia, even though a few years ago the two might have seemed quite incompatible. We have chosen to place Oxenham and Boyd's Chapter 17 in Part III on clinical issues rather than in Part I on policy, ethics and evidence. This is not because we see euthanasia as an everyday professional challenge, but rather because we want to acknowledge that terminal suffering and distress – real or anticipated – do take place in many life-limiting conditions and the open communication that prevails in clinical situations nowadays will bring patients, family carers and clinicians more and more into an open but nerve-wracking dialogue. Euthanasia clearly needs to be discussed by ethicists (as one of our contributors here is), philosophers and legislators, but it is surely by the bedside that the theoretical arguments need to be exposed and tested.

Oxenham and Boyd start by acknowledging that the diversity of views held about euthanasia – what they call 'cognitive dissonance' – easily leads clinicians into polarized debates but ask if this is not appropriate, as it would be more worrying if we found the issues easy. They propose a set of definitions which helps to reduce uncertainty, as least as far as the terms are concerned, if not the moral arguments underlying them. In discussing these arguments, both for and against, they present two types of philosophical statements: the consequentialist, and the deontological. The former is plain to understand – the morality of euthanasia depends on the consequences arising from allowing it, or forbidding it. On the other hand, the reader may not be familiar with 'deontology' – put simply, it denotes the ethical theory which takes duty as the basis of morality and the view that some acts are morally obligatory, regardless of their consequences.

One of the well-known consequentialist arguments against euthanasia is the 'slippery slope'; a deontological position against it is that doctors are duty bound to cure, relieve and comfort – and not kill. Arguing for it, the consequentialist would say that if euthanasia is not allowed then some people would suffer needlessly. The corresponding deontological argument in favour of legalized euthanasia is that the patient's right for autonomy is supreme. It is clear that posing one argument against another in this way, while intellectually stimulating, is unlikely to change minds and less likely to alter practice and law.

The authors therefore wisely move away from this theoretical stance and discuss at length the more modern topic of the doctor–patient relationship from the point of view of consumerism versus paternalism. There are echoes in this of the anti-establishment views of Corner and Dunlop developed in Chapter 18. Oxenham and Boyd are careful not to take one or other side, but rather they try to ask why patients may seek euthanasia as a release from their suffering. Often it comes down to loss of independence, and of hope, coupled with a dread of further suffering. They acknowledge that a small number of people will persist in asking for doctors to kill them, even after psychiatric assessment and a 'pause' to allow both sides to reflect on the underlying distresses. However, against this minority, they suggest that a much larger number who originally ask to be killed can be helped by other means.

In an interesting section of this chapter, the authors offer some ideas on responding to a patient's request for euthanasia. The issues they suggest that the clinician should consider include investigating the reasons for the request, correcting the correctable, returning control to the patient, and attending to spiritual concerns. An important message, to doctors in particular, is to admit one's own powerlessness in the face of unremitting suffering in another. Ultimately, they do admit that often there will be no ideal ethical solution to such a tricky clinical problem, and society will continue to struggle with these issues – and with the minority of patients who demand euthanasia today.

Corner and Dunlop, who contribute the final chapter of our volume, write from a hospital and hospice base respectively, and one wonders how that influences the position they adopt. Their starting point is reflective, concerning the historical development of palliative care and its apparent obsession with hospices and cancer. Their remarks about the lost radicalism of the early hospice movement and the accompanying medicalization and institutionalization have already been flagged by George and Sykes. In this chapter, however, the authors develop the theme of maturation and change in a substantially different way. Instead of focusing on diagnostic groups and generic delivery of palliative care, here we are confronted with a hearty exploration of the nature and purpose of palliative care itself. More than that, we are led through a lively critique of the biomedical model of illness with respect to terminal disease.

Corner and Dunlop ask us to consider the prevalent thinking of symptoms being equated with suffering, the focus on the malfunction of organs, the constant perceived need for pharmacological control, and they question if all these are appropriate premises for palliative care. They particularly challenge the current attitude of health care workers in wanting to 'manage' the symptoms of patients (or consumers, as Corner and Dunlop prefer to see the recipients of care). In their view, palliative care is in danger of following mainstream medicine in perpetuating the Cartesian splitting of mind and body, and of seeing the body as its only legitimate concern. Moreover, even the way that the biomedical model (and modern palliative care by implication) treats the latter is out of date with respect to current concepts of the sociology of 'the body', which the authors summarize here.

It may be surprising, even shocking, for those brought up on the now classic Saunders concept of 'total pain', to see this foundation stone of modern palliative care openly criticized. Even though it admits the existence of the physical, psychological, social and spiritual dimensions of pain, the very presence of this classification leads the system to envisage them as separate entities to be managed accordingly. The authors conclude that this prevents us from conceptualizing pain – and presumably, by extrapolation, other symptoms – as anything other than perceptions at the physical level which are to be manipulated by drugs. Expressing this theme at its most powerful level, the biomedical model, they argue, is in danger of denying the 'personhood, depersonalization and decontextualization of the problem, and denial of chronicity, suffering, distress and meaning as part of the experience'.

Lest the reader should feel hopeless for the future of the specialty, Corner and Dunlop do suggest a way of redressing the balance and reinvigorating palliative care, by a process which they call 're-framing'. By this is meant the deconstruction and reconstruction of the problem in such a way that its context, meaning and impact on patients is actively considered. A logical extension of this approach is to reconstruct the palliative care services themselves. Furthermore, the role of professionals could also be 'recast as servant to the consumer, rather than carer for the patient'.

To exemplify this radical approach, we are led to examine the reframing of pain and breathlessness, two common and significant problem areas of terminal disease. The example given of reconstructing services is of increasing the nurse input into assessments for, and in particular into admissions for palliative care. Finally, the reader is given the development of nurse-led clinics for breathlessness, developed by Corner herself, as a clear way of tying all these principles together into a comprehensive package of care. The authors therefore conclude on a note which challenges all involved in palliative care to think more radically about the current way in which problems are framed.

New themes and key questions in Part III

- *Diagnostic groups*: Is palliative care to remain linked almost exclusively to care of cancer patients, or should it start to spread its beneficial influences wider, to other life-limiting and chronic diseases? If it does this, do the models of care need to be revised? For example, is there a case for moving care away from hospice services, which are fully geared to cancer care, and into more 'generic' teams? Should palliative care even restrict itself to life-limiting diseases as has always been the case?

- *Therapies*: There is increasing interest in non-pharmacological interventions for symptom control, particularly those which may be initiated and supervised by nursing staff. In parallel with this move, palliative care is adopting psychological therapies which may be used alongside conventional drug interventions. On the other hand, some high-tech procedures such as endobronchial laser or stenting are also being incorporated in palliative care – what are the limits of technological encroachment into what was previously seen as a low-tech, high touch specialty?

- *Teamwork*: Although palliative care has always claimed to be based on multidisciplinary teamwork, this rhetoric has mainly applied to the inpatient hospice units of the UK. Elsewhere, such as in the USA, physicians are being reminded of both their duties, and also opportunities for increased job satisfaction, if they positively integrate themselves into end-of-life care of their terminally ill patients. What will be the consequences of broadening the base of palliative care – out of cancer to other end-stage diseases – for the composition of the multidisciplinary team? For example, will respiratory physicians, cardiologists, neurologists and rheumatologists all need retraining and be expected to contribute to such teams, or will they defer, as with cancer, to the palliative medicine specialists? Similar questions presumably face other specialties such as nursing and professions allied to medicine which are heavily involved in palliative care.

- *Euthanasia*: Palliative care has always distanced itself from euthanasia, seeing itself as an antidote to patients' terminal distress. From an ethical and societal point of view, this is being reviewed: evidence is accumulating that pain and other uncontrolled symptoms are less likely to be reasons for requesting euthanasia than perceived loss of independence and dignity. Although only a minority of patients in most communities persistently request to be mercifully killed, palliative care should not be expected to relieve all degrees of suffering. Is it legitimate to allow some patients to remain in a 'no-hope' state, in which their distress is acknowledged but not acted on?

- *Methods of assessing outcome*: The new interest in non-pharmacological and psychological therapies, and the spreading of palliative care into non-malignant populations, are calling into question the traditional outcome measures that have been used for evaluation. Are randomized controlled trials necessarily the gold standard for palliative care, as they are in other branches of medicine? How can the development of whole new types of generic services be costed and evaluated?

- *Needs of chronically ill and elderly patients*: If palliative care is going to be increasingly involved in non-malignant conditions, this could have major implications on the length of involvement with chronically ill patients, and hence on the costs of care. Similarly, making palliative care available to cancer patients from the time of diagnosis could have significant consequences on planning the allocation of resources for oncology. To what extent will the largely volunteer and charity-driven hospice movement in countries like the UK respond to these new needs? In countries where health insurance could be a major player in funding palliative care, to what extent could financial considerations override the clinical desirability to extend the benefits to dementia, chronic respiratory or cardiac patients?

14 Therapeutic innovations

CAROL L. DAVIS AND FRANCES SHELDON

There is one thing stronger than all the armies in the world: and that is an idea whose time has come.

(Victor Hugo, 1802–1885)

The main challenge in writing this chapter was to define what is meant by 'therapeutic innovation'. This chapter is about changes in the professional practice of palliative care, which are bound to interact with, and have implications for, organizational change and service development which are dealt with elsewhere in this book. How will a particular change in professional palliative care practice be classified as an innovation for inclusion in this chapter? Is an example in only one place sufficient? How long should it have been practised? Should procedures and practices well established in other fields of health and social care, but newly applied in palliative care, count?

The definition of innovation used in this chapter is that developed by Rogers:

An innovation is an idea, practice, or object that is perceived as new by an individual or other unit of adoption. It matters little, so far as human behaviour is concerned, whether or not an idea is 'objectively' new as measured by the lapse of time since its first use or discovery. The perceived newness of the idea for the individual determines his or her reaction to it. If the idea is new to the individual it is an innovation.

(Rogers 1983: 11)

This is developed by Angle and Van de Ven,

Invention is the creation of a new idea, but innovation is more encompassing and includes the process of developing and implementing a new idea.... As long as the idea is perceived as new to the people involved, it is an 'innovative idea' even if it may appear to others to be an 'imitation' of something that exists elsewhere.

(Angle and Van de Ven 1989: 2)

This chapter hopes to identify some of the exciting changes in contemporary palliative care practice. It cannot hope to identify them all. By the time this book appears in print some of the innovations discussed here will have flourished and become part of conventional practice, others will have sunk without trace.

Palliative care as a specialist area of care is itself relatively new. Professionals have been preoccupied with setting up the service and responding to the needs of patients and carers. Relatively few are writing books and journal articles. There is no easy way to obtain a reasonably true and inclusive picture of innovation. This is all the more difficult when work is still going on to define the boundaries between palliative care and specialist palliative care and to work out the role of specialist palliative care in relation to non-malignant disease. In this chapter, we consider innovations only in the field of specialist palliative care for patients with cancer and their carers. We felt unable to do justice to the many innovations in other fields including HIV and AIDS.

This chapter will have achieved its objective if it encourages others to build on what is reported here, to develop their own innovative ideas and to think critically about both.

Innovations in psychological therapies

The use of counselling, whether in using counselling skills in communication or more formally and explicitly as an intervention, has been well established in palliative care from the beginning (Vachon 1988). This is rooted in the holistic approach of palliative care. Faulkner and Maguire (1994), particularly, have focused on the needs of patients with malignant disease and developed a model of communication which has been widely taught. Practitioners are now beginning to develop a more varied repertoire of psychological therapies to respond more appropriately to different problems and to patients and carers who may prefer different ways of tackling the same problem.

Cognitive and behavioural therapies originated in the field of mental health, used most frequently with patients suffering from anxiety and depression. Psychologists have been at the forefront of developing these techniques. Moorey and Greer (1989) describe how they have adapted these therapies for use with cancer patients who may not necessarily be mentally ill, but are suffering severe stress. The underlying assumption is that it is not the objective effects of the disease which determine how a person reacts, but the way that individual interprets the disease and those effects. These therapies attempt to enable individuals to understand how their thoughts contribute to their distress, and encourage them to develop new strategies such as relaxation, reality testing and interruption of automatic thoughts to deal with this. Through these means the person may establish a greater sense of control. Moorey and Greer suggest that the focus in palliative care may be less on developing a fighting spirit and more on maintaining self-esteem and reality testing fears about dying. Jones *et al.* (1989) have given an account of the use of this approach with a young woman with breast cancer in despair as she approached death. Keeping a diary of thoughts, mood and activities enabled the patient to understand and answer some problems herself and, with her support nurse, to plan more appropriately. The nurse worked under the supervision of a psychologist and together with the chaplain. As more psychologists are appointed to palliative care services there is likely to be an increase in the use of these innovative techniques. Further positive evidence of their value may emerge from Cocker *et al.* (1994) who, in a pilot study, showed that women with advanced breast cancer had less anger and depression following a programme of cognitive therapy.

Imagework has been developed by Kearney (1992) as part of a psychotherapeutic approach to relieving distress. He describes it as 'working through the medium of imagery to facilitate a bridging between the conscious and unconscious self'. Again it recognizes the power of the emotions to affect physical distress. In the case reported the patient was a 33-year-old man with metastatic malignant schwannoma whose pain had not responded to pharmacological or physical treatments. Guided visualization made it possible to work with him on the fears that were increasing his pain without fully breaching his protective defence of denial. His psychological and physical distress were relieved and medication reduced. Kearney cautions that this technique should not be embarked upon unless the therapist has had training and has ongoing supervision, and that it is not suitable for some patients, such as those with a history of psychosis. Like many innovations in these types of therapies, imagework too could be of real benefit to many patients but it requires further evaluation and development.

Those approaching the end of their lives may want to review and reflect on their experiences and achievements. Since Butler's seminal article (1963) the formal use of reminiscence, usually a group activity, and structured life review with individuals (Haight and Webster 1995) have developed in the field of elderly care. Structured life review has been shown to enhance psychological well-being and life satisfaction in elderly people. Although there has always been much informal discussion between dying people and professionals about the course of their lives, these more formal approaches are now being adapted for use in palliative care. Lester (1994) has piloted a revised form of Haight's Life Review and Experiencing questionnaire, adapted for use in the different culture of the UK and shortened to take account of the reduced energies of dying people. She used it with three patients who were exhibiting severe emotional distress and demonstrated reduced anxiety and increased sense of self-esteem in all cases. Lichter (1993) has established a biography service in a hospice in New Zealand as a way of helping patients to discover a sense of meaning in life.

The technique of life story work is well established in the field of child care as a means of helping children facing separation from their families of origin to establish a sense of their past history and to foster self-esteem. This approach has been drawn on in palliative care by young parents who are dying and who leave letters or tapes for their children. A. Macmurray (personal communication, 1995) has used a structured life story approach with a young woman whose child had died and who was now dying herself. This therapeutic method enabled her both to explore the many painful events in her own life and to leave an account for her surviving daughter and husband. The common thread in all these approaches is a conscious attempt to mobilize the normal, informal activity of reviewing the past in a more formal way which addresses 'total pain' and contributes to a reduction of distress and a more satisfying ending.

Non-pharmacological symptom management

Until recently, there has been relatively little interest in research into non-pharmacological symptom management but this is no longer the case. A study evaluating a nursing approach to the management of breathlessness in lung cancer is of particular note. Established techniques have been adapted, expanded and used in a different setting, namely that of patients with malignant rather than non-malignant lung disease. The approach revolves around exploring the meaning of breathlessness on an individual basis and teaching breathing retraining techniques and practical coping strategies to patients and their families. Results of a pilot study suggest that it is beneficial and enhances quality of life (Corner et al. 1995). A multicentre study is in progress.

Lymphoedema represents end-stage failure of lymphatic drainage and can be problematic in patients suffering from a wide variety of tumours (Mortimer et al. 1993). Patients with breast cancer are particularly prone to lymphoedema of an upper limb caused either by disease progression or as a result of radiotherapy induced tissue damage. The importance of early intervention comprising conservative treatment including treatment and care of the skin, external support or compression such as bandaging, movement and massage has been highlighted by Badger (1987) and the techniques employed are becoming increasingly sophisticated. Other workers have demonstrated the, sometimes devastating, psychosocial implications of lymphoedema (Woods 1995) and suggest appropriate strategies to deal with them. These therapeutic innovations are already driving changes in multidisciplinary service delivery.

Innovations within other specialities can have a profound effect on the provision of palliative care. The treatment of choice for isolated bone pain is radiotherapy, providing the prognosis is long enough for the treatment to take effect. Radiotherapy techniques are constantly evolving. Of particular importance in the palliative care setting is the relatively recent recognition that single fractions of radiotherapy can provide good palliation of bone pain in certain circumstances (Price et al. 1996). Other innovative approaches to the treatment of bone pain include the use of selected radioactive isotopes which will target osteoblastic activity. One isotope, strontium–89, has been shown to provide effective palliation of pain in patients with multiple bone metastases from prostatic cancer (Lewington et al. 1991).

Recognition that the endobronchial component of many lung tumours is not only the cause of many symptoms, but also accessible to direct examination and intervention has triggered the development of a range of endobronchial therapies. These include brachytherapy (localized radiotherapy), laser photoresection, cryotherapy and the placement of stents.

Bronchoscopic placement of encapsulated radiation sources has been utilized as a method of delivering intense, localized radiotherapy without the problem of 'scatter' inherent in external beam radiotherapy for many years. Technological advances including the development of flexible bronchoscopy, miniature high dose radioisotope technology and remote afterloading systems have prompted increasing sophistication and safety of these techniques. Brachytherapy can now be administered as outpatient or day care therapy. Relief of cough, breathlessness and haemoptysis has been described as well as improvement in performance status (Burt et al. 1990; Dattatreyudu et al. 1993; Speiser and Spratling 1993). On the other hand, toxicity, particularly fistula formation and haemorrhage, can be life-threatening. Endobronchial laser therapy (Colles 1988) and cyotherapy (Walsh et al. 1990) have also been shown to bring about good symptom relief in selected patients. Combined techniques such as the use of Neodymium-yttrium aluminium garnet (Nd-YAG) laser followed by brachytherapy are advocated by some, but run the risk of increased toxicity particularly haemoptysis. A tracheal or bronchial stent can be inserted bronchoscopically. The successful use of both expanding metal (Simonds et al. 1989) and moulded silicone (Cooper et al. 1989) stents has been described. Unless combined with some form of anti-tumour therapy, however, tumour re-growth is inevitable and can be rapid.

These endobronchial techniques can bring about good relief of symptoms caused by endobronchial tumour. Further research needs to address the effect of these techniques on quality of life and hence to define the characteristics of those patients most likely to derive worthwhile benefit.

Research has demonstrated that 16 per cent (65/415) of a large sample of patients receiving conventional treatment for cancer also used complementary therapies and that patient satisfaction with them was high (Downer et al. 1994). The response rate to the questionnaire was 69 per cent. It is not easy to decide which aspects of complementary therapy should be considered as innovative. For instance, homeopathy as an approach to treatment is well established, so much so that the National Homeopathic Hospital in London was opened in the mid-nineteenth century and functions within the National Health Service. Acupuncture is widely used for the management of pain in pain clinics and specialist palliative care settings (Thompson and Filshie 1993). Other therapies are not so closely integrated into conventional care nor so well evaluated.

Aromatherapy services are not infrequently provided for patients receiving specialist palliative care, but attempts at formal evaluation of their effectiveness are uncommon. The interim results, in cancer patients receiving palliative care, of a comparison between massage with a carrier oil and aromatherapy massage with carrier oil and 1 per cent Roman Chamomile essential oil have been published. Aromatherapy massage, but not massage, was shown to have a statistically significant beneficial effect on quality of life and yet both interventions were regarded as beneficial by the patients in reducing anxiety, tension, pain and depression (Wilkinson 1995). The subjects were self-selected and predominantly female and so the results may not be generalizable to the wider population of patients receiving palliative care. Results from a larger number of patients are awaited.

To date, in the UK, complementary therapies have been made available to patients receiving palliative care in both inpatient and day care settings, frequently through the use of trained volunteers. When available, they are offered alongside conventional management. Ultimately, all treatments, even when provided by volunteers, have financial implications. It has been suggested that complementary therapists need to prove that their interventions can be used not as well as but instead of other approaches to treatment in palliative care (Smith 1995). This may not be necessary so long as it can be demonstrated that complementary therapies are efficacious, safe and improve the effectiveness of more orthodox interventions and/or add to the quality of care. More studies are urgently needed to answer these fundamental questions. Other questions including how they might work must wait.

Pharmacological symptom management

The development of novel drugs, different routes of administration and new indications for the use of established drugs could each lead to innovation in the pharmacological management of symptoms. Rather than attempt to review all the recent potential innovations in pharmacological symptom control, a few have been selected to illustrate specific points.

The pharmacological management of cancer pain is often hailed as one of the successes of the palliative care movement. While there is no doubt about the truth of this claim, it is also true that since the mid-1980s there have been few advances in the range of drugs available and that current, best possible pharmacological management allows pain control in only 80–90 per cent of patients (Hanks and Justin 1992). Undoubtedly, psychological, spiritual and cultural factors play a role in all cases and may be of overriding importance in some and a multidisciplinary approach possibly encompassing some of the innovations in psychological therapies, discussed earlier, has the potential to improve this rate. Nevertheless, in a proportion of patients particularly those with complex pains of different aetiologies, pain remains refractory to carefully individualized interventions. Some patients with cancer-related pain do not respond well to opioid analgesics and, in general, these 'opioid poorly responsive' pains are under-diagnosed. A large proportion of these patients will have at least a degree of neuropathic pain. A wide range of adjuvant analgesics, including anti-depressants, anti-convulsants and anti-arrhythmics, are employed in the management of neuropathic pain. Evidence to support the use of these drugs in patients with non-malignant pain is relatively good but in chronic cancer pain scientific studies are sparse and inconclusive. The management of neuropathic pain is in need of urgent rationalization and there is scope for the development of new agents.

Laboratory advances have highlighted the complexity and plasticity of the nervous system and, in particular, drawn attention to the importance of the N-methyl-D-aspartate (NMDA) receptor (Dickenson 1994). Antagonists at this receptor have been studied and have been found to have therapeutic potential in the treatment of neuropathic pain. Ketamine, a drug that has been used in general anaesthetic regimens for many years, is an NMDA receptor antagonist. Initial studies in animals (Chapman and Dickenson 1992) and humans (Łuczak et al. 1995; Edmonds and Davis 1996) suggest that sub-anaesthetic doses of parenteral ketamine can be efficacious in the management of neuropathic pain. Toxicity can be dose-limiting. Oral NMDA antagonists are being developed. Similarly, preclinical studies have revealed that antagonists of cholecystokinin, a natural opioid antagonist, also hold therapeutic promise. Over the next few years labratory research is likely to trigger the development of new drugs tailored specifically for the treatment of neuropathic pain. The therapeutic innovations generated by this convergence of basic science and clinical practice should hold the key to a more rational and, it is hoped, more successful approach to the management of neuropathic pain of whatever cause.

There have been recent developments in the class of opioid analgesics. Tramadol is an interesting, pharmacologically novel drug. It is a selective μ opioid agonist, like morphine, but in addition it inhibits neuronal release of noradrenaline and enhances release of 5-hydroxytryptamine. It has been available since the late 1970s but has only been licensed since the early 1990s, as a weak opioid, in the UK. Its opioid potency is one-tenth that of morphine. The registered indication for its use is the management of moderate to severe pain. Tramadol may be associated with a lower incidence of side-effects than equianalgesic doses of other opioids. Clinical trials of tramadol are well reviewed by Budd (1995). Further research is required in patients with chronic cancer pain particularly since tramadol may have therapeutic potential in the management of neuropathic pain which has not, yet, been investigated. Another therapeutic innovation in pain control has come about through the development of a new route of administration for an old drug, fentanyl. Fentanyl has been used for many years in general anaesthetic regimens. It is a strong opioid with an analgesic potency 75–100 times that of morphine but it has a short duration of action of between one and two hours. Prior to the early 1990s this has precluded its use in the management of chronic pain. Using well-established technology, fentanyl has been incorporated into a transdermal therapeutic system, the fentanyl patch which, once a steady state has been achieved, allows constant release of the drug over 72 hours. Open studies in patients with chronic cancer pain suggest that transdermal fentanyl is as efficacious as equianalgesic doses of morphine and may cause fewer side-effects (Zech et al. 1992; The TTS-Fentanyl Multicentre Study Group 1994). In a large randomized trial comparing transdermal fentanyl and slow release oral morphine sulphate, pain control was equivalent in the two arms of the study but constipation was significantly less troublesome during the transdermal fentanyl arm (p<0.001) (Ahmedzai and Brooks 1996). The trial was not blinded. Evidence to date suggests that transdermal fentanyl is efficacious in the management of chronic pain, that its side-effect profile is different from morphine and that, in particular, constipation is less of a problem. This requires further investigation in both the laboratory and the clinical setting. In addition, studies addressing its safety and efficacy in children and issues around conversion from a weak opioid to transdermal fentanyl are required. A learning curve accompanies the introduction of any new therapeutic strategy. So long as it is prescribed and used properly, transdermal fentanyl appears to be an innovation which is a useful addition to the therapeutic options for relatively stable cancer pain.

Intestinal obstruction is a fairly common complication of advanced malignancy, particularly colonic and ovarian carcinoma. Treatment traditionally includes fasting, nasogastric suction, intravenous fluids and consideration of surgery. These interventions are not appropriate in all patients and should be reserved for those in whom there is a possibility that surgery will be of benefit. The medical management of inoperable intestinal obstruction comprises treatment directed at relieving the symptoms rather than the signs or the cause of the obstruction (Baines et al. 1985). It is employed frequently within specialist palliative care but, sadly, not so frequently within acute, general settings where its increased use could be regarded as innovative. This underlines the problem that innovations in specific areas of health care are not always widely publicized or applied elsewhere. It is important to remember that palliative care has much to offer other specialties but it also has much to learn from them.

Somatostatin analogues, such as octreotide and vapreotide, stimulate water and electrolyte absorption, inhibit water secretion in the small bowel and reduce gastrointestinal motility (Nott et al. 1990). Preliminary evidence supports their use as an adjunct in bowel obstruction (Mercadanto and Maddaloni 1992; Khoo et al. 1994) and in the management of enterocolic fistulae (Mulvihill 1996). These agents, particularly octreotide, are being used in many centres as part of the management of intestinal obstruction. There seems little doubt that some patients benefit from this therapeutic innovation but there is an urgent need for information on which patients are most likely to benefit and what constitutes an adequate therapeutic trial as well as comparative studies with other agents, particularly hyoscine butylbromide. The fact that octreotide is an expensive drug may well ensure that these questions are answered quickly. The antisecretory actions of octreotide are also being employed in the treatment of other problems including sweating and exudative cutaneous breast cancer. These constitute truly novel indications for this drug.

Breathlessness is recognized as a difficult symptom to manage, particularly in patients with very advanced cancer. There has been a surge of interest in this symptom and its pharmacological and non-pharmacological management. Oral and parenteral opioids are an established part of the drug treatment of breathlessness in patients with malignant disease (Ahmedzai 1993). There is a current vogue for the use of inhaled opioids in the management of these patients, despite an increasing body of scientific evidence against it. The first study, in patients with chronic obstructive pulmonary disease (COPD), was published in 1989. It showed a significant improvement in bicycle endurance time after a small dose of nebulized morphine compared to nebulized normal saline (Young et al. 1989). Since then, four studies have been conducted, three in COPD patients (Beauford et al. 1993; Davis et al. 1994; Thomas et al. 1994) and one in patients with cancer-related breathlessness (Davis et al. 1996). All failed to show any statistically significant effect of nebulized morphine on breathlessness compared with nebulized normal saline. The design of these studies varied considerably and this highlights the difficulty of assessing breathlessness particularly in the setting of a clinical trial. None the less, to date, the scientific evidence does not support the use of nebulized morphine in the management of breathlessness.

Arts therapies in palliative care

A holistic approach must take account of the spiritual and creative aspects of each individual and palliative care has been enthusiastic about drawing on the arts to address this aspect of care. There is a long history of the use of these therapies in the field of mental health. The Palliative Care Unit at the Royal Victoria Hospital in Montreal was an early pioneer (Munro and Mount 1978) with a music therapist on the staff. She reports both a sense of spiritual comfort and reduced physical symptoms and use of medication in patients treated. The 'Partage' meeting in the same unit offered a model of using the arts to foster a sense of community and creativity. Staff, patients, volunteers and family members could all participate equally in exploring a particular theme through music, pictures or words. In the UK, the Royal Marsden Hospital was the first NHS hospital to establish an art therapy service linked to its Rehabilitation Centre (Connell 1992) and many hospices have developed some aspect of arts therapies, sometimes in association with the charitable initiative Hospice Arts. Frampton (1993) has described the range of initiatives that may be attempted, but warns that experience with a sculpture project at St John's Hospice, Lancaster, shows that unless patients are involved right from the start in developing projects they are unlikely to be effective. Arts therapies is an area where therapeutic innovation and service development often go hand in hand.

Work with children facing bereavement

Treating patients within their family as the unit of care is a basic principle of palliative care. St Christopher's Hospice produced a model for this, as for so much else, with its early use of genograms and the establishment of a bereavement service. There have been a number of initiatives directed at including and informing children who face the death of a parent. These may be working with children on a one-to-one basis, including them in family work or developing groups for them. A series of articles in the *European Journal of Palliative Care* (Baulkwill and Wood 1994; Firth and Anderson 1994; Hemmings 1994; Sheldon 1994) set out principles and provide examples of innovative work in this area. One particular intervention now being evaluated is the board game 'All about me' (Hemmings 1994). This game is played by the worker and child together and involves travelling along a board and at certain points turning over cards which ask for responses about opinions and feelings. The professional can select these cards according to the child's particular needs, and by answering the questions as well, demonstrates that the child is not the only one to experience feelings like sadness and anger.

A number of hospices and local bereavement services are now developing groups for children. Sometimes these run for one day only (Burroughs *et al.* 1992), sometimes for a series of sessions (Pennells and Kitchener 1990). One of the largest programmes for bereaved children is the Winston's Wish programme, developed from an American idea by Stokes and her colleagues in the Gloucester Palliative Care team. This started in a small way with a weekend camp for bereaved children and has now grown into a range of community-based initiatives. Sufficient experience has been accumulated so that the time is ripe to evaluate the whole programme.

Evaluation of innovation

Traditionally, conservatism has been widespread in medicine; history has often shown that innovative ideas and unconventional ways of thinking are usually rejected by the mainstream and its institutions (Kuhn 1970). It may be that palliative medicine and specialist palliative care are different. Perhaps new specialities which are keen to establish themselves and to prove their importance to the mainstream of health care, are more likely than others to welcome new ideas and nurture innovation. On the other hand, it may be that in the current climate, innovation in any field has become fashionable. Either way, specialists in palliative care must strike the right balance between the 'new' and the 'old' and be prepared to evaluate both approaches.

There is a trend in symptom control, in common with many other situations, towards increasingly sophisticated interventions sometimes requiring high technology. This quest for the 'new' is appropriate and, on the whole, should be encouraged but it needs to be balanced against the fact that 'old' methods are not necessarily passé. The resurgence of interest in the non-pharmacological management of breathlessness (discussed earlier) illustrates this well. Within the wider field of cancer care, the trend towards increasingly sophisticated, and sometimes toxic, anti-cancer therapies continues as is appropriate in a setting where cure, if at all possible, is the aim. At the same time, however, trials of palliative chemotherapy against best supportive care are being developed. These changes in oncological practice take us back to the original principles of palliative care – being alongside the patient and recognizing the patient's problems and needs rather than regarding them as a series of symptoms and signs that require intervention. Even in specialist palliative care, we need to remember that we do not need 'to do' rather than 'to be' in order to be acknowledged as credible health care professionals in the eyes of colleagues and of patients and their families.

In symptom management, non-pharmacological and pharmacological interventions are often employed simultaneously. This seems a logical and appropriate model of care but requires further evaluation. Before this can happen, appropriate methods of evaluation including outcome measures need to be devised and the clinical effectiveness of the individual interventions has to be assessed. This will be challenging. For instance, there is great public support for complementary therapy and increasing demand to assimilate its techniques into mainstream medicine. The demand for rigorous evaluation of complementary therapies is driven by several groups including those working in mainstream health care, commissioning health authorities and those practising complementary medicine. It has been argued that the same criteria now applied to evaluation of new therapeutic strategies in mainstream medicine must also be applied to both established and new complementary techniques (Smith 1995). This is difficult to countenance because it is unlikely that the same methodologies will be appropriate to both. In the palliative care setting, the difficulties of evaluating complementary therapies scientifically may be compounded by the problems of longitudinal evaluation of any intervention in a dynamic situation when relentless disease progression means that the goalposts are constantly shifting.

Methodological rigour is required in the assessment of any innovation. The multifactoral and changing nature of many of the problems encountered in the palliative care setting mean that study design is often challenging. Indeed, as Lichter (1993) observes, when total patient care is provided, with attention to physical, emotional and spiritual well-being, it is difficult to ascribe benefit to one particular intervention. Health care professionals are being urged to seek evidence of effectiveness through systematic review, which comprises the expert, systematic collation of research evidence on a specific subject (Haines and Iliffe 1995). This is commendable but is possible only if there is a sufficient critical mass of evidence available for scrutiny which is seldom the case in palliative care.

There is a real and urgent need for research into all aspects of palliative care including those discussed in this chapter. In general, randomized controlled trials remain the gold standard for testing new drugs and devices but many are flawed, usually in design. It is increasingly being recognized that even in this area of research, a range of methodological approaches including quality of life assessment are essential for well-rounded evaluation. Other aspects of palliative care research may require a purely qualitative approach but methodological rigour is still crucial. In some instances, neither pure quantitative nor pure qualitative methodology but a composite of the two is required, although this raises issues about the philosophical bases of the two methodologies. The challenge is to foster a flexible approach to research in palliative care while ensuring that new ideas are subjected to rigorous scrutiny that is as sensitive, specific and appropriate as possible. The implications of funding such research must be recognized and monies set aside. This is particularly pertinent for research into the non-symptom control areas of palliative care and the non-pharmacological aspects of symptom control especially when qualitative methods are the most appropriate, where research funds are usually difficult to obtain. There is potential to create a workable, integrated system for the evaluation of therapeutic innovation in palliative care which, in itself, may be innovative.

Conclusion

Innovations are usually regarded as being 'a good thing'. They also carry potential for harm not least because they can divert both interest and scarce resources from other areas. Therapeutic innovations may cause direct harm to patients and their families. New ideas tend to catch the imagination and generate enthusiasm. It is our responsibility to channel such enthusiasm into the appropriate evaluation of therapeutic innovations. The methods employed will vary but must be chosen and used with rigour. There is an enormous range and richness of new therapeutic ideas in palliative care, only some of which are discussed in this chapter. Undoubtedly, many will fall by the wayside but, none the less, they will have contributed to the development of effective palliative care. Others will be able to withstand scrutiny from those inside and outside the speciality and will be adopted into practice. In this way, evidence-based palliative care will develop and, ultimately, come of age.

References

Ahmedzai, S. (1993) Palliation of respiratory symptoms, in D. Doyle, G.W.C. Hanks and N. MacDonald (eds) *Oxford Textbook of Palliative Medicine*. Oxford: Oxford University Press.

Ahmedzai, S. and Brooks, D. (1996) Transdermal fentanyl versus oral morphine in the treatment of cancer pain. *Palliative Medicine*, 10(1): 60 (abstr).

Angle, H.L. and Van de Ven, A.H. (1989) Suggestions for managing the innovation journey, in A.H. Van de Ven, H.L. Angle and M.S. Poole (eds) *Research on the Management of Innovation: The Minnesota Studies Grand Rapids*. Ballinger/Harper Row for the University of Minnesota.

Badger, C. (1987) Lymphoedema: management of patients with advanced cancer. *Professional Nurse*, 2(4): 100–2.

Baines, M.J., Oliver, D.J. and Carter, R.L. (1985) Medical management of intestinal obstruction in patients with advanced malignant disease: a clinical and pathological study. *Lancet*, ii: 900–3.

Baulkwill, J. and Wood, C. (1994) Groupwork with bereaved children. *European Journal of Palliative Care*, 1(3): 113–15.

Beauford, W., Saylor, T.T., Stansbury, D.W., Avolos, K. and Light, R.W. (1993) Effects of nebulised morphine sulfate on the exercise tolerance of the ventilatory limited COPD patient. *Chest*, 104: 175–8.

Budd, K. (1995) A step towards the ideal analgesic? *European Journal of Palliative Care*, 2(2): 56–9.

Burroughs, A., Tyler, J., Moat, I. and Pye, S. (1992) Griefwork with children: workshop days at Pilgrims' Hospice, Canterbury. *Palliative Medicine*, 6(1): 26–33.

Burt, P., O'Driscoll, B., Notley, H., Barber, P. and Stout, R. (1990) Intraluminal irradiation for the palliation of lung cancer with high dose rate Micro-Selectron. *Thorax*, 45: 765–8.

Butler, R.N. (1963) The life review: an interpretation of reminiscence in the elderly. *Psychiatry*, 26: 65–73.

Chapman, V. and Dickenson, A.H. (1992) The combination of NMDA antagomism and morphine produces profound antinocieptions in the rat dorsal horn. *Brain Research*, 573: 321–3.

Cocker, K.I., Bell, D.R. and Kidman, A. (1994) Cognitive behaviour therapy with advanced breast cancer patients. *Psycho-oncology*, 3(2): 233–7.

Colles, M.J. (1988) What is a laser and how is it applied for therapy? *British Journal of Hospital Medicine*, 40: 111–14.

Connell, C. (1992) Art therapy as part of a palliative care programme. *Palliative Medicine*, 6: 26–33.

Cooper, J.D., Pearson, F.G., Patterson, G.A., Todd, G.R. and Ginsberg, R.J. (1989) Use of silicone stents in the management of airway problems. *Annals of Thoracic Surgery*, 47: 371–8.

Corner, J., Plant, H. and Warner, L. (1995) Developing a nursing approach to managing dyspnoea in lung cancer. *International Journal of Palliative Nursing*, 1(1): 5–11.

Dattatreyudu, N., Allison, R., Kaplan, B., Samala, E., Osian, A. and Karbowitz, S. (1993) High dose-rate intraluminal irradiation in bronchogenic carcinoma. *Chest*, 104: 1006–11.

Davis, C.L., Hodder, C.A., Lowe, S., Shah, R., Slevin, M.L. and Wedzicha, A. (1994) Effect of nebulised morphine and morphine 6-glucuronide on exercise endurance in patients with chronic obstructive airways disease. *Thorax*, 49: 393P (abstr).

Davis, C.L., Penn, K., A'Hern, R.P., Daniels, J. and Slevin, M.L. (1996) Single dose randomised controlled trial of nebulised morphine in patients with cancer related breathlessness. *Palliative Medicine*, 10(1): 64–5 (abstr).

Dickenson, A.H. (1994) Neurophysiology of opioid poorly responsive pain, in G.W. Hanks (ed.) *Palliative Medicine: Problem Areas in Pain and Symptom Management*, Cancer surveys series, vol. 21. New York: Cold Spring Harbor Laboratory Press.

Downer, S.M., Cody, M.M., McCluskey, P., Wilson, P.D., Arnott, S.J., Lister, T.A. and Slevin, M.A. (1994) Pursuit and practice of complementary therapies by cancer patients receiving conventional treatment. *British Medical Journal*, 309: 86–9.

Edmonds, P. and Davis, C.L. (1996) Experience of the use of subcutaneous ketamine in patients with cancer-related neuropathic pain. *European Journal of Palliative Care*: Abstracts of the Fourth Congress of the European Association for Palliative Care, 06 (abstr).

Faulkner, A. and Maguire, P. (1994) *Talking to Cancer Patients and their Families*. Oxford: Oxford University Press.

Filshie, J., Penn, K., Ashley, S. and Davis, C.L. (1996) Acupuncture for the relief of cancer-related breathlessness. *Palliative Medicine*, 10(2): 145–50.

Firth, P. and Anderson, P. (1994) Teamwork with families facing bereavement. *European Journal of Palliative Care*, 1(4): 157–61.

Frampton, D. (1993) Creative arts and literature, in D. Doyle, G.W.C. Hanks and N. MacDonald (eds) *Oxford Textbook of Palliative Medicine*. Oxford: Oxford University Press.

Haight, B.K. and Webster, J. (1995) *The Art and Science of Reminiscing: Theory, Research Methods and Application*. Washington: Taylor and Francis.

Haines, A. and Iliffe, S. (1995) Innovations in services and the appliance of science. *British Medical Journal*, 310: 815–16.

Hanks, G.W. and Justins, D.M. (1992) Cancer pain: management. *Lancet*, 339: 1031–6.

Hanks, G.W.C., Portenoy, R.K., MacDonald, N. and O'Neill, W. (1993) Difficult pain problems, in D. Doyle, G.W.C. Hanks and N. MacDonald (eds) *Oxford Textbook of Palliative Medicine*. Oxford: Oxford University Press.

Hemmings, P. (1994) Working with children facing bereavement as individuals. *European Journal of Palliative Care*, 1(2): 72–7.

Jones, K., Johnston, M. and Speck, P. (1989) Despair felt by the patient and the professional carer. *Palliative Medicine*, 3: 39–46.

Kearney, M. (1992) Imagework in a case of intractable pain. *Palliative Medicine*, 2(6): 152–7.

Khoo, D., Hall, E., Motson, R., Riley, J., Denman, K. and Waxman, J. (1994) Palliation of malignant intestinal obstruction using ocreotide. *European Journal of Cancer*, 30: 28–30.

Kuhn, T.S. (1970) *The Structure of Scientific Revolutions*, 2nd edn. Chicago: University of Chicago Press.

Lester, J. (1994) 'Life review with the terminally ill', unpublished MSc dissertation. University of Southampton.

Lewington, V.J., Ackery, D.M., Bayley, R.J., Keeling, D.H., McLeod, P.M., Porter, A.T., Zivanovic, M.A. and McEwan, A.J.B. (1991) A prospective randomised double-blind crossover study to examine the efficacy of strontium–89 in pain palliation in patients with advanced prostate cancer metastatic to bone. *European Journal of Cancer*, 27: 954–8.

Lichter, I. (1993) Biography as therapy. *Palliative Medicine*, 7(2): 133–7.

Luczak, J., Dickenson, A.H. and Kotlinska-Lemieszek, A. (1995) The role of ketamine, an NMDA receptor antagonist, in the management of pain. *Progress in Palliative Care*, 3(4): 127–34.

Mercadanto, S. and Maddaloni, S. (1992) Octreotide in the management of inoperable gastrointestinal obstruction in terminal cancer patients. *Journal of Pain and Symptom Management*, 7: 496–8.

Moorey, S. and Greer, S. (1989) *Psychological Therapy with Cancer Patients: A New Approach*. Oxford: Heinemann Medical.

Mortimer, P.S., Badger, C. and Hall, J. (1993) Lymphoedema, in D. Doyle, G.W.C. Hanks and N. MacDonald (eds) *Oxford Textbook of Palliative Medicine*. Oxford: Oxford University Press.

Mulvihill, S., Pappas, T.N., Passero, E. and Debas, H.T. (1996) The use of somatostatin and its analogue in the treatment of surgical disorders. *Surgery*, 100: 467–76.

Munro, S. and Mount, B. (1978) Music therapy in palliative care. *Canadian Medical Association Journal*, 119(9): 3–8.

Nott, D.M., Ellenhager, S., Yates, J., Nos, J. and Jenkins, S.A. (1990) Effects of SMS 201–995 (ocreotide) in ameliorating the complications of small bowel obstruction in rats. *Gut*, 31: A591.

Pennells, M. and Kitchener, S. (1990) Holding back the nightmares. *Social Work Today*, 1 March.

Price, P., Hoskin, P.J., Easton, D., Austin, D., Palmer, S. and Yarnold, J.R. (1996) Prospective randomised trial of single and multifraction radiotherapy schedules in the treatment of painful bone metastases. *Radiotherapy and Oncology*, 6: 247–55.

Rogers, E.M. (1983) *Diffusion of Innovations*, 3rd edn. New York: The Free Press.

Sheldon, F. (1994) Children and bereavement as individuals. *European Journal of Palliative Care*, 1(1): 42–4.

Simonds, A.K., Irving, J.D., Clarke, S.W. and Dick, R. (1989) Use of expandable metal stents in the treatment of bronchial obstruction. *Thorax*, 44: 680–1.

Smith, I. (1995) Commissioning complementary medicine. *British Medical Journal*, 310: 1151–2.

Speiser, B.L. and Spratling, L. (1993) Remote afterloading brachytherapy for the local control of endobronchial carcinoma. *International Journal of Radiation, Oncology, Biology and Physics*, 25: 579–87.

The TTS-Fentanyl Multicentre Study Group (1994) Transdermal fentanyl in cancer pain. *Journal of Drug Development*, 6(3): 93–7.

Thomas, S.H.L., Masood, A.R. and Read, J.W. (1994) Lack of effect of nebulised morphine on ventilation, breathlessness and exercise endurance in patients with chronic obstructive lung disease. *British Journal of Clinical Oncology Pharmacol*, 37: 515 (abstr).

Thompson, J.W. and Filshie, J. (1993) Transcutaneous nerve stimulation (TENS) and acupuncture, in D. Doyle, G.W.C. Hanks and N. MacDonald (eds) *Oxford Textbook of Palliative Medicine*. Oxford: Oxford University Press.

Vachon, M. (1988) Counselling and psychotherapy in palliative/hospice care: a review. *Palliative Medicine*, 2: 36–50.

Walsh, D.A., Maiwand, M.O., Nath, A.R., Lockwood, P., Lloyd, M.H. and Saab, M. (1990) Bronchoscopic cryotherapy for advanced bronchial carcinoma. *Thorax*, 45: 509–13.

Wilkinson, S. (1995) Aromatherapy and massage in palliative care. *International Journal of Palliative Nursing*, 1(1): 21–30.

Woods, M. (1995) Social factors and psychosocial implications of lymphoedema. *International Journal of Palliative Nursing*, 1(1): 17–20.

Young, I.H., Daviskas, E. and Keena, V.A. (1989) Effect of low dose morphine on exercise endurance in patients with chronic lung disease. *Thorax*, 44: 387–90.

Zech, D.F.J., Grond, S.U.A., Lynch, J. *et al.* (1992) Transdermal fentanyl and initial dose-finding with patient-controlled analgesia in cancer pain: a pilot study with 20 terminally ill cancer patients. *Pain*, 50: 293–301.

15 Beyond cancer?

■ ROB GEORGE AND JO SYKES

In this chapter we shall look beyond cancer at the types of illnesses that merit palliative care, evidence of demand for this type of service, the generic approach that may be suitable and some of the difficulties in providing it. We also offer a way through anxieties about deluge of work, and dilution of basic palliative philosophy.

We need to start, however, with an important question. If we believe, alongside Sir Kenneth Calman, that people with cancer should have the right to decent palliative care, is there any reason to justify our failure to extend this to other diagnoses? Colin Douglas (1992) wrote that the hospice movement is too good to be true and too small to be useful. Is he right?

History

Palliative medicine cuts across the grain of late-twentieth-century medicine. Among many colleagues, and within the medical schools, there still remains a dogged belief in nosology and the perception that answers will be found to diseases and death in cellular biology and genetics. The hospice movement entered the arena with uncomfortable and disarming views about the reality of death, the futility of invasive and curative medicine and how to deal with the person *behind* the pathology. Notwithstanding the historical roots of the hospice movement in the care of the 'generically' dying and destitute (Saunders 1987), there has been a very limited move so far into the mainstream of medicine. One may speculate as to the reasons:

1 Most can accept cancer as fatal. For a new discipline dealing with suffering and death, it was the obvious place to start.
2 New caring initiatives start, almost by definition, out of charity (an act of benevolence beyond what is accepted as a person's right). To generate support, they must be explicit and capture the heart of society. Cancer is a paradigm: pain, suffering, indignity and death concern us all. The early champions were charismatic and focused on this.
3 The striking impact of the movement upon suffering and pain in particular has led within the professional lives of its founders to the acceptance of palliative medicine as a mainstream speciality alongside oncology and radiotherapy. Within the narrow confines of cancer, their job is therefore complete.

However, returning to Douglas, why should only the minority who die of malignancies – and precious few even of them – be singled out for de luxe dying? He makes an argument for palliative care support units offering consultations, home care services, and a few beds for difficult cases, in all places where the serious dying is done: district general hospitals and teaching hospitals. Davis and Hardy (1994) state that clinical application of the principles of palliative care need not and should not be limited to patients suffering from malignant disease. Optimal symptom control and care of the whole person are an integral part of the comprehensive care of any patient and deserve to be considered as such. Ahmedzai (1993) feels that the assumption of hospices that the large majority of people who die of non-malignant causes are not frightened should be challenged by direct evidence. There is ready support by the public for children's hospices, which take predominantly non-malignant cases, and also hospice-type services for AIDS patients; care of the dying may even rank second after caring for children in the eyes of the public.

Coming of age is a painful and often sobering experience. The egocentricity of youth, with its fads and independence, is less tolerable and uncomfortable when responsibilities begin to emerge. For palliative medicine, this is the wide world of the distressed, 'dis-eased' and dying who do not have the luxury of a cancer diagnosis that entitles them, historically, to good palliative care. While development of new things can be likened impertinently to the maturing of a child, business and organizational theory recognize this as familiar and characteristic of a consolidating initiative.

One principle of change, however, stands out and should be heard by the speciality: the obstruction to a new development usually comes most strongly from the protagonists of the most recent and successful innovation. Palliative care in cancer, thanks to the pioneers, has been moved successfully from an act of charity to a matter of justice. Going beyond cancer – generic palliative care, if you like – must be the speciality's next goal and falls to this generation of specialists.

Palliative care for all: justice or charity?

Questions of justice refer to needs without which the person would be harmed or detrimentally affected. Paraphrasing Aristotle, Beauchamp and Childress (1994) have suggested that no person should be treated unequally, despite all differences with other persons, unless some difference between them is relevant to the treatment at stake. From this viewpoint, decisions, rules and laws tend to be unjust when they make distinctions between classes of persons who are actually similar in relevant respects. The various theories of justice do not differ significantly in this view. However, we do need to explore the argument briefly here; it is discussed in detail elsewhere (George 1997).

Given that palliative care is ever justified – a self-evident fact in the UK with respect to cancer is its acceptance by both society through donation and state through funding – intuition drives one to see no moral difference between patients dying or suffering symptoms from any terminal disease. But to say this we must establish that need (as opposed to want) clearly exists.

The evident extent of palliative need

A survey of palliative care services in Britain and Ireland in 1990 revealed that of 95 units with five or more beds, 67 per cent cared for patients with motor neurone disease (MND), 40 per cent multiple sclerosis (MS) patients, 40 per cent persons with AIDS, 21 per cent patients with Parkinson's disease, 23 per cent patients with heart or chest disease, 14 per cent stroke sufferers, and 8 per cent Alzheimer's sufferers (Smith *et al.* 1992). Five units took all of the patient groups apart from AIDS, and one unit took all groups. Three excluded only patients with Alzheimer's disease. We have no idea of the number of patients this involves.

In an update in 1991, the same investigators revealed that of 139 inpatient units (88 per cent of the 158 units listed in the 1991 Directory of Hospice Services), over 50 per cent cared for MND patients, and almost as many mentioned AIDS (Eve and Smith 1994). Only 6 (less than 4 per cent) said they would care for a patient with any terminal illness. Of 129 day care units replying to a questionnaire, 82 cared for patients with MND, and 56 for patients with AIDS. They state that a significant number would care for patients with other diagnoses, but we are not told how many. Hospital support teams were surveyed and asked whether they accepted patients with diseases other than cancer. Almost all the teams who replied to this part of the questionnaire accepted patients with MND and AIDS. About two-thirds would accept patients with heart disease or MS. Almost half of the services said that they would care for any terminally ill patient and some specifically mentioned chronic pain problems, renal failure, diverticular disease, ischaemic problems, rheumatoid arthritis, and vascular disease. Again, there is no evidence on how many such cases are actually referred.

Doyle, Hanks and MacDonald include in the introduction to the *Oxford Textbook of Palliative Medicine* the fact that programmes assisting AIDS patients are in place, and some palliative care groups also enrol patients with MND and allied neurological disorders. They go on to point out that all these disorders are characterized by constantly changing physical symptoms, increased risk of psychosocial distress, societal misunderstanding, and a relatively short period of final illness (Doyle *et al.* 1993). As well as making these conditions suitable for the principles of palliative care, some of the above factors can make it difficult to know when palliative care becomes appropriate and when the terminal phase of the illness has arrived.

Wilson *et al.* (1995) attempted to estimate the number of non-cancer patients requiring inpatient palliative care in the Thames Valley by sending questionnaires to general practitioners. There was a reasonable consensus about the non-malignant conditions most in need of palliative care, the largest groups of patients being those with strokes, cardiovascular disease, MS, and rheumatoid arthritis. They make the point that this reflects the distribution of these non-cancer patients in an average practice and not necessarily their suitability for hospice-type care, using the example that MND is very appropriate but a relatively rare condition. The final figure that they come up with is 11 non-cancer patients per practice/year in need of respite or continuing care in the Thames Valley, and this works out to be more bed-days per year than were available at that time for mainly cancer patients. This accords with our own surveys in central London, where the perceived needs of general practitioners (GPs) showed cancer to be equal to chronic organ failures, degenerative diseases and HIV (we are in a high incidence area). GPs for example perceive themselves to need as much help with cardiorespiratory disease as with cancer (Camden and Islington Palliative Care Team 1996).

In 1992, the Standing Medical Advisory Committee, Standing Nursing and Midwifery Advisory Committee report on Palliative Care argued that palliative care services are appropriate, and should be developed, for those dying from causes other than cancer (SMAC/SNMAC 1992). Little is known about the needs of or appropriate service provision for these patients (Addington-Hall and McCarthy 1995). Clark (1994) argues that while the philosophy of 'hospice' can be extended, available resources are less elastic, and goes on to recommend encouraging purchasers to undertake need assessments and then develop appropriate services in response.

In a random sample of 639 adults dying in 1987, 44 people received hospice services, of which 2 had a diagnosis other than cancer (Seale 1991).

In summary, there is clearly a disadvantaged group and this is probably in a majority. On the grounds of justice, one either regulates up so that all receive palliative care, or society decides that the dying do not merit this and no one receives palliative care. If there is a case for palliative care in cancer, the ethical case for palliative care beyond cancer is resounding and restricted practice is indefensible.

Generic palliative care

Several themes are common to 'generic' palliative care.

Practical problems with facilities

For understandable reasons, the vast majority of services are bound up with buildings. How do we adapt to the needs of other diseases in institutions familiar only with cancer? There are three legitimate anxieties:

1 Severely incapacitated patients through slowly progressive disease require much personal attention and may also require specialized equipment and skills. It may be difficult to support the training and equipment needed to care for a particular type of patient if the numbers being referred to a service are small.
2 The prognosis in these patients is usually less clear-cut than with cancer. The palliative care centres which do admit these patients tend to provide respite admissions for periods of two to three weeks to relieve the burden on the carers (Wilson *et al.* 1995).
3 The integration of non-cancer patients into palliative care facilities for those with cancer has been controversial. The difficulties concerning the inpatient care of sufferers from Alzheimer's disease is a case in point, and it may be that special centres or better care in the community is required.

Philosophy of care

Palliative care is quite open in declaring that whole person care is the order of the day with terminally ill and dying people. It is not reductive, but divergent, exploring the roots and branches of a person's suffering, pain or distress. It is therefore labour intensive, time consuming and based in trusting relationships with patient and family. We need to be clear therefore about whether this approach is needed or appropriate for all patients with palliative needs – especially if they are merely symptomatic and not yet dying. If it is, then we shall rapidly find we have too much work and our standards will suffer without major injections of funds. How can we tune our philosophy of practice to accommodate this but protect the essence of our approach? This is not wishful thinking, but is already upon us, as Calman (1994) is actually taking us down this road with cancer already. The requirements for involvement of palliative care in teamwork from the point of diagnosis will be expected of the new cancer centres and there is no doubt that some patients will have episodic needs relating to physical problems prior to being pronounced 'incurable' and in need of full palliative care.

Our own experience with a generic caseload supports the case for dividing our practice into three broad categories: consultative work, full multidisciplinary palliative care and terminal care in the last days.

Broad principles of managing generic caseloads

Consultative work

This is high turnover, sharp and focused. Two points need emphasis:

- These are short-term contacts with defined endpoints. Maintenance of the case is down to Primary Health Care or the Inpatient staff.
- There is a role for the palliative physician much earlier on in disease than is historically agreed, namely involvement in the management of iatrogenic symptomatology, assistance with side-effects and matters surrounding pain control, gut management, and so on.

Support

Support is directed towards colleagues with broader single joint consultations, e.g. ethical dilemmas, teaching and assistance on living wills; or a quick overview of cases where clear direction and the change to or mix of therapeutic and palliative approaches is being considered.

Case examples

1 A young woman from the caring professions developed complicated neurological complications of HIV. The matter of placement arose. She was adamant about staying in the acute facility, which was about to discharge her. Palliative care was asked to consult on the ethics of these plans and ways to communicate the dilemma to the family. Two meetings resolved the matter.
2 A woman with advanced Alzheimer's disease, disabled to the point of vegetation, needed a replacement gastrostomy tube. Her husband was

adamant about acute treatments and refused additional assistance in care. Primary health care was at the end of its tether. Palliative care took the case for three weeks' respite for the professionals with the task of advocating for improving overall symptom control and practical care.

Symptom control

This takes the classical reductive medical model and explores this area of pathology and practical solution, e.g. within the acute units, oncology, care of elderly people and general medicine. In essence the approach is problem solving with respect to symptomatology focusing on diagnostic and therapeutic algorithms where the view in mind is one explicitly of symptom relief. The advisory role is circumscribed, focused and short term akin to the request for a neurological or dermatological opinion. Patients and family may be seen only a couple of times, with fresh referrals when needed.

Case examples

1 An elderly woman with ischaemic leg ulcers was referred for pain control. This was difficult to achieve immediately and needed regular review (every two to four weeks) for three months. The main role was support of the district nurse in her decision making.
2 A male haemophiliac with chronic leg pain related to arthroscopy was referred for an opinion on opiate use. The pain was neuropathic and responded to appropriate adjustments of the regime. Four single consultations have been needed over six months jointly with the haematologists.
3 A girl with 'refractory vomiting' following chemotherapy for leukaemia was referred for advice. A single consultation resolved the problem.

Full palliative care

For patients whose lives are going to end in the short to medium term, the need for a complete service is clear. Their needs with respect to symptom control, psychosocial and spiritual care is the same, although again there will be cases – just as with malignancy – where clinical improvement or stability is unexpected and specialist palliative care can withdraw for a time.

Case example

A patient with fibrosing alveolitis was referred for assistance with breathlessness. He was frail and frightened. The GP was at a loss. The patient was supported with full palliative care until his death six months later. His estranged family was reconciled to some degree and he was able to prepare for his death appropriately.

Terminal care

A major area of need concerns those imminently dying. Just as patients with chronic relapsing diseases have the habit of stabilizing when all expected them to die, so the time comes when 'yet another acute exacerbation' becomes the time of death. Cardiorespiratory disease is the typical example. Inpatient clinicians are then faced with the need for rapid, effective symptom control, assistance with talking to a family with whom they have personal relationship and support at the death of a longstanding patient. Demonstrating that we can be just as effective in these acute situations builds bridges, enriches hospital practice and restores the art to medicine.

Case examples

1 A houseman referred a dying male patient with chronic airflow limitation. Acute treatment was failing and he was breathless and confused. The inpatient clinicians were afraid to use opiates or sedatives and the family and nurses were increasingly distressed. The houseman was taught how to use medication in the last 48 hours of life and the nurses helped to console the family.
2 A GP referred a cantankerous, octogenarian recluse who was dying: cause unknown. He resolutely refused investigation, was in squalid surroundings, had pain and an elderly, exhausted sister. The district nurse was the only professional given access at the time of referral. We were asked to help her keep him comfortable and support his sister through the remaining days.

Specific problems

We conclude with the literature on relevant, specific problems.

Elderly people

With increasing numbers of aged people, the challenge of caring for this population will increase. A number of papers suggest that elderly patients have needs in provision of their terminal care which are somewhat different from those recognized in younger patients (Wilson *et al.* 1987; Seale 1991; Severs and Wilkins 1991).

Blackburn (1989) has attempted to identify and describe the special needs of elderly patients in hospital. Case records of 27 patients aged over 66 years who died on a mixed function male geriatric ward were analysed. Principal causes of death were chest infection, chronic bronchitis, dementia,

Parkinson's disease, ischaemic heart disease, and carcinoma. He draws the following conclusions:

- Elderly patients have multiple clinical diagnoses involving multisystem pathology.
- Diagnosis of dying is often made only by exclusion, i.e. after failure of response to standard treatment. Thus the moment at which death can be predicted with certainty is often closer to the actual event and there is a shorter time for the provision of good terminal care when compared to cancer patients.
- Communication is more difficult due to a combination of the higher incidence of confusion in elderly patients than in younger cancer patients, expressive problems associated with cerebrovascular accidents (CVAs), and impaired senses of hearing and vision.
- Reduced social networks leading to reduced care and support from family and friends.

Seale (1991) confirmed that the diagnosis of dying is more difficult in elderly people. The incidence, duration, intensity and type of symptoms follow a different pattern in cancer compared to other illnesses. Long-term mental confusion and disability, as well as other symptoms related to age are more common in non-cancer patients. Non-cancer patients tend to be older and people aged 75 and over who do not die from cancer are more likely to have outlasted their spouses, brothers and sisters and even their children. They are predominantly women and many live alone or in residential care.

This will clearly have an impact on some established practices in current cancer oriented palliative care. Emphasis on family involvement and support may be less appropriate than in cancer. Grief in the relatives of the elderly non-cancer patient may be less intensely focused on the actual bereavement, and more on the distress of coping with long-term dependency, where practical help and support are paramount. Specialist home care teams tend to emphasize emotional support and advice rather than practical nursing tasks, and bereavement services set up by many hospices are more appropriate in cases of cancer.

In another study looking at appropriateness and acceptability of conservative care of terminally ill elderly patients in a geriatric unit, agitation was identified as the commonest cause of distress in dying patients (Wilson *et al.* 1987). A significantly higher proportion of patients with a respiratory diagnosis were recorded as being distressed, highlighting the inadequacy of managing breathing problems. Only 20 out of 150 patients received intravenous fluids, and there were no complaints from relatives about this. They suggest that relatives often find it easier to resist such measures than care staff. Among other problems picked up were the prescription of inappropriate drugs despite poor compliance, and the use of diuretics in 25 per cent of patients, most of whom did not have cardiac or renal failure.

Severs and Wilkins (1991) reviewed a 12-bedded palliative care ward created within a district general hospital. The aim was to provide a setting for elderly people to die with dignity and with psychological and counselling support for themselves and their relatives. The assumption was that the long-stay geriatric ward is suitable for the final days of some elderly patients but also has to cater for the more long-term needs of chronically ill people who are not expected to die in the near future. The initial admission policy was for patients with a two to four week prognosis. This was soon abandoned; although we are not told why, one can speculate on the difficulties of predicting this due to the factors already discussed. Of interest is that 19 out of 128 patients stayed longer than 40 days, 15 out of 128 stayed less than 24 hours and 4 out of 128 required long-stay care. The main reasons given for admission were physical dependency, social isolation, need for adequate pain control, feeding problems, fear and uncertainty, and mental confusion. They felt that the ward did achieve its aim, although more formal assessment of this was planned.

Alzheimer's disease and dementia

A number of papers deal with the perceived difficulties of providing palliative care for patients with Alzheimer's disease, other causes of primary dementia, and of secondary dementia (Brechling and Kuhn 1989; Ahmedzai 1995; Hanrahan and Luchins 1995). Alzheimer's disease affects 400,000 people in the UK and as such is the commonest cause of dementia (Rossor 1993). The major concerns seemed to be the difficulty in predicting survival time, and the worry that families of dementia patients needed more extensive support and respite than they could provide. The need for extra staff training, and patient behaviour problems in an inpatient setting were also discussed.

The Alzheimer's Disease Society in the UK and the Alzheimer's Association in the USA produce information leaflets on care in Alzheimer's disease. A list of possible poor prognostic signs are as follows:

- speech ability limited to about half-a-dozen words;
- intelligible vocabulary limited to a single word;
- ambulatory ability lost;
- ability to sit up lost;
- ability to smile lost;
- ability to hold head up lost;
- difficulty swallowing;
- faecal and urinary incontinence;
- score of three or less on Mini Mental State Examination.

While these markers may be of help, in reality, diligent, reactive support has to be the order of the day and a palliative approach should be the foundation of that. Specialist care is likely to be needed only periodically and in the terminal phase.

Terminal renal failure

In a commentary in the *Lancet*, Oreopoulos (1995) recommends that competent patients who decide to withdraw from dialysis should be assured that they will not be abandoned but will continue to be cared for. He continues that such care includes a palliative care plan to address psychological and physical symptoms and that consultation with 'our colleagues in palliative care' should occur more often. A survey of 22 hospices and hospital-based palliative care units within the Thames region revealed seven which admitted patients with any terminal disease (Andrews 1995). Thirteen had never been referred a patient with uncomplicated renal failure and said they would not be prepared to consider such a referral for a variety of reasons including uncertainty about lifespan, and policy. However, 11 units had managed renal failure in the context of other illnesses and only three of these had problems specifically related to the renal disease: myoclonic jerks, hallucinations, opioid sensitivity, and emotional issues relating to stopping dialysis. None of these is unique or beyond the clinical scope of credible palliative care units.

A further limitation on referrals into palliative care are the strong, established links that patients develop with their renal unit (an issue for all specialist centres) and in most cases it will be appropriate for them to remain there. Cohen *et al.* (1995) studied 18 patients dying from discontinued dialysis; suffering was not absent and the advisory role of the palliative care team would seem to have an important place here. After discontinuation of dialysis, the patients survived between 2 and 34 days. The oft used statement that death from renal failure is a relatively 'quick and painless way to go' may be falsely reassuring for some patients and their families.

Terminal cardiac failure

There is little in the literature regarding the palliative care of terminal cardiac failure, and what there is focuses on lack of provision and the reasons why hospice care may not be appropriate (Beattie *et al.* 1995; Gannon 1995; Jones 1995). Personal experience from work within hospital and community-based palliative care teams suggests these to be the most likely settings where the palliative care team can advise on refractory symptoms such as nausea and breathlessness. The prognosis for these patients is poor, with half of the patients with severe, and approximately one-quarter with moderate heart failure requiring palliative care within one year (Forbes and Davis 1996). Although low dose opiates can ease breathlessness, it must be remembered that active treatment of heart failure needs to be continued until late in the patient's illness to avoid rapid worsening of symptoms. The psychological impact of heart failure should not go unmentioned and will need to be addressed and dealt with.

Chronic respiratory disease and other causes of dyspnoea

Chronic obstructive pulmonary disease (COPD) is the commonest chronic lung disorder and chronic respiratory disease accounts for 5 per cent of all deaths but 13 per cent of adult disability in the UK. By the time advanced hypoxia is present, prognosis is of the order of less than three years if long-term oxygen is not given (Shee 1995). The management of patients with COPD usually consists of a combination of medical management (stopping smoking, the use of inhaled bronchodilators, and a trial of steroids with or without antibiotics), oxygen therapy in appropriate patients (which can prolong life but not necessarily improve reported quality of life) and pulmonary rehabilitation to try and slow down the vicious cycle of increasing inactivity and decreased fitness which occurs in these patients and leads to increased isolation and low self-esteem.

Dyspnoea is experienced by all of us at some time, but when chronic, and mediated by a life-threatening illness, it becomes a frightening symptom. Psychological support and allowing patients to express their fears becomes very important in this situation. It is also sometimes a very difficult symptom to treat (Ahmedzai 1993). Most chest physicians do not prescribe opioids and benzodiazepines for chronic stable dyspnoea, but Shee (1995) advocates that some breathless patients with severe COPD or lung fibrosis are helped by opioids given initially in low doses. He also proposes that the principles of the treatment of dyspnoea in dying patients are similar, whether one is dealing with end-stage lung disease or cancer. We agree with that.

There are many other non-malignant causes of dyspnoea which may require different types of medical management (Regnard and Ahmedzai 1991). However, the holistic approach to patient care is still applicable.

Motor neurone disease

This disorder, characterized by the progressive loss of alpha motor neurones in adult life with no known cause or specific treatment, has been cared for in some UK hospices for a number of years (Norris 1992; O'Brien et al. 1992). The resultant increasing muscle weakness leads to increasing immobility and difficulties with feeding, speech, and breathing, eventually leading to respiratory failure and death. Death occurs within three years from diagnosis in over half of all patients. When deterioration does occur, it does so suddenly and death can occur within 24 hours in over half of cases. There is great scope for good symptom control throughout the course of the illness, e.g. muscle cramps, drooling, severe fatiguability, sleep problems, incipient contractures, dysphagia and neuralgia. There are also many ethical decisions to be made during palliative care of a patient with motor neurone disease (Oliver 1993). This, along with the uniformly poor prognosis and relatively small numbers of patients affected by this non-malignant condition, may be what has made it so amenable to the principles of hospice and palliative care. The involvement of hospices in the care of these patients has helped to confirm that the use of opiates in the terminal stages is safe, non-addictive, and effective (Norris 1992).

In addition to terminal care, there is evidence that periods of respite care in hospices provide opportunities for symptom control and coordination of future community care (Hicks and Corcoran 1993). Most patients were discharged home after respite admissions and the median stay in the hospice of 15 days was identical to that of cancer patients.

Other chronic progressive neurological diseases

Multiple sclerosis sufferers experience a plethora of symptoms throughout the course of their illness. Stiffness, tightness, muscle spasms, and cramping pains due to spastic muscle weakness need a combination of physiotherapy, anti-spasticity drugs and rehabilitation where possible. Fatigue can be very disabling, particularly when the disease is active, and precipitating factors need to be avoided (Obbens 1993). Bladder dysfunction occurs in at least two-thirds of patients later in their disease. Pain can occur at any stage; it is mainly neurogenic or musculoskeletal and 55–82 per cent of multiple sclerosis patients complain of this (Payne and Gonzales 1993). Also of relevance is the increased incidence of depression among patients with MS compared to patients with other chronic neurological diseases; unrelated to this is the occurrence of significant cognitive dysfunction.

Parkinson's disease requires management in a similar way to the already mentioned disorders. Recognition of psychological needs is poor in these patients and one study revealed almost half of patients being significantly anxious or depressed (Forbes and Davis 1996). Specialist palliative care may have something to add to the care of some of these patients.

Rheumatoid arthritis

Rheumatoid arthritis is an incurable, systemic disease which is best treated by a multidisciplinary team (Galasko 1993). Pain is a common symptom in these patients and is not always relieved by conventional analgesics as was highlighted by an infamous court case (Dyer 1992). Ideally, a combination of medical management, occupational and physiotherapy, orthopaedic surgery and psychosocial care should all be considered.

Conclusions

Society is in favour of palliation. It seems that palliative care for all is the only moral, intellectual and practical way forward for the speciality and medicine. Provided clinicians recognize the three 'stages' of death their dialogue will reflect the uncertainty with patients, relatives and colleagues in 'grey' cases. One would like to think that a movement born out of a motive to relieve suffering would *ex hypothesi* be at the forefront of rectifying the continued lack of access among the disadvantaged dying to adequate palliation. With the health service reforms, our history of restrictive practice will have to recede if funds are to be made available from the public purse. This is the legacy of the pioneers who have put palliative care on the agenda of health care.

The new generation of practitioners who inherit this achievement now have to take the speciality forward and address the needs of the disadvantaged dying. We have been given the chance to be seen as a serious and credible discipline. Instead of being too good to be true and too small to be useful, let us be too good to ignore and too useful to be small. Otherwise we will have squandered an inheritance, euthanasia will win the day and Douglas will have proved to be right.

References

Addington-Hall, J. and McCarthy, M. (1995) Regional study of care for the dying: methods and sample characteristics. *Palliative Medicine*, 9: 27–35.

Ahmedzai, S. (1993) Palliation of respiratory symptoms, in D. Doyle, G.W.C. Hanks and N. MacDonald (eds) *Oxford Textbook of Palliative Medicine*. Oxford: Oxford University Press.

Ahmedzai, S. (1994) The medicalization of dying: a doctor's views, in D. Clark (ed.) *The Future for Palliative Care*. Buckingham: Open University Press.

Ahmedzai, S. (1995) Palliative care for all? (editorial). *Progress in Palliative Care*, 3(3): 1–3.

Alzheimer's Disease Society and Alzheimer's Association (n.d.) *Care for Advanced Alzheimer's Disease*. Alzheimer's Association, 70 East Lake Street, Chicago, IL 60601–5997; Alzheimer's Disease Society, Gordon House, 10 Greencoat Place, London SW1P 1PH.

Andrews, P.A. (1995) Palliative care for patients with terminal renal failure (letter). *Lancet*, 345: 506–7.

Beattie, J.M., Murray, R.G., Brittle, J. and Catanheira, T. (1995) Palliative care in terminal cardiac failure. Small numbers of patients with terminal cardiac failure may make considerable demands on services [letter, comment]. *British Medical Journal*, 310: 1411.

Beauchamp, T.L. and Childress, J.F. (1994) Justice, in their *Principles of Biomedical Ethics*, 4th edn. Oxford: Oxford University Press.

Blackburn, A.M. (1989) Problems of terminal care in elderly patients. *Palliative Medicine*, 3: 203–6.

Brechling, B.G. and Kuhn, D. (1989) A specialised hospice for dementia patients and their families. *Journal of Hospice Care*, May/June: 27–30.

Calman, K. (1994) *Expert Advisory Group on Cancer: A Policy Framework for Commissioning Cancer Services: Consultative Document. Chairman: K. Calman.* London: Department of Health.

Camden and Islington Palliative Care Team (1996) *Camden and Islington Palliative Care Team Annual Review 1994–6.* Camden and Islington Community NHS Trust, 26 Nassau Street, London W1N 7RF.

Clark, D. (1994) At the cross-roads: which direction for the hospices? (editorial). *Palliative Medicine*, 8: 1–3.

Cohen, L.M., McCue, H.D., Germain, M. and Kjellstrand, C.M. (1995) Dialysis discontinuation: a 'good' death? *Archive of Internal Medicine*, 155(1): 42–7.

Davis, C. and Hardy, J. (1994) Palliative care. *British Medical Journal*, 308: 1359–62.

Douglas, C. (1992) For all the saints. *British Medical Journal*, 304: 579.

Doyle, D., Hanks, G.W.C. and MacDonald, N. (1993) Introduction, in *Oxford Textbook of Palliative Medicine*. Oxford: Oxford University Press.

Dyer, C. (1992) Rheumatologist convicted for attempted murder. *British Medical Journal*, 305: 731.

Eve, A. and Smith, A.M. (1994) Palliative care services in Britain and Ireland – update 1992. *Palliative Medicine*, 8: 19–27.

Forbes, K. and Davis, C. (1996) Conference report: managing terminal illness. *Journal of the Royal College of Physicians*, 30(3): 257–9.

Galasko, C.S.B. (1993) Orthopaedic principles and management, in D. Doyle, G.W.C. Hanks and N. MacDonald (eds) *Oxford Textbook of Palliative Medicine*. Oxford: Oxford University Press.

Gannon, C. (1995) Hospices cannot fulfil such a vast and diverse role. *British Medical Journal*, 310: 1410.

George, R.G.D. (forthcoming) Palliative Care for all: justice or charity? European Journal of Palliative Care.

Hanrahan, P. and Luchins, D.J. (1995) Access to hospice programs in end-stage dementia: a national survey of hospice problems. *Journal of the American Geriatric Society*, 43(1): 56–69.

Hicks, F. and Corcoran, G. (1993) Should hospices offer respite admissions to patients with motor neurone disease? *Palliative Medicine*, 7: 145–50.

Jones, S. (1995) Palliative care in terminal cardiac failure (letter). *British Medical Journal*, 310: 805.

Norris, F.H. (1992) Motor neurone disease: treating the untreated. *British Medical Journal*, 304: 459–60.

O'Brien, T., Kelly, M. and Saunders, C. (1992) Motor neurone disease: a hospice perspective. *British Medical Journal*, 304: 471–3.

Obbens, E.A.M.T. (1993) Neurological problems in palliative medicine, in D. Doyle, G.W.C. Hanks and N. MacDonald (eds) *Oxford Textbook of Palliative Medicine*. Oxford: Oxford University Press.

Oliver, D. (1993) Ethical issues in palliative care: an overview. *Palliative Medicine*, 7(suppl. 2): 15–20.

Oreopoulos, D.G. (1995) Commentary. Withdrawal from dialysis: when letting die is better than helping live. *Lancet*, 346: 3–4.

Payne, R. and Gonzales, G. (1993) Pathophysiology of pain in cancer and other terminal diseases, in D. Doyle, G.W.C. Hanks and N. MacDonald (eds) *Oxford Textbook of Palliative Medicine*. Oxford: Oxford University Press.

Regnard, C. and Ahmedzai, S. (1991) Dyspnoea in advanced non-malignant disease: a flow diagram. *Palliative Medicine*, 5: 56–60.

Rossor, M. (1993) Alzheimer's disease. *British Medical Journal*, 307: 779–82.

Saunders, C. (1987) What's in a name? *Palliative Medicine*, 1: 57–61.

Seale, C. (1991) Death from cancer and death from other causes: the relevance of the hospice approach. *Palliative Medicine*, 5: 12–19.

Severs, M.B. and Wilkins, P.S.W. (1991) A hospital palliative care ward for elderly people. *Age and Ageing*, 20: 361–4.

Shee, C.D. (1995) Palliation in chronic respiratory disease. *Palliative Medicine*, 9: 3–12.

SMAC/SNMAC (Standing Medical Advisory Committee, Standing Nursing and Midwifery Advisory Committee) (1992) *The Principles and Provision of Palliative Care*. London: HMSO.

Smith, A.M., Eve, A. and Sykes, N.P. (1992) Palliative care services in Britain and Ireland 1990: an overview. *Palliative Medicine*, 6: 277–91.

Wilson, I.M., Bunting, J.S., Curnow, R.M. and Knock, J. (1995) The need for inpatient palliative care facilities for non cancer patients in the Thames Valley. *Palliative Medicine*, 9: 13–18.

Wilson, J.A., Lawson, P.M. and Smith, R.G. (1987) The treatment of terminally ill geriatric patients. *Palliative Medicine*, 1: 149–53.

Teamwork in end-of-life care:
a nurse–physician perspective
on introducing physicians to
palliative care concepts

JANE M. INGHAM AND NESSA COYLE

Although death and grieving are normal parts of life, advanced illness is frequently characterized by distress and suffering. In addition to being associated with many physical symptoms and limitations, advanced illness predisposes individuals to a diverse range of psychological, social, ethical and spiritual dilemmas and problems. Each of these problems has the potential to impact upon the experience of distress and perception of quality of life. With an appreciation of the complexity of these issues it becomes apparent that, to maximize quality of life for people with advanced illness, a team approach to health care that combines professional expertise and humane concern is optimal (Corr and Corr 1983).

Although there is a growing recognition of the benefits to be derived by the implementation of a team approach to the provision of end-of-life care, existing health care systems do not always foster team development. Traditionally, physicians have not been trained to collaborate in a team approach and, in many instances, have not been extensively exposed in their hospital training to either hospice or home care issues. While in some countries systems have been developed to facilitate the development of a team approach to end-of-life care, in others the responsibility for the shaping of a team may fall to an individual, for example, a physician, nurse, family member or even patient.

Although the absence of structured palliative care services within the hospital systems of many countries may be a barrier to care, evidence exists that suggests other barriers may also be significant. For example, data from US surveys indicate that physicians' awareness of basic symptom management techniques is frequently poor (VonRoenn *et al.* 1993; Cleeland *et al.* 1994), and their ability to provide end-of-life care in concordance with patients' wishes is limited (The SUPPORT Principal Investigators

1995). Further, significant limitations have been described relating to physicians' awareness of the key ethical guidelines and concepts concerning end-of-life patient care (Solomon *et al.* 1993).

This chapter, although in part modified for this volume, has been previously published as a paper within an educational resource document produced by the American Board of Internal Medicine End-Of-Life Patient Care Project (American Board of Internal Medicine 1996). By widely distributing our original paper, along with other papers focused on key palliative care concepts, the intent of the American Board of Internal Medicine was to assist physicians in leadership positions within training institutions to play a key role in fostering a 'broad view' of the physician's role. The fostering, from early in medical training, of such a view may assist in the development of a health care system more attuned to the needs of those with far advanced illness. Our intent in the original paper was, therefore, to introduce emerging concepts in end-of-life health care to physicians-in-training, and to emphasize their vital role as a part of a team providing palliative care (Ingham and Coyle 1996). In this chapter our intent remains the same. For those with more experience in palliative care many of the concepts discussed will be familiar, yet we hope to provide a useful example of the spectrum of issues that may need to be addressed in the training of physicians and others for end-of-life care. While not aiming to understate the role of other health care professionals, we emphasize the role of the physician in recognizing the needs of individual patients and families, and in initiating a team approach to the end-of-life health care.

Specifically, this chapter addresses the concept of teamwork in palliative care with particular emphasis on the opportunities for providing optimal, team-based palliative care in developed countries. We provide a practical, nurse/physician perspective of the physicians' role in end-of-life health care and in the health care team; outline the current framework upon which the model of the interdisciplinary team approach is built; and describe, in broad terms, the increasingly important concepts of 'team', 'continuity' and 'collaborative practice'. Included is a discussion of some models of end-of-life care, and various approaches to their implementation in the complex spectrum of health care environments. Finally, we present a practical approach by which physicians may participate in a team-oriented system of care with the aim of addressing the health-related needs of patients with far advanced illness.

The physician's role in end-of-life patient care both before and after the implementation of a 'team' approach

An awareness by physicians of the key components of palliative care is essential in the process of optimizing health care for patients who are nearing the end of life. Although many patients may benefit from the input of a specialty-trained palliative care physician, it is vital that primary physicians, regardless of their area of specialty practice, have an understanding of the issues involved in the care of this group of patients. Trends in medical training have often led to a focus on curative strategies; however, the potential for improvement in end-of-life health care is significant if physicians begin to view this aspect of medical care as an important challenge.

To facilitate the delivery of optimal end-of-life care it is important for physicians to take a broad view of their role in patient care. Specifically, such a broad view must acknowledge the physician's role as it relates to the implementation of therapeutic strategies; it must also emphasize aspects of the role that encompass the assessment and recognition of a wide spectrum of patient needs. Physicians must be aware of, and trained for, their role in the mobilization of health care resources; the provision of continuity of care; and in the education, and provision of advice, for patients, families and other professionals.

Implementation of therapeutic strategies

The development of palliative care as a medical specialty has been associated with an attempt to emphasize the physician's role in the implementation of a diverse array of therapies directed towards minimizing distress and improving quality of life. To achieve this goal it is necessary to accept a medical perspective that prioritizes palliation in addition to cure.

Chronic debilitating disease is an increasingly common cause of death. World Health Organization (1993) data indicate that, worldwide, although infectious and parasitic diseases account for the highest percentage of deaths, 34 per cent, circulatory diseases and chronic obstructive pulmonary diseases account for 26 per cent and cancer causes approximately 10 per cent. It is predicted that shifts in patterns of disease and an aging population will increase the proportion of individuals dying from chronic diseases (World Health Organization 1989; Bulatao 1993). Each chronic disease may be associated with the development of both acute and chronic pathophysiological processes as the end of life approaches. Each may be associated with a plethora of symptoms; numerous levels of disability and functional impairment; widely varied requirements for medical, nursing and other interventions; and multiple degrees of individual and family distress. ('Family' will be used in this chapter as a broad term referring to the individuals who are closely bonded, socially, to the patient. The nature of close relationships varies widely and these persons may not be next of kin or immediate relatives. In the home care setting these individuals are frequently also the patient's caregivers.) The diversity of these issues points to the range of skills and therapies that may be necessary for the provision of end-of-life health care.

With specific regard to the physician's role in the implementation of pharmacological therapies, numerous therapeutic advances have impacted on the management of both specific disease processes and individual symptoms. Therapies directed at the specific disease process, in addition to therapies directed at specific symptoms, may have an important role in minimizing symptom distress. Improved patient care and more effective symptom management in the setting of both curable and incurable illness is likely to result from the fostering of a dialogue between the physicians involved in day to day patient care, those who are expert in the management of specific pathological conditions, and those expert in the provision of palliative interventions.

In addition to emphasizing the physician's role in implementing symptom-directed pharmacological therapies, palliative medicine aims to encourage physicians to take a broad view of 'therapies' and become skilled in recognizing and anticipating the need for expertise and resources from both inside and outside of the medical realm. Other professionals may, for example, assist in the implementation of specific therapies, the assessment of needs, and the provision of services. Patients and families will benefit if physicians are cognizant of their own skills and limitations, and are willing and able to harness the skills of others.

Continuity of care

In many societies, the relationship between the patient and the physician has been established well before the period immediately prior to death. Frequently, although not always, the physician has had the opportunity to build a trusting relationship, to develop an understanding of the patient's and family's priorities and goals, and to witness some of the family and social dynamics that surround the patient. The involvement of a knowledgeable and trusted physician with an established background of continuity with the patient and family is optimal in the team approach to care. Such involvement can assist in minimizing the fear of abandonment by the physician that is often a major source of worry for the dying patient and their family. In addition, the trust that has developed over time is a key factor in a patient's willingness to allow the introduction of other health professionals into their system of care. The physician who has been involved with the patient over time is therefore in an important position to both initiate a team approach and to share knowledge and insights with other team members so as to insure that the spectrum of physical, social, psychological concerns are addressed as disease progresses.

Mobilization of resources: the health care team

The role of the physician in the changing longitudinal framework of illness, is frequently pivotal in the recognition of needs and the mobilization of resources aimed at assisting the patient and family as the end of life approaches. This important triage role cannot be understated, as the initial implementation of a team approach to health care often hinges on the physician's recognition of a need for an interdisciplinary approach to care. Recognition of these needs can be facilitated by a comprehensive patient and family assessment that explores the factors that are contributing to distress. The mobilization of other resources and expertise can offer patients and their families tremendous benefits that would otherwise be unavailable to them. Varying aspects of care may be provided by other professionals and include specific therapeutic interventions; monitoring of therapies; nursing skills; counselling, support and spiritual advice; and after hours and crisis coverage.

When the specific needs of the patient and family require ongoing input from one or more professionals, optimal medical care is facilitated when the health care providers collaborate as a coordinated team. This approach is particularly important as the disease process becomes more complex, as the patient becomes more frail, as the needs of the patient and family become more pronounced, and as the number of professionals involved in the provision of care increases. Collaboration is essential to maximize therapeutic efforts; minimize the confusion that often arises when many professionals provide information and advice; and facilitate the provision of a reliable system of health care. A team of reliable professionals within a structured system of care will provide most patients and families with a sense of security, consistency and comfort.

Educational role: medical issues for patient, family and other professionals

As a patient nears the end of life, a skilled and knowledgeable physician can be a valuable source of education and advice for the patient, family and other professionals. As has been eloquently discussed by Corr (1993), care for the dying in modern society has been 'moved away from the family and out of the home' and 'death . . . has become a less familiar feature of life, and a more alien event'. Patients, family members and professionals vary tremendously in their knowledge of the medical, cultural and other issues involved in the care of dying people. As a consequence of this, education and advice becomes an important aspect of the medical role in end-of-life care.

The patient, family, and those counselling them, need to possess an understanding of the nature of the disease process and options for therapy so that informed decisions can be made regarding goals of care and subsequent therapeutic interventions. These important decisions require an understanding of the likelihood of therapies being curative or palliative, and the likely impact of treatment options on disease progression and on quality of life. The input of a physician who is able to communicate, in terms that the patient and family can understand, insights into the patho-physiology of symptoms, the nature of the disease process and, important-antly, the palliative options for therapy, can be invaluable. In addition, the physician is often in a position to give specific and practical advice regarding the nature and implications of current and anticipated symptoms, the dying process and the care of the dying. More broadly, a know-ledgeable physician may have an invaluable educational role in fostering the implementation of community-specific strategies aimed at improving the health care for those with far advanced disease.

Although there is increasing emphasis on palliative care in both medical education and the medical literature, the reality of the present situation is that physicians themselves may not have had significant exposure to the care of dying patients in their training. As this aspect of patient care is an integral part of medical practice, physicians may need to specifically seek to acquire skills appropriate to their practice population. It should be noted that, frequently, a useful educational resource for the physician will be the other skilled professionals within the practice environment and team structure.

The interdisciplinary team for end-of-life care

Team definitions, principles of team functioning and common problems

Given the recognition that end-of-life health care for chronic disease is most effective when provided by a team, it is important to recognize also that a group of professionals does not, in itself, equate with a 'team'. A team has been defined as 'two or more persons working together' with 'team-work' defined as 'the combined action of a team, . . . especially when effect-ive or efficient' (*Concise Oxford Dictionary of Current English* 1992). When individuals from different disciplines approach a similar situation as a team a more comprehensive perspective is likely to evolve than would have done if each individual had considered the situation alone. Importantly, the forma-tion of a team must imply a common purpose and unified identity. The common purpose must be defined, and on occasions redefined, as knowledge and information is shared among the individual team members, the patient and family. In a team, areas of responsibility are clarified and defined by each individual's particular expertise and training. Each individual's latitude for decision making within his or her area of responsibility should be under-stood by all professionals involved. An understanding of this definition and approach will assist in the development of a cohesive team structure.

The interdisciplinary team approach to health care has been widely accepted as the most appropriate in the palliative care setting (Ajemian 1993). Although health care is frequently provided by a multidisciplinary group, there are important differences between that approach to care and the approach provided by an interdisciplinary team. A multidisciplinary approach involves care provided by a number of professionals whose individual professional identities supersede that of a 'team' identity, whereas in the interdisciplinary approach the 'team' identity is paramount. Frequently patients have their health care provided by a multidisciplinary group without formalized communication, in the interdisciplinary team decision making and the sharing of information by means of efficient, consistent and reliable communication strategies are considered to be a key component of cohesive and effective team functioning.

The interdisciplinary team for end-of-life care is comprised of professionals from differing disciplines who assist the patient and family in defining the goals of care, and effectively mobilize each other's skills to meet the changing needs of the patient and family. It is important to establish clearly who comprises the interdisciplinary team. In the case of a patient nearing the end of life, the team should, preferably, include personnel who had previously been a part of the patient's multidisciplinary group of health care providers.

In an effective and efficient interdisciplinary team each member will have an understanding of the skills, capabilities and roles of other members. Team leadership, authority and responsibility are vested in the person whose expertise is most appropriate to the particular clinical situation and, given this, the most appropriate skills for the team leader are likely to vary depending on the specific task (Ajemian 1993). The team approach may incorporate elements of 'collaborative practice' (Mullaney et al. 1974; Dudgeon 1994; Kedziera and Levy 1994), a method of practice characterized by conjoint problem solving, task interdependence, shared record keeping and shared accountability (Kedziera and Levy 1994). Not unexpectedly, it is common for problems to arise in the many grey areas where the skills of team members overlap. For team members to feel confident, rather than threatened, in areas where expertise and decision making capabilities overlap there must be a mutual respect among the professionals from differing disciplines. All team members must be secure in their understanding each professional's expertise and limits.

Vachon (1987), in a study of occupational stress, found that occupational stressors in individuals providing hospice care were most commonly related to team dynamics and issues concerning individual occupational roles. The common problems cited as triggers of stress included communication problems with others in the team, together with role ambiguity and role conflict. For the interdisciplinary approach to be effective, it is important that efforts be made to anticipate and address these factors and that mechanisms for dealing with conflict recognition and resolution be incorporated routinely into team practice (Rubin and Beckhard 1972; Lowe and Herranen 1978; Ajemian 1993; Kedziera and Levy 1994).

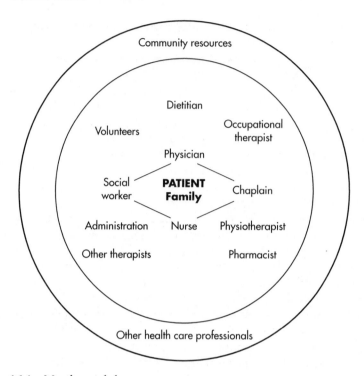

Figure 16.1 Members of the team
Source: Ajemian, I. (1993) The interdisciplinary team, in D. Doyle, G.W.C. Hanks and N. MacDonald (eds) *Oxford Textbook of Palliative Medicine*. Oxford: Oxford University Press.

The composition of the interdisciplinary team

The composition of teams providing health care for dying patients may vary tremendously. The needs and goals of both the patient and family dictate the requirements for skilled resource personnel and should guide decisions regarding team composition. Although it is generally acknowledged that the patient is central in the unit of care, it is important to recognize that family members, particularly in the home care setting, are frequently providers of care at the same time as being in need of health care resources. Family members, for example, may benefit if given access to skilled resources for guidance, teaching and support.

Most teams will contain core personnel, frequently a physician, nurse, social worker and chaplain, who will consult and utilize the skills of others as needed (Figure 16.1) (Ajemian 1993). As indicated above, a team may contain as few as two members and in such cases the professionals are most likely to be a physician and a nurse. The team may, routinely or in selected cases, include other physicians, nursing personnel, social workers, physical and occupational therapists, clergy, patient advocates, pharmacists, dietitians, other therapists, volunteers, and others (Downie 1983; Brown and Hoffman

1990; Dicks 1990; Lapeer 1990; Schulz and Brushwood 1991; Mandel 1993; Marcant and Rapin 1993; Bollwinkel 1994; Fusco-Karmann and Tamburini 1994; McWhinney and Stewart 1994; Monroe 1994; Smith and Yuen 1994). Although it is beyond the scope of this chapter to include a specific discussion of the role of each discipline in end-of-life care, a comprehensive review of this area has been provided by Ajemian (1993).

In many cases, the ideal approach involves the physician and other professionals who have been integral in the patient's system of long-term care, to be members, or at least consultants for, the team. Most patients, particularly those with chronic conditions, consider continuity of medical care a priority. It is important to note that continuity of medical care does not necessarily imply that primary physicians remain involved in day to day contact with patients. The role of the physician may vary and will depend on the physician's skills, interest and other commitments. In addition, it will be influenced by the availability of other resources in terms of team personnel. Some physicians may fill the role of the core physician for end-of-life care and others may have a more peripheral role (Figure 16.1). Even when the physician is a core member of the team, day to day contact with the patient may be through the team nurse and continuity is maintained by communication within the team structure.

Although some patients will shape their own team according to their needs and priorities, clinical experience indicates that, for the most part, patients and their families rely on their physician for advice and guidance at this difficult time. It is important for physicians to possess a working knowledge of the methods available in their practice environment to access the skills and resources of other professionals to assist the patient and family.

Types of interdisciplinary teams

Various models exist for teams to assist in patient care at the end of life and in many communities a range of options exists for the provision of home care (Ford 1993). Although in some settings a team may need to be created specifically to meet the needs of an individual patient or a particular practice, in many communities, established interdisciplinary teams exist for the provision of end-of-life care. Hospice services, and the less common hospital-based supportive care teams, symptom assessment teams, or palliative care teams, provide an established team approach to end-of-life care and referral to such services may be appropriate in many cases. As indicated above, decisions regarding referral will be dictated by the patient and family's needs and goals, in addition to practical and financial factors.

The term 'hospice' implies a philosophy of care aimed at maximizing quality of life as death approaches (Corr and Corr 1983; Mor et al. 1988; Ford 1993). Hospice teams aim to address the patient's physical, emotional and spiritual needs and, most commonly, focus care in the home. Hospice care aims also to provide families with assistance and support so that they may be able to care for the patient in the home. To achieve this goal most hospice programmes employ an interdisciplinary approach to care. In the USA, hospice teams are structured according to Medicare regulations and include physicians, nurses, home health aides, social workers, chaplains and volunteers. Other health care workers and community resources are brought in as necessary. In settings outside the USA the components of hospice teams are frequently similar, although their structure is often less regulated. In many settings the primary responsibility for the patient's medical care is assumed by a specialized hospice-associated physician; however, to provide continuity of care many hospice programmes allow the referring physician to be part of the team. Although many physicians want to be involved in the provision of terminal care for patients dying at home, some do not, either because of lack of perceived expertise or lack of time. Many hospice teams accommodate both these perspectives and the hospice physician will frequently, if required, assume medical responsibility for the patient's care.

Referral to hospice is likely to be appropriate when palliation rather than curative therapy is the primary intent and family support is required. Physicians should be encouraged to familiarize themselves with the availability of hospice services in their area of practice and methods of accessing information regarding hospice care. For example, in the USA, hospice coverage is widely available and provided by Medicare nationwide, by Medicaid in many states, and by most private insurance companies. Information about services can be obtained from the National Hospice Organization, the Academy of Hospice Physicians, the American Cancer Society, the American Association of Retired Persons, and the Social Security Administration. Similar organizations in other countries can be contacted for information related to hospice availability and accessibility.

Specialist teams, based within the hospital setting, are known by various names including palliative care team, supportive care team, symptom control team, or symptom assessment team. Such teams began to evolve in the 1970s; however, as a specialty area this is a relatively new field. The development of hospital-based teams, in part, reflects a recognition of the need for palliative care in the hospital setting. In the USA, for example, almost 2.2 million deaths occur annually; of these, approximately 62 per cent occur in hospitals (National Center for Health Statistics 1994). Interest in the development of hospital-based palliative care services has grown and such teams are now common in some areas, particularly in Canada, Australia, the UK and other European countries (Bates *et al.* 1981; Coyle 1989; Kramer and Dwyer 1989; Walsh 1990; Hockley 1992; O'Neill *et al.* 1992; Pannuti and Tanneberger 1992; Lickiss *et al.* 1994; Lassauniere and Zittoun 1995).

Hospital-based palliative care teams usually aim to coordinate and, in some cases, provide in-hospital and home care services to address the disease-related, physical and psychological needs of the hospital associated population with far advanced disease. Such teams mobilize, as appropriate, institutional and external resources for patient care and consider close liaison with home care services and hospice programmes as a vital aspect of the service. Teams vary in their structure and approach. Some consist of a specialist palliative care physician and a nurse providing a consultation service alone. Others provide a more structured, interdisciplinary team approach with a range of types of care including both inpatient palliative care and home care (Walsh 1990). In some the nurse will be the team member who initially provides the consultation and coordinates care (Coyle 1989), whereas in others the physician will provide the initial assessment.

Most palliative care teams become involved in patient care in response to a request for a consultation from the patient's primary physician. Many of these consultations are requests for assistance in controlling pain, dyspnoea, nausea or other challenging symptoms. Other requests are for help in discharge and home care planning for patients nearing the end of life. Depending on the needs of the patient and the resources available, the inpatient consultation team may suggest referral of the patient to a home nursing agency, a hospice home care team or to a long-term care facility that specializes in the care of dying persons. On occasions, the outcome of the consultation is the development of a team approach to end-of-life care that involves collaboration between the referring physician, the palliative care team and other selected professionals. Often the input of the social worker is vital for clarifying the feasible options considering the family dynamics, financial situation, available benefits and existing community resources.

Specialized teams can be specifically created to provide end-of-life care in various environments and communities. Teams that primarily exist for other purposes, assuming they are coordinated and have the appropriate skills and resources, may be able to facilitate the provision of end-of-life care. Such teams may include those providing community interventions for specific populations, for example in the geriatric or HIV-infected population. As indicated above, although in the current health care environment there are frequently several health care professionals involved in the care of the patient, this does not necessarily equate with a team approach to health care delivery. Coordination of care is imperative particularly as the patient's condition deteriorates. Poorly coordinated care is likely to increase the difficulties and confusion experienced by the patient and family.

Practical issues in implementing a 'team' approach

Assessing needs

To shape a system of care that will address the current and anticipated needs of the patient a comprehensive assessment is essential. A practical approach to comprehensive symptom assessment has been discussed in numerous texts (Foley 1993; Cherny and Portenoy 1994; Sui *et al.* 1994; Ingham and Portenoy 1996). Approaches to the assessment of specific needs for the home care of patients with advanced disease have also been reviewed (Coyle *et al.* 1990; Doyle 1993). In addition, instruments exist for the evaluation of home care needs (Coyle *et al.* 1996). Of major importance in the assessment of patients with advanced disease is the physician's ability to communicate effectively and to assess difficult and distressing areas of concern. A useful and practical approach to communicating in the setting of advanced illness has been described by Buckman (1993).

Assessment of the needs of patients nearing the end of life requires an understanding that patients often signal levels of distress to the physician with the complaint of a symptom or complex of symptoms. Although symptoms may be triggered by pathophysiological processes that subsequently impact on quality of life, an understanding of the patient's distress and needs hinges on a recognition of the factors that modify this process by augmenting or tempering the expression and experience of distress. These modifying factors include physical condition; psychological state; coping and personality variables; family, social and financial supports and burdens; and spiritual and existential resources and concerns. The diversity of these factors serves to emphasize again that a range of professional skills is required for the assessment of needs and for the provision of effective end-of-life care (Ajemian 1993).

In summary, a comprehensive and ongoing assessment is necessary to illuminate the details of patient and family worries, and specific symptom and disease-related concerns. Although physicians should be skilled in assessment, the input of other professionals may be important specifically for this assessment, for example the skills of social workers may assist in clarifying the patient's needs. A comprehensive assessment will help to clarify the nature of the additional resources that are required; ascertain the need for the implementation of a team approach to care; and assist in decisions regarding the selection of an appropriate team.

When to consider a team approach to end-of-life care

The nature of the disease and the manifestations of distress are the most important indicators of when it is appropriate to implement a team approach for the care of an individual with advanced disease. Although an event, a specific prognosis or change in prognosis, or a statement of intent such as a 'Do not resuscitate' order may prompt a review of the goals of care, these factors should not be necessary to prompt consideration of a team structure to facilitate the delivery of care. Certain factors may signal that referral to a specialized team may be appropriate. These factors include the presence of advancing disease not responding to disease-directed therapies; evolving and/or poorly controlled symptoms; multiple symptoms; deteriorating functional status and increasing debility and/or nursing requirements. In addition, the presence of significant family distress should prompt reassessment of the patient's needs. Importantly, it must be recognized that distress may be manifest by the expression of many diverse concerns including difficulty coping physically, emotionally or financially, and specific symptoms such as difficulty sleeping or fatigue. It is also important for physicians to be sensitive to the less direct indicators of increasing distress, such as multiple calls or missed appointments, and alert particularly to the needs of the patient who is isolated with few social or family supports.

In addition to patient-related factors, indicators of caregiver burden should prompt consideration of the implementation or expansion of team support. The impact of patient distress on family members can be considerable, particularly in the home where family responsibility for caregiving is significant. Caregiver burden may impact negatively on patient care and is increased by upsetting or poorly controlled symptoms; the need for administration of frequent medications; time demands related to the illness; physical strain and interrupted sleep; confinement and isolation; emotional adjustments; work adjustments, and numerous other factors (Ferrell *et al.* 1991).

In addition to the immediate caregivers and family, physicians may also experience stress and sense an increasing burden of care associated with caring for a patient who is nearing the end of life. The sense of burden and stress should signal the need to consider a team approach to care so that the patient and family may have the opportunity to receive support from more than one source. The care of dying people and their families is often very time consuming; in many situations, a major limitation for physicians will relate to the time constraints imposed by a busy practice. Time constraints should not be viewed as a failure on the part of the physician but rather a reality. For these and other reasons outlined above, most patients nearing the end of life will benefit from the input of several professionals who combine their individual skills and resources to provide care.

Common needs and requirements

Numerous factors associated with advanced illness may impact on the patient and family and result in suffering (Cherny *et al.* 1994, 1996). To assess the needs of patients and families, it is useful to have a familiarity with the common causes of concern and distress. In addition, issues specific to particular disease states may be relevant, as are practice-specific issues that may relate to either a particular population or geographical area. For example, a practice may particularly provide care for patients with HIV-related, oncological, geriatric or paediatric problems, or it may be located in an isolated area with few services.

Common to the patients and families experiencing advanced disease is a sense of overall burden, in addition to numerous disease-specific burdens and concerns. Exploration of this sense of overall burden may reveal areas of concern where interventions may be useful. Worries may reflect a current, or an anticipated problem, and exploration of these, in a timely manner, may assist to alleviate some troublesome concerns. Both current and anticipated problems may require interventions, that may include therapeutic interventions, counselling, and clarification or implementation of support systems. The plethora of issues that can arise in patients with advanced illness results in a common requirement for ongoing advice, instruction and support. This is important in all health care settings but particularly when care is being provided in the home.

Numerous practical issues contribute to the common fears of patients and their families as the end of life nears. Worries that arise with advanced illness frequently reflect the lack of familiarity of the dying process and, in this regard, the input of various professionals can be very helpful. Patients and families are often uncertain about appropriate interventions. These interventions may be diverse and include, for example, how often to turn a patient in bed; how much to feed an anorexic patient; and whether to, or how to, explain to a child about a parent's illness. The skills of various professionals may be useful in addressing this diverse range of concerns.

In addition to having concerns regarding these interventional issues, it is common for both patients and families to be concerned or fearful about the disease process and the meaning of symptoms or events. Again these concerns may be diverse and may include, for example, whether a particular symptom, or exacerbation of a symptom, is an indicator of impending death; and what constitutes an emergency or a warning of an impending emergency. Fears as to what the future may hold and the possible mode of death often weigh heavily on the minds of those living with advanced illness. A patient or family member may have no understanding of what to expect with advancing illness and may perceive a minor symptom, such as a bleeding haemorrhoid, as indicating the beginning of the acute dying process. Often, the concept of an emergency must be redefined and clarified for the patient and caregivers based on their goals of care. For example, a dying patient with refractory leukaemia who has elected to remain at home for palliative care may have been in the habit of rushing into the hospital if a fever developed in the middle of the night, this may no longer be appropriate. The development of severe dyspnoea or pain may, however, require an urgent intervention for palliation. The clinician should be cognizant of the disease as a process, anticipate the likely spectrum of evolving symptoms and distress, and establish a method for dealing with emergencies accordingly.

In summary, knowledgeable and sensitive input from a skilled health care team can be tremendously helpful in identifying and addressing the needs,

Table 16.1   Health-related requirements for the prevention and management of distress in patients with far advanced disease

---

Essential requirements
- Access to an informed and knowledgeable resource to clarify concerns regarding, and the implications of, the disease status and process
- Reliable and easy access to skilled assessment
- Communication aids, e.g. telephone, medi-alert alarm
- 24-hour resource for emergency intervention

Common requirements
- Pharmacological therapies
- Physical aids, e.g. commode chair
- Counselling and pastoral support
- Assistance with health care system-related or financial and insurance concerns

Required in selected cases
- Specific psychological and/or psychiatric therapies
- Physical, rehabilitative and other therapies
- Other interventions

---

clarifying the many concerns of patients and families, and providing guidelines for patients and families as the end of life approaches.

Selecting a team

Table 16.1 contains a broad outline of the requirements necessary to address current and anticipated concerns in this population and may provide a useful reference when considering the requirements for personnel. Ideally, the system of care that is recommended should incorporate personnel capable of addressing the essential requirements listed and provide a reliable method for accessing other skills and resources as required. As skills often overlap and access to resources is variable, Table 16.1 does not dictate the inclusion of specific disciplines. Access to medical and nursing expertise should be available and, as indicated above, continuity is ideal. Commonly, an existing hospice team or palliative care team may be accessed.

A useful approach for physicians to consider, having assessed the needs of their practice population and the existing local resources, is the possibility of establishing a practice-specific method for implementing a team approach to end-of-life care. In a particular practice environment a physician may refer regularly to a specific hospice or palliative care team. Another approach may involve the development of a team. If this latter approach is taken, a significant amount of thought and planning is crucial. Effective team functioning will be enhanced with continuity, consistency and commitment, and depends upon the ongoing experience of working together as a team facing a spectrum of problems and cases. For these reasons, a dedicated, specialized team is recommended. To achieve this, some team members may need to seek training in specific areas, through a course or perhaps by spending some time with an established service. Such training may address, for example, symptom management, communication, or counselling.

Regardless of the specific type of team considered to be most suited to the patient's needs, a coordinating figure is ideal for the care of each patient. This individual serves as the primary liaison between the team, patient and family, and to bring the team plan to the bedside, whether that is in the home or the hospital. Patient and family preference may influence this issue; however, the team nurse, who is often in close proximity to the patient and family through day to day observation and care, is well situated to fill this role. In teams where the nurse is the team leader, decisions will commonly necessitate guidance from the physician and other team members, however, in the development of such a role there is often a shift in the balance of decision making from the physician to the nurse. With this approach, an understanding of the principles of collaborative practice is imperative (Dudgeon 1994; Kedziera and Levy 1994).

Key elements for effective team functioning

A great deal has been written describing practical approaches to effective team functioning, both in relation to general heath care (Rubin and Beckhard 1972; Lowe and Herranen 1978) and to health care for those with advanced disease (Ajemian 1993; Kedziera and Levy 1994). Physicians may find a review of this information useful when consideration is being given to participating in, or establishing, a team for the provision of end-of-life care. As indicated above, it is important to consider carefully issues relating to staff selection, clarification of roles, decision making methods, communication strategies, goals of care, staff support, and conflict management and resolution (Ajemian 1993).

Most importantly, the goal of the team is to function to meet the end-of-life health care needs and goals as defined by the interaction with each patient and family. Professional expertise that is concerned, skilled and reliable is vital in the provision of this care. The patient and family are likely to benefit from regular and consistent contact with the team. The scheduling of regular calls or visits, as well as intermittent family meetings, can be helpful and provide some structure and organization to what may otherwise seem to be a somewhat chaotic situation. From the patient and family perspective, the clarification of the availability of resources and, specifically, of a method for accessing the team will frequently provide a sense of comfort and support. Ideally, as the end of life approaches, the team should provide the patient and family with the opportunity to have the burden of medical decision making and triage minimized. To facilitate this, a consistent, 24-hour method of accessing the team is most important. This approach will assist with the triage of problems and allow the task at hand to be referred to the most appropriate personnel.

Conclusion

That the physician need be less involved as the goal of health care shifts from cure to comfort is a myth. The involvement of a knowledgeable and trusted physician can be invaluable for both patients and their families. An understanding of techniques for assessing and anticipating patient and family needs, and a knowledge of the resources available for the care of patients with far advanced illness is crucial for physicians if they are to provide assistance and guidance for these patients and their families. In addition to the input of a physician, patients who are nearing the end of life are likely to benefit from a team approach to end-of-life health care. Such an approach serves to extend the range of care that can be offered and, given the complexities of advanced disease and the diversity of concerns that arise as the end of life nears, is most often the ideal. Access for patients and families to a range of skilled health care professionals who understand each other's complementary roles, and possess the skills necessary to work in collaboration, will greatly facilitate the provision of optimal health care.

The concepts discussed in this chapter, while not new in themselves, are frequently unfamiliar concepts for physicians trained in the acute hospital setting. In the course of their training physicians need to become familiar with the needs of those nearing the end of life. To optimize care, physicians must be introduced to the knowledge and skills necessary for the provision of end-of-life care, including skills that enable them to participate in a team approach to care. Globally, the challenge that confronts health care providers is to develop community and practice-specific systems of care that will, in time, improve the quality of life of the population with far advanced disease. This process of system development mandates both an understanding by physicians of the issues that surround end-of-life care, and a collaborative exploration of the options for care in each practice environment.

Acknowledgements

This chapter was originally compiled as part of the American Board of Internal Medicine Pilot Project on End-of-Life Patient Care Educational Resource Document, *Caring for the Dying: Identification and Promotion of Physician Competency*. The Board's permission to reproduce the chapter is gratefully acknowledged.

References

Ajemian, I. (1993) The interdisciplinary team, in D. Doyle, G.W.C. Hanks and N. MacDonald (eds) Oxford Textbook of Palliative Medicine. Oxford: Oxford University Press.

American Board of Internal Medicine (1996) Care for the Dying: Identification and Promotion of Physician Competency. Philadelphia: American Board of Internal Medicine. (This material was published in conjunction with the ABIM End-of-Life Patient Care Project.)

Bates, T., Hoy, A., Clarke, D. and Laird, P.P. (1981) The St Thomas' Hospital Terminal Care Support Team, Lancet, 30 May, 1(8231): 1201–3.

Bollwinkel, E. (1994) Role of spirituality in hospice care. Annals of the Academy of Medicine, Singapore, 23(2): 261–3.

Brown, J. and Hoffman, L. (1990) The dental hygienist as a hospice care provider. American Journal of Hospice and Palliative Care, 7(2): 31–5.

Buckman, R. (1993) Communication in palliative care, in D. Doyle, G.W.C. Hanks and N. MacDonald (eds) Oxford Textbook of Palliative Medicine. Oxford: Oxford University Press.

Bulatao, R. (1993) Mortality by cause, 1970–2015, in J.N. Gribble and S.H. Preston (eds) Epidemiological Transition: Policy and Planning Implications for Developing Countries, Workshop Proceedings. Washington, DC: National Academy Press.

Cherny, N. and Portenoy, R. (1994) Cancer pain: principles of assessment and syndromes, in P.D. Wall and R. Melzack (eds) Textbook of Pain. Edinburgh: Churchill Livingstone.

Cherny, N., Coyle, N. and Foley, K. (1994) Suffering in the advanced cancer patient: a definition and taxonomy. Journal of Palliative Care, 10(2): 57–70.

Cherny, N.I., Coyle, N. and Foley, K.M. (1996) Guidelines in the care of the dying cancer patient, in N.I. Cherney and K.M. Foley (eds) Hematology/Oncology Clinics of North America. Philadelphia, PA: W.B. Saunders.

Cleeland, C., Gonin, R., Hatfield, A., et al. (1994) Pain and its treatment in outpatients with metastatic cancer. New England Journal of Medicine, 330: 592–6.

Concise Oxford Dictionary of Current English (1992) Oxford: Clarendon Press.

Corr, C. (1993) Death in modern society, in D. Doyle, G.W.C. Hanks and N. MacDonald (eds) Oxford Textbook of Palliative Medicine. Oxford: Oxford University Press.

Corr, C. and Corr, D. (1983) Hospice Care: Principles and Practice. New York: Springer.

Coyle, N. (1989) Continuity of care for the cancer patient with chronic pain. Cancer, 63(11 suppl.): 2289–93.

Coyle, N., Loscalzo, M. and Bailey, L. (1990) Supportive home care for the advanced cancer patient and family, in J.C. Holland and J.H. Rowland (eds) Handbook of Psychooncology. New York: Oxford University Press.

Coyle, N., Layman-Goldstein, M., Passik, S., Fishman, B. and Portenoy, R. (1996) Development and validation of a patient needs assessment tool (PNAT) for oncology clinicians. Cancer Nursing, April, 19(2): 81–92.

Dicks, B. (1990) The contribution of nursing to palliative care. *Palliative Medicine*, 4: 197–203.

Downie, P. (1983) The place of physiotherapy in hospice care, in C.A. Corr and D.M. Corr (eds) *Hospice Care: Principles and Practice*. New York: Springer.

Doyle, D. (1993) Domiciliary palliative care, in D. Doyle, G.W.C. Hanks and N. MacDonald (eds) *Oxford Textbook of Palliative Medicine*. Oxford: Oxford University Press.

Dudgeon, D.J. (1994) Physician/nursing roles and perspectives in relationship to delivery of palliative care. *Annals of the Academy of Medicine, Singapore*, 23(2): 249–51.

Ferrell, B., Rhiner, M., *et al.* (1991) Family factors influencing cancer pain management. *Postgraduate Medical Journal*, 67(1): 9.

Foley, K. (1993) Pain assessment and cancer pain syndromes, in D. Doyle, G.W.C. Hanks and N. MacDonald (eds) *Oxford Textbook of Palliative Medicine*. Oxford: Oxford University Press.

Ford, G. (1993) The development of palliative care services, in D. Doyle, G.W.C. Hanks and N. MacDonald (eds) *Oxford Textbook of Palliative Medicine*. Oxford: Oxford University Press.

Fusco-Karmann, C. and Tamburini, M. (1994) Volunteers in hospital and home care: a precious resource. *Tumori*, 80(4): 269–72.

Hockley, J. (1992) Role of the hospital support team. *British Journal of Hospital Medicine*, 48(5): 250–3.

Ingham, J. and Coyle, N. (1996) The role of the health care team, in *Caring for the Dying: Identification and Promotion of Physician Competency*. Philadelphia, PA: American Board of Internal Medicine. (This material was published in conjunction with the ABIM End-of-Life Patient Care Project.)

Ingham, J. and Portenoy, R. (1996) Symptom assessment, in N.I. Cherney and K.M. Foley (eds) *Hematology/Oncology Clinics of North America*. Philadelphia, PA: W.B. Saunders.

Kedziera, P. and Levy, M. (1994) Collaborative practice in oncology. *Seminars in Oncology*, 21(6): 705–11.

Kramer, J. and Dwyer, B. (1989) Palliative care in the teaching hospital. *Cancer Forum*, 13(1): 4–8.

Lapeer, G. (1990) The dentist as a member of the palliative care team. *Journal of the Canadian Dental Association*, 56(3): 205–7.

Lassauniere, J. and Zittoun, R. (1995) The Palliative Care Centre of Hôtel-Dieu Hospital. *Support Care Cancer*, 3(1): 7–10.

Lickiss, J., Wiltshire, J., Glare, P., *et al.* (1994) Central Sydney Palliative Care Service: potential and limitations of an integrated palliative care service based in a metropolitan teaching hospital. *Annals of the Academy of Medicine, Singapore*, 23(2): 264–70.

Lowe, J. and Herranen, M. (1978) Conflict in teamwork: understanding roles and relationships. *Social Work in Health Care*, 3: 323–30.

McWhinney, I. and Stewart, M. (1994) Home care of dying patients: family physicians' experience with a palliative care support team. *Canadian Family Physician*, 40: 240–6.

Mandel, S. (1993) The role of the music therapist on the hospice/palliative care team. *Journal of Palliative Care*, 9(4): 37–9.

Marcant, D. and Rapin, C. (1993) Role of the physiotherapist in palliative care. *Journal of Pain and Symptom Management*, 8(2): 68–71.

Monroe, B. (1994) Role of the social worker in palliative care. *Annals of the Academy of Medicine, Singapore*, 23(2): 252–5.

Mor, V., Greer, D. and Kastenbaum, R. (1988) *The Hospice Experiment*. Baltimore, MD: Johns Hopkins University Press.

Mullaney, J., Fox, R. and Liston, M. (1974) Clinical nurse specialist and social worker: clarifying the roles. *Nursing Outlook*, 22(11): 712–18.

National Center for Health Statistics (1994) General Mortality, 1990. Unpublished data from the National Center for Health Statistics, United States Department of Health and Human Services.

O'Neill, W., O'Connor, P. and Latimer, E. (1992) Hospital palliative care services: three models in three countries. *Journal of Pain and Symptom Management*, 7(7): 406–13.

Pannuti, F. and Tanneberger, S. (1992) The Bologna Eubiosia Project: hospital-at-home care for advanced cancer patients. *Journal of Palliative Care*, 8(2): 11–17.

Rubin, I. and Beckhard, R. (1972) Factors influencing the effectiveness of health care teams. *Milbank Memorial Fund Quarterly*, 3: 317–35.

Schulz, R. and Brushwood, D. (1991) The pharmacist's role in patient care. *Hastings Center Report*, 21: 12–17.

Smith, M. and Yuen, K. (1994) Palliative care in the home: the GP/home hospice team. *Australian Family Physician*, 23(7): 1260–5.

Solomon, M. Z., O'Donnell, L., Jennings, B., *et al.* (1993) Decisions near the end of life: professional views on life-sustaining treatments. *American Journal of Public Health*, 83(1): 14–23.

Sui, A., Reuben, D. and Moore, A. (1994) Comprehensive geriatric assessment in W.R. Hazzard (ed.) *Principles of Geriatric Medicine and Gerontology*, 3rd edn. New York: McGraw-Hill.

The SUPPORT Principal Investigators (1995) A controlled trial to improve care for seriously ill hospitalized patients: SUPPORT. *JAMA*, 274: 1591–8.

Vachon, M. (1987) Team stress in palliative/hospice care. *Hospice Journal*, 3(2–3): 75–103.

VonRoenn, J., Cleeland, C., Gonin, R., *et al.* (1993) Physician attitudes and practice in cancer pain management: a survey from the Eastern Cooperative Oncology Group. *Annals of Internal Medicine*, 119: 121–6.

Walsh, T. (1990) Continuing care in a medical center: the Cleveland Clinic Foundation Palliative Care Service. *Journal of Pain and Symptom Management*, 5(5): 273–8.

World Health Organization (1989) *Health of the Elderly*, Technical Report Series 779, Geneva: WHO.

World Health Organization (1993) Global health situation. *Weekly Epidemiological Record*, 68(6): 33–6.

17 Voluntary euthanasia in terminal illness

DAVID OXENHAM AND KENNETH BOYD

Euthanasia is a complex but also emotive topic. Debate on it tends to polarize into strongly held views, for and against. Many doctors and nurses, for example, may have sympathy for euthanasia in certain circumstances (Di Mola 1994) but their anxiety about possible abuses can lead to what psychiatrists call 'reaction formation'. Any withdrawal from an entrenched anti-euthanasia position, they fear, threatens an inevitable slide down the 'slippery slope' towards involuntary euthanasia, so they state the anti-euthanasia position all the more forcefully. The problem with this approach is that it tends to confirm the fears of members of the public, including potential patients, who feel that there may sometimes be a case for euthanasia. It also hardens the attitudes of those who argue politically for voluntary euthanasia, resulting in unhelpful confrontation rather than constructive discussion.

Against this background, it is important to recognize our own sense of cognitive dissonance when faced with the complexities of this issue. What is appropriate in one situation may not be so in another, and determining what is best for a particular patient can be both intellectually and emotionally demanding. Yet the fact that we have to struggle with these decisions demonstrates that they and the patients involved are important, and that we are acting as moral agents. It would be far more worrying if we found these decisions easy. Recognizing their difficulty, moreover, should make us more open minded and generous towards others, in other circumstances or countries, who also have struggled with these issues, but have come to different conclusions. The underlying problem we all face, is that advances in medical technology not only provide more life-prolonging treatments, but also demand more overt decisions about ending life. These may include euthanasia, but even in countries where the law allows it, it is only one

Table 17.1 Definitions

- The term **euthanasia** should be reserved for the 'compassion-motivated, deliberate, rapid, and painless termination of the life of someone afflicted with an incurable and progressive disease' (Roy and Lapin 1994: 57).
- Euthanasia is **voluntary** if it is performed at the dying person's request or with that person's consent. If it is performed without a person's consent it is **non-voluntary**; if against a person's consent it is **involuntary**.
- '**Treatment limiting decision**' is a description of any action concerning withdrawing or withholding treatment which is deemed to serve no purpose, even if life is shortened. This is generally held to be ethically correct. This description has replaced the terms '**active**' and '**passive**' **euthanasia** which are ambiguous and should be avoided.
- Occasionally in the course of a terminal illness a drug used to control a symptom is thought to contribute to or hasten the death of a patient. This treatment can be justified by the principle of '**double effect**'. Relieving, by appropriate measures, a patient's pain and suffering even if it shortens life is not euthanasia.

---

of a number of possibilities. In the Netherlands, for example, 40 per cent of non-sudden deaths involve some kind of decision (Van der Maas *et al.* 1991): euthanasia (3.6 per cent), withholding treatment (17 per cent), giving treatment which will relieve symptoms but shorten life (17 per cent). In discussing euthanasia therefore, it is important to recognize the diversity of end of life decisions and the different issues they raise. It is also important, for reasoned discussion of these issues, to agree on and be clear about the terms we use. Table 17.1 contains some generally accepted definitions (House of Lords 1994; Keown 1995; Pijnenborg 1995). It is best, for example, to reserve the term 'euthanasia' for 'active' voluntary euthanasia; the issue about which there is most disagreement.

Ethical considerations

Arguments against euthanasia

Arguments against euthanasia can take either consequentialist or deontological forms. The consequentialist arguments predict that allowing euthanasia will have unacceptable results. Randall (1993), for example, argues that legalizing it will lead to a profound alteration in the doctor–patient relationship, in effect removing patients' trust in doctors not to kill them. Others argue that if euthanasia is legalized in cases where it is generally agreed to be appropriate, it will inevitably be extended to those for which its justification is far less obvious. This might ultimately lead to euthanasia on demand or even involuntary euthanasia (abortion is often cited as a precedent for this).

Another consequentialist argument is that giving some people the right to ask for death will lead others to feel that they have a duty to ask for it. Thus respecting the autonomy of some will become a way of reducing the autonomy of others. A current worry is that elderly patients, having lost their entitlement to 'cradle to grave care' they believed they had paid for, may prefer their life savings to go to their children rather than be used up on expensive nursing home care. Or again, it may be argued that the more powerful members of an increasingly uncaring society will use euthanasia to sanitize death and to devalue sick, disabled or disadvantaged people.

Such fears, on the other hand, are shared by many people who are not necessarily opposed to euthanasia in principle. A major difficulty in trying to weigh up these consequentialist arguments is that however plausible their predictions may be, the very fact that they are predictions means that they cannot be proven.

Deontological arguments against euthanasia are based not on consequences but basic convictions about the duties of doctors and other health professionals. Their duty is to cure, relieve and comfort, but not deliberately to kill. These arguments are stronger than consequentialist ones in so far as for those who hold them, they are unarguable. Their weakness, however, is the obvious one – that not all doctors and other professionals hold (or indeed in the past held) these basic convictions about the nature of their duty.

Arguments in favour of euthanasia

Arguments in favour of euthanasia also have consequentialist and deontological strands. A major consequentialist argument is that if euthanasia is not allowed, those patients whose suffering cannot otherwise be relieved, will suffer for reasons which at least in principle could be avoided. Palliative care specialists may feel that this applies to very few patients. The strength of the argument, however, is in whether the exception should be prohibited to defend a principle – whether some must suffer, not necessarily by their own choice, for the general good.

Deontological arguments for euthanasia focus on patients' rights and patient autonomy. 'Prominence of autonomy in medical ethics dictates that patient control must include choice regarding the timing, circumstances and method of death' (Campbell *et al.* 1995: 37). Strong advocates of respect for autonomy argue that the patient and not the doctor has the right to choose what treatment is appropriate. The doctor's only role is to judge whether the patient is capable of making an informed choice, and if so, to provide the necessary information.

The prominence of the principle of respect for autonomy in medical ethics is of fairly recent origin, however, and most ethicists argue that it is not an absolute but a prima facie principle. In other words it has to be weighed up against the traditional duties of beneficence (serving the patient's best interests) and non-maleficence (above all, avoid harm), and the no less basic principle of justice or fairness (Gillon and Lloyd 1994).

Respect of autonomy may have arisen from a justifiable rejection of old-fashioned medical paternalism (when doctors simply did what they thought was best for their patients without asking them). There may now be a danger of society moving directly from rejecting paternalism in health care to embracing a naive consumerism. This would be to overlook the fact that the doctor is a moral agent – the patient's partner or sometimes even opponent in their medico-moral choices – with a duty 'not to be merely a fact-provider but also an argument-provider' (Savulescu 1995). In this context it is worth noting that in the Netherlands 80 per cent of patients, judged competent to make an informed choice, were involved in their end-of-life decisions, and that two-thirds of patients did not pursue their initial request for euthanasia (Van der Maas et al. 1991). The duty to respect a patient's autonomy, in other words, need not entail going against what the doctor believes to be in the patient's best interests, particularly if end-of-life decisions are discussed with patients while they are still competent to make their own decisions.

Rights, duties and judgements

Deontological arguments for euthanasia are sometimes framed in terms of the patient's 'right to die'. When this argument is applied to treatment-limiting decisions, it has compelling moral force. Patients clearly have a right to decline treatment which may prolong life. They may also elect to have treatment which will relieve their symptoms but may shorten their life. The principle of 'double effect' makes this justifiable to the professional conscience of most doctors. A patient's 'right to die', however, does not extend to a 'right to be killed', since that would imply that someone has a duty to kill them. Even the strongest advocates of voluntary euthanasia do not argue that all doctors should be obliged to assist death on request. What they envisage rather is that doctors who can do so in good conscience should be allowed to.

Many doctors are understandably reluctant to assume the burdens of conscientious decision making about euthanasia which weigh very heavily on many of their colleagues in the Netherlands, for example. With this in mind, some ask, need doctors or nurses be involved at all? Randall (1993), for example, predicting harmful consequences for doctor–patient relationships, suggests that if euthanasia were to be allowed, the initial assessment could be made by two lawyers and the act itself performed by a suitably trained technician.

This proposal, however, seems unlikely to get around the problem of medical involvement if euthanasia were to be legalized. An important practical objection, for example, is the need to safeguard patients with treatable depression from receiving inappropriate euthanasia. As Madeley (1994) argues (and as recent legislation in the Northern Territories of Australia provides), a minimum safeguard in these circumstances may be an independent psychiatric assessment. But, arguably, even psychiatric judgement may be more technical, less holistic, and so less morally appropriate to such momentous decisions than an interactive, intersubjective judgement formed in the context of an established patient–doctor relationship.

A key feature of such holistic judgements is Gillett's (1994) concept of the 'pause'. He argues that the more difficult an ethical decision, the greater the chance that a significant conflict between our arguments and our intuitions will cause us to pause before deciding. The pause results from a sense that something important in the situation has not been taken into account. It may relate to unidentified and unmet needs of the patient or it may reflect the doctor's awareness of the dangers of acting as both life-bringer and death-bringer. But whatever it brings to awareness, the crucial contribution of the pause is that it does this when a doctor who knows the patient and has experience of terminal illness attends to intuitive and unconscious elements in the decision making process.

There is more to such decisions, in other words, than can be clearly stated in legal or even psychiatric terms. Those for whom there is no pause, for whom such decisions are easy or at least obvious, thus seem less likely to make what is morally the most appropriate decision. To say this is not to diminish the value of legal judgement, which has its proper place. But so too has the clinical wisdom and personal knowledge of the patient's 'own' doctor.

Many general practitioners in the UK seem prepared to carry out euthanasia in certain circumstances, were it to be legalized (Ward and Tate 1994). Euthanasia decided by two lawyers and performed by a technician would be morally a very different act than euthanasia decided with and performed by such doctors. It would be less personal and more at risk of being morally inappropriate. If euthanasia were to be legalized therefore, there seems no way to escape the conclusion that a doctor (particularly one who knows the patient well) would both morally and practically be the most appropriate person to be involved in the decision making process and in carrying out the act of euthanasia.

Factors affecting requests for euthanasia

Compared to the amount of writing on the ethical and moral aspects of end-of-life decisions there are few good data about why people ask for euthanasia. In order to understand and place in perspective the abstract arguments it is useful to summarize the studies of patients requesting for euthanasia and examine the reasons behind these requests.

The most comprehensive study of the practice of euthanasia and other end-of-life decisions was that undertaken in the Netherlands in the early 1990s (Pijnenborg 1995). Doctors performing euthanasia were asked what were their patients' reasons for the request.

The most important were:

- unbearable situation (70%);
- dread of future suffering (50%);
- 'unworthy dying'(46%);
- loss of dignity (57%);
- dependency on others (33%);
- tiredness of life (33%).

Pain was mentioned as a reason by 46 per cent of patients but was the sole reason for only 3 per cent. The distinctions between the categories are not sufficiently clear to draw very definite conclusions but they do show that patients request euthanasia for many reasons other than physical suffering.

This observation is supported by Seale and Addington-Hall (1995a, b). Their study in the UK reported relatives' recollection of patients' requests and found that 3.6 per cent of patients had asked for euthanasia at some point in the last year of life. They assessed symptom severity, dependency, and other cultural factors and found that requests for euthanasia were more closely correlated with dependency rather than pain or other distressing symptoms.

Chochinov and his colleagues (1995) interviewed 200 terminally ill patients in North America and assessed their desire for death, as well as measuring their degree of pain, level of social support, and whether or not they were depressed. They found that 8.5 per cent of patients acknowledged a persistent and pervasive desire to die. This desire correlated with ratings of pain and poor social support but most closely with the presence and level of depression. Of those expressing a strong desire to die, 60 per cent were depressed, compared to 8 per cent of those not wishing to die. They concluded that a potentially treatable condition was present in the majority of terminally ill patients wishing to die. Madeley (1994) suggests that the 23 per cent of patients in the Remmelink study who requested euthanasia because of 'tiredness of life' may have been displaying a symptom of depression.

Chochinov et al. (1995) also suggested that the intensity of the desire to die may vary with time. At the end of two weeks two-thirds of the non-depressed patients who had expressed a wish to die no longer wished to do so.

Dependency and control

Dependency is perhaps the most difficult problem for many patients, especially those who have been used to the idea of complete independence of action. 'No-one's ever had to do anything for me', 'I can't stand asking the nurses when I want to do anything'. Many people, despite optimal control of their physical symptoms, find a life of dependency intolerable. They may feel that the only aspect of their life they have potential control over is the timing and manner of their dying.

Patients' sense of personal control improves their ability to cope with stressful events. In particular patients who use behavioural control (taking concrete action to reduce the impact of a stressor) and cognitive control (being able to use thought processes or strategies to modify the impact of a stressor) show better adjustment to serious illness (Sarafino 1994).

These forms of control are generally useful tools in adjusting to illness. For patients coping with the dependency brought on by terminal illness, unable to influence events, they may no longer be so helpful. It may be that people who use control to cope with life and illness have particular difficulties when confronted with irresolvable dependency. Some requests for euthanasia can be seen as an attempt to continue to use coping mechanisms that have served the person so well in the past but are no longer functional.

Spiritual issues

Kearney (1992) suggests that some patients request euthanasia because of deep spiritual pain. He feels that patients need to be able to see a common thread running through their lives. People dying in pain or distress may lose this sense of identity and suffer disconnection and alienation from the deep level of their psyche. These people may request or demand for death as a result of the alienation from self that they are experiencing. Recognizing the problem as essentially a spiritual one is important as particular skills and interventions may be needed.

To sum up then, it seems though that between 3 and 8 per cent of terminally ill patients either request euthanasia or have a sustained and pervasive wish to die. People have many different reasons for their request. Some will have unrelieved physical symptoms or be in fear of future suffering. A large proportion may be depressed. These problems may respond to explanation or medical and psychological interventions. An important factor in many requests for euthanasia is increasing dependency and loss of dignity. These issues are much more difficult to resolve. If the practice and extent of palliative care improves, requests for euthanasia because of unrelieved physical problems should decrease. As autonomy and personal control become more important in our society dependency may become the most common reason why people request euthanasia.

Responding to a request for euthanasia

So far in this chapter we have discussed the ethical arguments for and against euthanasia and have examined some of the reasons why people ask to die. In clinical practice one of the most important issues is how to respond to a patient who asks for euthanasia. It is of little practical benefit if carers understand the ethical issues surrounding end-of-life decisions but do not know what to say or do when faced with a patient who asks to die. Here are some ways of responding to euthanasia requests:

- ask about it;
- acknowledge the request;
- investigate the reasons;
- correct the correctable;
- return control to the patient;
- think about spiritual problems;
- admit your own powerlessness.

In hospices a request for euthanasia is particularly distressing both because it demonstrates the depths of the patient's suffering and because of a perceived failure on the part of the hospice staff to relieve that suffering. Where euthanasia is not an acceptable option caregivers need some ideas about how to respond to these requests. In order to do so they need to suspend their own feelings about the morality of a request for euthanasia and be able to acknowledge the reality of the pain that has led a patient to ask to die (Cole 1993). Many health professionals find it difficult to address these issues (Di Mola 1994) but patients need to be able to talk about their fears about death and continuing living. Some reasons why patients request euthanasia may be remediable. Therefore even though euthanasia is illegal it is still important to ask patients whether they have thought about it. In the same way that psychiatrists ask depressed patients specifically about suicidal ideas, it is sometimes necessary to ask terminally ill patients whether they have had thoughts about euthanasia. An affirmative response to a question such as 'Do you sometimes wonder whether it's worth going on?' can be followed by 'Have you ever thought about asking someone to end things for you?' It can be a tremendous relief for a patient to find someone with whom they can discuss this difficult and confusing subject. Far from shocking patients or reaffirming a tentative thought about euthanasia asking can allow them to express fears and worries they might otherwise keep to themselves. Patients find thoughts about a deliberate act of dying upsetting. If they sense disapproval or upset from their carers they will become more distressed and may avoid further discussion. Acknowledging the validity of patients' feelings allows them to talk openly about progressively more difficult subjects (Maguire and Faulkner 1994). Acknowledging each problem as it is disclosed ('That sounds important and I would like to come back to it; I wonder if there is anything else?') allows a fuller disclosure of the patient's problems. It is better not to correct misconceptions, or give reassurance or advice until all the problems are expressed. In this way a carer can formulate a more complete understanding of the reasons behind a request for euthanasia.

Once all the reasons have been identified it will be possible to address or correct some or all of them. Unresolved physical symptoms need to be treated before patients can make appropriate informed decisions about their future. If a depressive illness has been identified this needs to be explained to the patient and treatment offered. A combination of adequate symptom relief and appropriate use of the principle of double effect will mean that many common physical symptoms (such as pain or breathlessness) can be adequately managed without resort to euthanasia.

Many patients have misapprehensions and misunderstandings about their illness and do not have good enough information on which to base their decisions. Like many professionals they may not be clear about the distinction between euthanasia and other end-of-life decisions. They may believe that the doctor must continue to strive to prolong life and will be comforted by the reassurance that treatment will be directed at symptom control even if this were to shorten life. For some patients there is a belief that the suffering is unending and that death is many months away. Giving patients a clearer idea of the course of their illness may remove the 'dread of future suffering' and give them hope.

Many patients do not understand the amount of control they already can have in treatment decisions. Involving patients in these decisions is one way to return control to them. Allowing patients to make fully informed decisions about their treatment can reduce the health professionals' control of a clinical situation. This may leave the caregiver feeling vulnerable but allow the patient a greater sense of control. There may be other ways of giving the patient more control, for example by altering the ward environment. Spiritual problems may be at the root of a few patients' requests for euthanasia and will be a factor in many more. Relief of physical suffering, the development of a relationship of trust between patient and carer, will allow most patients the opportunity to find inner consolation and peace (Mount and Kearney 1996). A few patients will remain stuck in a painful and distressing 'spiritual prison'. There is a group of patients who, despite adequate symptom control and apparent psychological stability, remain committed to requesting euthanasia. Hockley (1991) describes their situation as being one of 'rational no-hope'. Both Hockley (1991) and Kearney (1992) describe patients who, despite presenting in this way, were helped to personal reconciliation; one by prayer and the other with the help of imagework. Both authors claim that these deaths were more meaningful and more peaceful than seemed possible if their requests for euthanasia had been met. Special skills such as imagework or visualization may help such patients to move to a different level of experience and bring the comfort they seek. This subject is further explored by Mount and Kearney (1996).

There will be some patients whose situation we can do little to improve. They will remain dependent and lacking in control; distressed by their inability to help themselves. It does not help to say 'Don't you worry about that; we're here to help you'. Patients would rather that we recognize their pain and acknowledge that their very dependency is what distresses them. We shall never be able to give some patients back their independence of action. We need to be prepared to share a patient's powerlessness by admitting our own. As Sheila Cassidy writes 'Slowly, as the years go by I learn about the importance of powerlessness. . . . The dying know we are not God. They accept that we cannot halt the process of cancer. . . . All they ask is that we do not desert them' (Cassidy 1988: 64). This approach does not solve every patient's problems nor does it stop every patient continuing to request euthanasia. It does help to identify specific problems and concerns, enabling these to be addressed. It also allows a patient to develop a trusting relationship with a caregiver and it is much easier from this basis for the patient to accept the moral and ethical problems facing the health care team.

Palliative care and legalized euthanasia

Palliative care professionals have, for a long time, been able to argue that the provision of good palliative care relieves suffering to such an extent that euthanasia is no longer wanted by many people, even those who have previously been its advocates. This has allowed them to opt for maintenance of the status quo where active euthanasia and assisted suicide are illegal. Today, however, opinions and legislation on euthanasia and other end-of-life medical decisions are evolving in various parts of the world. In some countries euthanasia is now decriminalized or legalized. In the Netherlands doctors helping with euthanasia or assisted suicide are now unlikely to be prosecuted if they comply with a code drawn up by the Royal Dutch Medical Association (KNMG) (Keown 1995). In the Northern Territories of Australia a bill legalizing euthanasia became law on 1 July 1996 (Zinn 1996). In Oregon a measure legalizing assisted suicide has been made law, although this has been challenged and a decision is awaited; the US federal appeals court has ruled that terminally ill patients have a right to a doctor's assistance in hastening their death (Macready 1996). Both Western Australia and Canada are actively debating 'right to die' legislation. Hospices in these countries now have to look at how they respond to the reality of euthanasia while still remaining true to their principles. In the future there are likely to be more attempts to legalize euthanasia, particularly in countries where autonomy and consumerism are important values. The challenge for the future will be how to respond to this new situation.

The Oregon Hospice Association set up an ethics task force to look at the problems that palliative care units might face should assisted suicide be legalized in Oregon (Campbell *et al.* 1995). It argues that the dilemma for hospices will be how to respect patient autonomy while not hastening death, and it defines the central controversy as one of conflicting meanings of patient control. The immediate result of the legal moves in Oregon was that hospices and their staff had to determine how and to what extent they were going to participate in what had become a lawful act.

In the presence of legalized euthanasia different palliative care units may respond differently, leading to a fragmentation of the 'hospice movement' where some units are seen to 'do' euthanasia while others do not. Although ultimately the chief doctor has responsibility for clinical decisions, palliative care units pride themselves on a team working with a set of similar attitudes and values. This common ethos is put under great strain by confronting issues around legalized euthanasia. Legalized euthanasia or assisted suicide would present new and very difficult challenges for hospices; the moral conflict between not hastening death and not abandoning the patient does not therefore have an easy solution.

Conclusion

There does not seem to be any ideal legal solution to the question of euthanasia, and in some cases no ideal ethical solution. There are, however, better or worse solutions in terms of ethics and communication. There is a difference between moral relativism (saying there are no right and wrong answers) and saying that each case is different. Given that persistent and justifiable requests are likely to be rare, each case has to be negotiated on its own merits and will never be easy. Acknowledging this is the most effective way of avoiding the slippery slope. Applying ethics intelligently and communicating well with patients will resolve some apparently intractable dilemmas and enable both professionals and patients to be more comfortable with decisions.

There will probably remain a small number of psychologically stable, physically asymptomatic but terminally ill patients who continue to wish to end their lives by euthanasia. We and the rest of society will continue to struggle with their right to do so. What is clear is that much larger numbers of patients who are said to want or need euthanasia, are in far greater need of understanding, explanation, and physical or psychological treatment.

References

Campbell, C., Hare, J. and Matthews, P. (1995) Conflicts of conscience: hospice and assisted suicide. *Hastings Center Report* 25(3): 36–43.

Cassidy, S. (1988) *Sharing the Darkness: The Spirituality of Caring.* London: Darton, Longman & Todd.

Chochinov, H., Wilson, K.G., Enns, M., Mowchun, N., Lander, S., Levitt, M. and Clinch, J.J. (1995) Desire for death in the terminally ill. *American Journal of Psychiatry,* 152: 1185–91.

Cole, R.M. (1993) Communicating with people who request euthanasia. *Palliative Medicine,* 7: 139–43.

Di Mola, G. (1994) Attitudes of health care professionals towards euthanasia. *European Journal of Palliative Care,* 1: 140–4.

Gillett, M. (1994) The principle and the pause, in R. Gillon and A. Lloyd (eds) *Principles of Health Care Ethics.* Chichester: John Wiley.

Gillon, R. and Lloyd, A. (eds) *Principles of Health Care Ethics.* Chichester: John Wiley.

Hockley, J. (1991) The concept of hope and the will to live. *Palliative Medicine,* 7: 181–6.

House of Lords (1994) *Report of the Select Committee on Medical Ethics.* HL Paper 21–1. London: HMSO.

Hunt, R. (1995) The incidence of requests for a quicker terminal course. *Palliative Medicine,* 2: 167–8.

Kearney, M. (1992) Palliative medicine: just another speciality? *Palliative Medicine,* 6: 39–46.

Keown, J. (ed.) (1995) *Euthanasia Examined.* Cambridge: Cambridge University Press.

Macready (1996) Assisted suicide is legal, says US judge. *British Medical Journal,* 312: 655–6.

Madeley, P. (1994) Role of depression ignored (letter). *British Medical Journal,* 309: 472.

Maguire, P. and Faulkner, A. (1994) *Talking to Cancer Patients and their Relatives.* Oxford: Oxford University Press.

Mount, B. and Kearney, M. (1996) Spiritual care of dying patients, in H. Chochinov and W. Breitbart (eds) *Psychiatric Dimensions of Palliative Medicine.* Oxford: Oxford University Press.

Pijnenborg, L. (1995) *End of Life Decision-Making in Dutch Medical Practice.* Den Haag: Cip-Gegevens Koninklijke Bibliotheek.

Randall, F. (1993) Two lawyers and a technician. *Palliative Medicine,* 7(3): 193–8.

Roy, D. and Lapin, C. (1994) Regarding euthanasia. *European Journal of Palliative Care,* 1: 57–9.

Sarafino, E. (1994) *Health Psychology: Biopsychosocial Interaction,* 2nd edn. Chichester: John Wiley.

Savulescu, J. (1995) Rational non-interventional paternalism: why doctors ought to make judgements of what is best for their patients. *Journal of Medical Ethics,* 21: 327–31.

Seale, C. and Addington-Hall, J. (1995a) Euthanasia the role of good care. *Social Science and Medicine,* 40(5): 581–7.

Seale, C. and Addington-Hall, J. (1995b) Dying at the best time. *Social Science and Medicine*, 40(5): 589–95.

Van der Maas, P.J., Van Delden, J.J.M., Pijnenborg, L. and Looman, C.W.N. (1991) Euthanasia and other medical decisions concerning the end of life. *Lancet*, 338: 669–74.

Ward, B.J. and Tate, P.A. (1994) Attitudes among NHS doctors to requests for euthanasia. *British Medical Journal*, 308: 1332–4.

Zinn, C. (1996) Australian doctors renew battle over euthanasia. *British Medical Journal*, 312: 1437.

18 | New approaches to care

JESSICA CORNER AND ROBERT DUNLOP

More than 30 years since the inception of the modern hospice movement, hospice care and the wider speciality of palliative care are undergoing something of a re-evaluation both from within and from without by sociologists and health planners. Not only must palliative care prove its own worth in improving the quality of care in all settings in which such services might be required, but also to continue to provide real leadership for the future direction of care. (Palliative care is used to denote the speciality devoted to the care of those whose disease is no longer responsive to curative treatment (WHO 1990), and therefore for the purpose of this discussion unless otherwise indicated encompasses hospice care.) As Eric Wilkes (1993: 5) points out, 'we can look back and see that the hospice movement has irreversibly improved the standards of care for the dying. Because of this, our easy great days may be behind us.'

This doubt over the direction of palliative care stems from a number of concerns over whether its current emphasis is necessarily right, and surrounds three central issues. First, whether palliative care has lost the radicalism so characteristic of its early years as it has increasingly become absorbed into mainstream health care, and as a consequence is less able to offer leadership and innovation. Second, the exclusive nature of hospice and palliative care has meant that a wide range of needs and disease groups have been neglected. Third, there has been criticism surrounding the impact of the process of medicalization within palliative care.

James and Field (1992: 1363) note that the hospice movement has been 'unashamedly reformist ... fired by the radically disruptive intention of altering the tenor of British society's care of the dying'. The hospice movement was a response to the increasingly institutionalized picture of death in the UK. Where the goal of 'cure' predominated using modern technology to artificially maintain life as long as possible, death was seen as failure, and symptoms of dying patients were inadequately controlled, while society effectively denied death as the 'last taboo'.

The hospice movement provided a charismatic alternative to this and hospices were radical, innovative institutions offering an alternative model of care. James and Field (1992), however, argue that the movement may be losing this radicalism in the face of it being reabsorbed into the mainstream of British health care services. In particular hospices and palliative care units are criticized as becoming bureaucratized with increasingly rigid hierarchies and management practices. A process of reprofessionalization is said to be taking place with a movement away from charitable and voluntary work predominating. With this reprofessionalization, the mainstream principles of biomedical care are re-emerging, and certain practices within palliative care are at risk of becoming routinized and controlled by policy and procedure.

McNamara et al.'s (1994) examination of the institutionalization of the good death provides a good example of this. Using ethnographic interview and participant observation of nursing in a hospice unit in Western Australia, they observed that certain features of the 'good death' ideal had become routinized so that such deaths were 'required' by staff in the interest of what might be considered socially acceptable and for the smooth running of the organization. Nurses were at risk, over time, of developing a rigidity in their views over what constituted a 'good death', so that those patients who did not conform to this ideal, for example by not accepting their death or hanging on to life, were felt to have 'problems'.

There is also evidence to suggest that hospices are no longer providing care which is radically different or of a higher quality than mainstream health services (Seale 1989). This may well be in part because of palliative care's influence on the quality of care more generally (for example in pain and symptom control), and the development of palliative care services within hospital and community services. The integration of palliative care within mainstream health care may mean that it will be difficult to continue to identify palliative care as unique or different.

Seale (1991) has questioned the relevance of the hospice and palliative care philosophy, since it has concentrated almost exclusively on the needs of people with cancer (representing only 24 per cent of all deaths) who are generally middle aged and therefore are more likely to have family support and who have problems and needs specific to their diagnosis. There is evidence that such a model of care cannot be neatly extrapolated to other patient groups. Palliative care's continuing emphasis on care for people with cancer has led to the accusation of a service based on exclusivity. Even among those with cancer, there is a problem with acceptability. While many patients and families are pleased to receive hospice or home care services, some are not. The prospect of a Macmillan nurse visiting will also be unacceptable to some patients, while the idea of referral to a hospice frequently evokes a feeling of hopelessness. Ethnic minorities are under-represented in the workload of specialist palliative care services. This may be because patients and families from other cultures pose problems because of different attitudes to truth-telling, patient autonomy, and accept-ance of a terminal illness. In the light of these problems what is clearly needed is a palliative care movement which continues to offer new and radical approaches to care and address some of these central concerns.

The trend towards medicalization within palliative care deserves particu-lar scrutiny since this is central to current debate surrounding the direction of the speciality. Medicalization is a term which was first used to describe the influence of medicine on the society's relationship with death. Over time, the expert at the bedside of the dying person ceased to be the priest and became the doctor; as this occurred the care of dying people was transformed from that of assisting the individual to identify meaning in his or her plight, to one of treatment, and the preservation of life at all costs by whatever means at the doctor's disposal (Walter 1993). The technical revolution in health care has increasingly meant that such care has taken place in hospitals, away from home and family. The use of artificial means of sustaining life has made it difficult to identify when the actual moment of death is about to or has occurred, thus often precluding a more gentle and meaning-centred approach to care. Hospice and more recently palli-ative care sought to provide an alternative to this, in particular facilitating home rather than institutional death.

Interestingly the accusation of 'medicalization' has been levelled at pal-liative care itself. Biswas (1993) and Field (1994) have argued that hospice and palliative care have now themselves become medicalized with a shift in emphasis away from care of dying persons to the rather more euphem-istic endeavours of symptom control and 'palliation'. These terms them-selves may have allowed the denial of the inevitability of eventual death to become 'built in' to specialist care. Criticisms also surround the increas-ing use of technical and invasive procedures in care. Medicine is felt to have become dominant over other health professionals working within palliative care so that a medical orientation towards care predominates, and with this a movement away from attending to the needs of the person as a whole may have occurred. While these accusations have been vehe-mently rejected as false (Ahmedzai 1993, 1994), in the face of a growing list of criticism, consideration needs to be given to the overall orientation of palliative care, and how new approaches to care might arise, since research and development are a strong *raison d'être* for the speciality.

The problem is perhaps embedded in the earliest origins of hospice care. The early success of the hospice movement in the management of cancer pain using powerful pharmacological means has unintentionally set a path for the construction of care which has increasingly placed heavy emphasis on a biomedical model. The ability to relieve cancer pain using these means led to the search for more and better drugs first for pain, and then for other symptoms found to be common in advanced disease. This endeavour was more heroic than perhaps other aspects of care such as distress, loss of function or spirituality and therefore were allowed to become dominant. The doctor as prescriber of pharmacologically dominated care was then the natural leader for services based on these approaches. The biomedical model of care is not solely the responsibility of the medical profession, however; it represents the whole construction of care, and is adhered to by all participants in palliative care, consumers and professionals alike, and has the following features:

- the assumption that pain and other physical symptoms are the predominant cause of suffering in the dying;
- a belief that these symptoms are best managed by establishing their root cause and by utilizing modern pharmacology and other biomedical innovations for their 'relief';
- psychological, social and spiritual aspects of these symptoms, though considered to be important and therefore should be addressed, are of secondary rather than primary importance;
- the employment of the biomedical model to manage these problems has a tendency to objectify the problem and in the process risks the denial of personhood, depersonalization and decontextualization of the problem, and denial of chronicity, suffering, distress and meaning as part of the experience of illness and dying.

As the speciality of palliative care becomes more established, the increasing adherence to this model is in danger of creating a narrow and rigid service, rather than fostering creativity and innovation.

While many working within palliative care would rightly argue that the philosophy of care is entirely centred on the person, and is lauded for its humanity in care, this care is still constructed against a background of the profound influence of the biomedical model (as are all established health services and health professionals' practice). Palliative care may need to move beyond the constraints of this to further understand the needs of consumers of care and their families.

The limitations of the biomedical model are now well rehearsed in the literature. A central problem surrounds the biomedical relationship to 'the body' because this

- regards the body as an external object to the enquiries that yield knowledge of it;
- assumes that the practitioner is in control of the body of the patient, and diagnosis and treatment therefore requires the patient to be subordinate to the practitioner;

- biomedicine deals with malfunctioning organs and its symptoms and not with the 'body' which constitutes the person as such.

(Lyon and Barbalet 1994)

The biomedical understanding is felt to be profoundly limiting of healing in its broadest sense and has contributed to the development of the counter-cultures of consumerism and alternative models healing.

A further limitation of the biomedical model lies in its foundations in the epistemology of Cartesianism. Descartes's influence on western thought has left us with the conception of the separate nature of mind and body and, according to Cassells (1982), left only the body in the domain of medicine. The mind remained the domain of the church (and later psychologists and psychiatrists), leaving medicine very narrow boundaries within which to work. The remnants of this are clear within the concept of 'total pain' which revolutionized the control of pain in palliative care. In using a 'total pain' approach physical, psychological, social and spiritual components of pain are recognized and dealt with (Saunders 1967). However, these are seen as separate entities to be managed accordingly. This does not easily allow for pain to be conceived as embodied (that is an experience of the inextricably linked self and body) or indeterminent (inexpressible or measurable) in nature (Lanceley 1995), or an experience which exists far beyond that of pain perception which can be manipulated by powerful drugs.

The definitions of palliative care adhere to this tradition, for example Twycross and Dunn (1994: 5) state that 'Palliative care provides relief from pain and other distressing symptoms. It also integrates psychological, social and spiritual aspects of care so that patients may come to terms with their own death as fully and constructively as they can.' Physical, psychological and social aspects of illness are considered separate compartments of the individual's illness experience, and any definitions of care seem to serve to remind practitioners not to forget any of these components. While this is a great improvement on the wider health care community's tendency not to address concerns that exist beyond the purely physical, it nevertheless risks placing profound limitations on the way illness and related problems are addressed. Palliative care has done much to improve and move forward the quality of care, but attempts now need to be made to overcome some of the fundamental limitations which arguably exist within its current construction.

Reframing care

This might be achieved through a process we have called reframing care. One approach to this is to undertake a radical deconstruction and

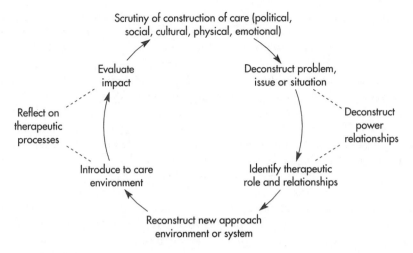

Figure 18.1   The process of reframing care

reconstruction of given health care situations or problems consumers of services face, using a cyclical approach such as that shown in Figure 18.1. During this process all the features of the problem and the context in which it arises, and is treated or cared for, are taken apart. All elements are examined for their usefulness or ability to hinder healing, adjustment or alleviation. This may require for example in the case of the management of breathlessness, an examination of the outpatient environment in which consultations are made with health carers about the problem, and the nature of interactions between health professionals and sufferers in exploring it. As well as specific interventions currently considered 'standard treatment'. This process encompasses the political, social, cultural as well as the physical and emotional, and understanding the nature of power relationships between carers and sufferers need also to be deconstructed. This may allow different approaches to care to be developed, suggest areas of health care that palliative care has not hitherto reached or establish totally new situations or methods by which palliative care can contribute. This process involves taking apart and shedding all aspects of the current content and context of the care of a given situation or problem, so that it can be looked at afresh without historical, philosophical or political constraint. By doing so freedom for innovation can be gained.

Beyond biomedicine: meaning-centred approaches to care

A scrutiny of the construction of biomedical approaches to care for example may begin to offer alternative perspectives on which developments may be based. Cassells (1982) rejects the dualistic position of biomedicine which separates mind from body, and argues that it leads to inadequate understanding of personhood, and therefore contributes to suffering. Suffering is the central issue to be addressed according to Cassells, and although it often occurs in the presence of pain and other symptoms, it extends beyond the purely physical and can occur in any realm of the person: social roles; self; family; beliefs; and life meanings. Good and Delvicchio Good (1980) argue for a meaning-centred approach to understanding clinical practice to replace the 'empiricist model of clinical reasoning' which assumes that symptoms are reflections of disordered somatic processes. In this model the central task of the physician is to decode patients' description of their symptoms in order to diagnose disease. In contrast a meaning-centred approach seeks to access patients' interpretations of their illness and assists them to construct new understanding of their illness. The therapeutic benefit in this context is the ability of the therapist to influence the patient's reality and construct a new reality. Kleinman (1988) has used this in the context of patients with chronic pain to develop a new model of practice in which the patient's narrative of the illness experience is used therapeutically to elicit the meaning and significance of symptoms, and the consequences of illness, to the patient's personal and social world. This is then used to assist the patient to overcome problems and disability associated with the illness and to rekindle hope through a process of re-moralization. It should also be possible to construct a model for palliative care which could take into account these issues, and could provide the basis for innovations in care.

In doing this, however, there are some core issues which may need to be addressed. For example this may require the abandonment of principles of care such as symptom management and patient acceptance of dying as the overarching goals of palliative care. Health professionals may need to lay aside paternalistic or maternalistic approaches to care since this can lead to the temptation to resolve problems that patients 'appear' to be suffering from, and in so doing undermine their sense of control by encouraging a dependence on professionals. Instead the role of health professionals could be recast as servant to the consumer, rather than carer for the patient. This may help focus attention on the different type of relationship which is required to preserve and embrace personhood.

In a consumer oriented relationship, rather than see themselves as providers of pain relief and symptom control, health professionals instead would see themselves as repositories of a knowledge base which is at the consumers disposal. They should be able to pick and choose the elements of such knowledge which suit their circumstances, their view of the world, and their way of maintaining control. This would require the professional carer to have a strong sense of personal and professional esteem, capable of withstanding any sense of being 'used' and not needing 'fulfilment' from 'grateful' clients. The professional's experience therefore is not used to promote acceptance of illness and dying but to maintain a calm demeanour for those who are struggling with the issues raised by terminal illness.

Reframing symptoms

As has already been noted in palliative care, great emphasis has been placed on the management of physical symptoms as the core of practice; however, in this context the term 'symptom' is highly problematic because of the assumption that this is universally defined and therefore managed beyond the person by the health carer with little reference to contextual, political, social or cultural influences. It also inherently excludes the patient's narrative and personal meanings from the therapeutic process. The terms 'problem' and 'need' might serve to change the orientation of care in the context of what has been understood as 'symptom management', since these suggest something that is difficult to deal with or understand which requires being overcome or accomplished. The power for action and ownership, however, remains with the person experiencing the problem. Looked at in this way it is possible to see that as health carers we have no right to 'manage' these problems, only to assist in their containment, and both the sufferer and health carer have a mutual need to understand them (Corner 1995). What needs to be explored is how this different understanding of concerns and problems might be applied to aspects of care for people with distressing symptoms?

Pain, breathlessness, fatigue, depression, anxiety and more: a constellation of states of mind and body

There are a whole constellation of symptoms and problems associated with advanced cancer that are known to be difficult to alleviate or address. These have tended to be compartmentalized as either 'mind' or 'body' problems and then treated accordingly. Currently, these problems are classified as 'mind' or 'body' related, the majority of interventions selected for these use a pharmacological solution in the first instance, as the most effective means of dealing with them. While in many instances these will be of value, all too often problems are only partially alleviated. Or for example in the case of anxiety or depression, they create many dilemmas as to when appropriate intervention should be instigated, or as to what is appropriate intervention.

These are problems which in the context of someone facing death in the not too distant future, take on significant meaning to the sufferer and those close to them. Because of this they frequently belie definition and clinical diagnosis along traditional biomedical lines. These are problems of the 'body' in the sociological and phenomenological sense. That is, they are certainly a result of physiological decline due to illness, but are experienced within the body and as part of that individual's social and cultural world. How this experience is played out will directly influence the nature of the experience of the particular constellation of problems and needs.

Each problem is related to another and may not be possible to separate out in the way that traditional diagnosis requires. Work is needed to explore these issues so that new approaches to care can be developed.

For example Lanceley (1995) argues that there is evidence to suggest care for pain in palliative care, despite the enormous strides which have been made in the effective alleviation of pain in advanced disease, is often anything but holistic and person-centred. The influence of the biomedical model neglects some important aspects of pain and its experience in particular:

- the indeterminate nature of pain (that is its inexpressibility by those suffering from it, and the impossibility of true understanding on the part of the non-sufferer);
- the importance of culture to pain meaning and understanding, and not simply to the style in which it is expressed;
- the need to develop and use in practice the notion of embodied pain (person, body and the experience of pain are one, pain is experienced physically and emotionally in an indistinguishable form);
- that the pain experience may be expressed by the sufferer as an object 'it' in an attempt to gain control over it: understanding of subject and object in pain talk may be one means of developing therapeutic approaches to it.

As Lanceley concludes,

> it is necessary for us to open our minds to different ideas which may conceivably influence our ways of being with people in pain. Only if we continue our explorations and claim responsibility for how we understand pain will we actively and consistently negotiate with pain sufferers to create situations which can interpret, alleviate and 'contain' the pain.
>
> (Lanceley 1995: 157)

The problem of breathlessness

The problem of breathlessness in advanced cancer is increasingly being seen as an intractable one. Despite a range of pharmacological options available (Ahmedzai 1993), there is evidence to suggest that even with the best palliative management the problem worsens rather than improves (Higginson and McCarthy 1989). This has led a team of nurses (Bailey 1995; Corner *et al.* 1995) to critically examine the nature of breathlessness care and reframe it. Early results indicate that this new approach may be valuable in enhancing the quality of life of patients with lung cancer who are suffering from breathlessness (Corner *et al.* 1996). An integrative model of breathlessness has been developed where the emotional experience of breathlessness is considered inseparable from its physical experience or the mechanisms by which breathlessness arises or is exacerbated. This leads to a model of care where breathlessness is understood holistically in the context of the individual's life, illness experience and its meaning. Therapeutic intervention is designed around a nursing clinic where sufferers are invited to attend on an outpatient basis reinforcing normality and health promotion, and where constraints on time can be kept to a minimum and privacy with patients maximized. In addition the clinic provides a focus for the further development of the therapeutic approach by reflecting on experiences gained. The intervention itself (Corner *et al.* 1995) consists of the following strategies:

- detailed assessment of breathlessness and factors which ameliorate or exacerbate it, taken from the sufferer's narrative;
- exploration with individuals of the meaning of breathlessness, their disease and their feelings about the future;
- advice and support for sufferers and their families on ways of managing breathlessness;
- breathing retraining techniques for sufferers and families;
- progressive muscle relaxation and distraction techniques;
- goal setting to complement breathing and relaxation techniques, to assist in the management of functional and social activities, and to support the development of coping strategies;
- early recognition of problems warranting biomedical intervention.

Evidence from a study of nurses using this approach (Bailey 1995) suggests that the deep emotional consequences of breathlessness have directed the nurses towards concentrating on emotional issues at least as much as breathing retraining. The nurse is called upon to apply the practical discipline of breathing retraining to a highly charged emotional situation such as night panic attacks, loss of function or social role, or distressing episodes of breathlessness in which sufferers fear they might die. The nurse is aware and involved in the predicament and has to work with a high level of distress. Bailey (1995) likens this to Fabricius's (1991) description of the psychotherapeutic role which resembles a mother 'holding' her infant, protecting it physically from harm and psychically from overwhelming distress. With this level of support and real understanding individuals are able to rebuild their confidence and functional level, while also facing realistically their advancing disease and its meaning to them. A small randomized study of 20 patients with lung cancer has shown significant improvements in ratings of breathlessness, distress caused by breathlessness, functional capacity and ability to perform activities of daily living in those attending the clinic using this approach, compared to a control group (Corner *et al.* 1996).

There are powerful parallels between Lanceley's (1995) description of potential for working with pain and the approach developed for the problem of breathlessness; they do not reject the need for powerful drugs to alleviate the pain of cancer or breathlessness but suggest a much broader approach with a less fixed response to its control. What is needed now is the development and rigorous evaluation of pain and breathlessness care programmes utilizing these concepts.

The potential for some of these principles to be extrapolated into other areas is being studied at the Centre for Cancer and Palliative Care Studies in London. A study which is exploring the problem of fatigue in advanced cancer patients using the sufferer's narrative, elicited during in-depth interviews, about the problem so that a detailed understanding of the nature of fatigue and what it is like to live with it is developed. The aim of this is then to develop an intervention strategy for working with individuals experiencing fatigue which can be evaluated. This work suggests that sufferers need to develop a deep understanding of the meaning of fatigue as a problem for themselves, and to be assisted to develop self-help strategies for living with it. Another study is examining self-management of the problem of ascites in women with ovarian cancer, in which they will work to delay reaccumulation of ascites through the use of a programme of breathing exercises and wearing an abdominal binder (Preston 1995). One of the interesting features of this approach is the desire to put the individual in charge of the management of the problem, rather than the health carer. It will be some time, however, before a substantial body of data is available to evaluate the impact these principles may have.

Reconstructing services to recover care

Innovation in care is not only required in relation to single or constellations of symptoms. Services themselves require reconstruction in order to allow a broader perspective to care to be adopted and implemented. If narrative, meaning and facilitated self-management are to be given higher priority in palliative care and health services more generally, then services need to be established which provide an environment in which these can thrive.

Increasingly the role of nursing in innovations in care are being explored and a number of exciting new initiatives are under way. The features of these new nursing services are to allow the extension of palliative care while also offering radical new innovative models of care or service delivery.

Nurse-led admissions

At St Christopher's Hospice, London, a pilot project is being used to evaluate the possibility of nurse-led admissions. The usual practice is for a doctor and nurse to work together when a patient is admitted to the inpatient unit. The doctor conducts a thorough history of the medical and psychosocial issues, followed by a physical examination, the nurse asks supplementary questions.

The nurse-led admissions project has given nurses the authority to conduct the initial interview and a limited physical examination, which is later reviewed with the doctor in discussion, with more detailed examination by the doctor if deemed necessary. This approach is not only providing opportunity for nurses to broaden their clinical skills but also streamlining the service.

Nurse-led clinics for patients with breathlessness

As a result of the approach developed for breathlessness care in lung cancer already described, Cancer Relief Macmillan Fund are funding a national multicentre study of the role of nursing in the management of breathlessness. Macmillan nurses are establishing nursing clinics along similar lines to those described by Corner *et al.* (1995). These will offer support and help to people with lung cancer suffering from breathlessness and will be evaluated in a clinical trial. These clinics are being established in settings where the Macmillan nurses may not have reached before, since they are being taken to chest clinics where it is possible to identify those in need. This means that palliative care will be made available to those who previously might not have accessed it.

Nurse-led follow-up in lung cancer

Primary lung cancer is the commonest form of cancer, with 32,500 new cases diagnosed in the UK each year (SMAC/SNMAC 1992). The disease has a poor prognosis with only 8 per cent of patients surviving five years from diagnosis and the majority of deaths occur within one year of diagnosis (Cancer Research Campaign 1992). Many present with advanced disease and therefore primary treatment is palliative.

A working party on the management of lung cancer identified a need to improve the organization and coordination of services for patients with lung cancer, both within and between primary, secondary and tertiary care (SMAC/SNMAC 1992). Symptoms and problems experienced by people with lung cancer are numerous and evidence from a survey of physicians, surgeons and oncologists responsible for the follow-up of patients with lung cancer revealed a reluctance to refer to palliative care services despite the fact that many had unrelieved symptoms and their consultants acknowledged that their prognosis was extremely short, suggesting that the transition between acute and palliative care services is not smooth (Bristol Myers Squibb 1991). This has led the Royal Marsden NHS Trust and the Centre for Cancer and Palliative Care Studies to propose a new model of service based on nurse-led follow-up, which would move post-treatment management away from a cancer surveillance model, which is of questionable efficacy and is costly, to a more client-centred, supportive model. Individuals with lung cancer who have completed first-line treatment will be invited to take part in an evaluation of the nurse-led service. This will involve an initial detailed assessment of their needs, then instead of routine follow-up appointments with the medical team or discharge back to the general practitioner (GP), an open access service will be offered through telephone clinics and appointment free drop in clinics at both the cancer centre and local trust hospitals. These will undertake disease surveillance for disease problems, but will focus on supporting the individual and family, and immediate fax communication with the GP. It is envisaged that this will avoid unnecessary outpatient visits while targeting in-depth support at those most in need, and facilitating early appropriate transition to palliative care and other community services, thus providing a bridge at the interface between hospital and primary care services. This approach will be evaluated in the context of a randomized controlled trial comparing this service with conventional medical follow-up, and is funded by Cancer Relief Macmillan Fund and the NHS Cancer Research and Development Programme.

Conclusion

Despite the proliferation of palliative care services and the therapeutic innovations that have occurred, limitations are evident. These may be related to fundamental philosophical issues which limit the practice of palliative care. In particular, palliative care needs to develop approaches to care which place less emphasis on the biomedical model of symptom management, and reverse the trend towards medicalization of death within the palliative care context. A process by which the reframing of care can take place is offered as an alternative, in which the individual and their own understanding is placed at the core of therapeutic intervention. Services based on these principles, may need radical reconstruction. This does not obviate the need for adequate symptom management using powerful drugs if necessary, but would explore many routes toward achieving the ends sought by the sufferer, and not those determined by the practitioner or clinician.

References

Ahmedzai, S. (1993) Respiratory symptoms, in D. Doyle, G.W.C. Hanks and N. MacDonald (eds) *Oxford Textbook of Palliative Medicine*. Oxford: Oxford University Press.

Ahmedzai, S. (1994) A defence of medicalisation. *Progress in Palliative Care*, 2(4): 121–5.

Bailey, C. (1995) Nursing as therapy in the management of breathlessness in lung cancer. *European Journal of Cancer*, 4(4): 184–90.

Biswas, B. (1993) The medicalization of dying: a nurse's view, in D. Clark (ed.) *The Future for Palliative Care*. Buckingham: Open University Press.

Bristol Myers Squibb Pharmaceuticals Limited/Cancer Research Campaign (1991) Lung cancer report. Unpublished research report.

Cancer Research Campaign (1992) *Cancer Research Campaign Statistics*. London: Cancer Research Campaign.

Cassells, E.J. (1982) The nature of suffering and the goals of medicine. *New England Journal of Medicine*, 306(11): 639–45.

Corner, J. (1995) Innovative approaches in symptom management. *European Journal of Cancer Care*, 4(4): 145–6.

Corner, J., Plant, H. and Warner, L. (1995) Developing a nursing approach to the management of dyspnoea in lung cancer. *International Journal of Palliative Nursing*, 1(1): 5–11.

Corner, J., Plant, H., A'Hern, R. and Bailey, C. (1996) Non-pharmacological intervention for breathlessness in lung cancer. *Palliative Medicine*, 10: 299–305.

Fabricius, J. (1991) Running on the spot or can nursing really change? *Psychoanalytic Psychotherapy*, 5: 97–108.

Field, D. (1994) Palliative medicine and the medicalization of death. *European Journal of Cancer Care*, 3(2): 58–62.

Good, B.J. and Delvicchio Good, M.J. (1980) The meaning of symptoms a cultural hermeneutic model for clinical practice, in I. Eisenberg and A. Kleinman (eds) *The Relevance of Social Science for Medicine*. Dordrecht and Boston, MA: Reidel.

Higginson, I. and McCarthy, M. (1989) Measuring symptoms in terminal cancer: are pain and dyspnoea controlled? *Journal of the Royal Society of Medicine*, 82: 264–7.

James, N. and Field, D. (1992) The routinization of hospice: charisma and bureaucratization. *Social Science and Medicine*, 12(3): 1363–75.

Kastenbaum, R. (1988) Safe death in the post-modern world, in A. Gilmore and S. Gilmore (eds) *A Safer Death: Multidisciplinary Aspects of Terminal Care*. New York: Plenum Press.

Kleinman, A. (1988) *The Illness Narratives: Suffering, Healing and the Human Condition*. New York: Basic Books.

Lanceley, A. (1995) Wider issues in pain management. *European Journal of Cancer Care*, 4(4): 153–7.

Lyon, M.L. and Barbalet, J.M. (1994) Society's body: emotion and the 'somatization' of social theory, in T.J. Csordas (ed.) *Embodiment and Experience*. Cambridge: Cambridge University Press.

McNamara, B., Waddell, C. and Colvin, M. (1994) The institutionalisation of the good death. *Social Science and Medicine*, 39(11): 1501–8.

Preston, N. (1995) New strategies for the management of malignant ascites. *European Journal of Cancer Care*, 4(4): 178–83.

Saunders, C.M. (1967) *The Management of Terminal Illness*. London: Hospital Medicine Publications.

Seale, C.F. (1991) Death from cancer and from other causes: the relevance of the hospice approach. *Palliative Medicine*, 5: 12–19.

Seale, C.F. (1989) What happens in hospices: a review of research evidence. *Social Science and Medicine*, 28(6): 551–9.

Standing Medical Advisory Committee/Standing Nursing and Midwifery Advisory Committee (1992) *The Principles and Provision of Palliative Care*. London: HMSO.

Twycross, R.G. and Dunn, V. (1994) *Research in Palliative Care: The Pursuit of Reliable Knowledge*. Occasional Paper 5. London: National Council for Hospice and Specialist Palliative Care Services.

Walter, T. (1993) Death and the new age. *Religion*, 23: 127–45.

Wilkes, E. (1993) Introduction, in D. Clark (ed.) *The Future for Palliative Care*. Buckingham: Open University Press.

World Health Organisation (1990) Cancer Pain Relief and Palliative Care, *Technical Report, Series B04*. Geneva: World Health Organisation.

Index